*The International Behavioural and Social Sciences Library*

# CURRENT TRENDS IN ANALYTICAL PSYCHOLOGY



TAVISTOCK

*The International Behavioural and Social Sciences Library*

## PSYCHOLOGY
In 11 Volumes

| | |
|---|---|
| I | Current Trends in Analytical Psychology<br>*Edited by Gerhard Adler* |
| II | Focal Psychotherapy<br>*Michael Balint, et al.* |
| III | Primary Love and Psycho-Analytic Technique<br>*Michael Balint* |
| IV | Attention and Interpretation<br>*W R Bion* |
| V | Themes in Speculative Psychology<br>*Nehemiah Jordan* |
| VI | Envy and Gratitude<br>*Melanie Klein* |
| VII | New Directions in Psycho-Analysis<br>*Edited by Melanie Klein, et al.* |
| VIII | A Study of Brief Psychotherapy<br>*D H Malan* |
| IX | Displacement of Concepts<br>*Donald A Schon* |
| X | Identity<br>*Edited by Kenneth Soddy* |
| XI | System and Structure<br>*Anthony Wilden* |

# CURRENT TRENDS IN ANALYTICAL PSYCHOLOGY

## Proceedings of the First International Congress for Analytical Psychology

EDITED BY GERHARD ADLER

Routledge
Taylor & Francis Group
LONDON AND NEW YORK

First published in 1961 by
Tavistock Publications (1959) Limited

Published in 2001 by
Routledge
2 Park Square, Milton Park, Abingdon, Oxfordshire OX14 4RN
711 Third Avenue, New York, NY 10017

First issued in paperback 2014

*Routledge is an imprint of the Taylor and Francis Group, an informa business*



The publishers have made every effort to contact authors/copyright holders of the works reprinted in the *International Behavioural and Social Sciences Library*. This has not been possible in every case, however, and we would welcome correspondence from those individuals/companies we have been unable to trace.

These reprints are taken from original copies of each book. In many cases the condition of these originals is not perfect. The publisher has gone to great lengths to ensure the quality of these reprints, but wishes to point out that certain characteristics of the original copies will, of necessity, be apparent in reprints thereof.

*British Library Cataloguing in Publication Data*
A CIP catalogue record for this book
is available from the British Library

Current Trends in Analytical Psychology
ISBN 0-415-26478-2
Psychology: 11 Volumes
ISBN 0-415-26515-0
The International Behavioural and Social Sciences Library
112 Volumes
ISBN 0-415-25670-4

ISBN 13: 978-1-138-87155-7 (pbk)
ISBN 13: 978-0-415-26478-5 (hbk)

# *Current Trends in Analytical Psychology*

PROCEEDINGS OF THE FIRST INTERNATIONAL CONGRESS FOR ANALYTICAL PSYCHOLOGY

Edited by
GERHARD ADLER

TAVISTOCK PUBLICATIONS

*First published in 1961 by*
*Tavistock Publications (1959) Limited*
*2 Park Square, Milton Park, Abingdon, Oxon, OX14 4RN*
*in 12 point Bembo*
*by J. W. Arrowsmith Limited, Bristol*

# Contents

# *Preface*

WITH this book we present to the wider public the papers read at the First International Congress for Analytical Psychology held in Zürich from the 7th to the 12th August 1958.[1] The Congress was a milestone in the history of Analytical Psychology. It was the first official function of the International Association for Analytical Psychology, which was founded in 1956.

The main function of the International Association is to provide a forum for the exchange of ideas. Over a period of sixty years the prodigious work of C. G. Jung has continuously inspired research in many fields both clinical and theoretical. The direction taken by this research has varied according to the interests of analysts and groups in different countries and at different times. As a result, the development of Analytical Psychology has produced a considerable variety of approaches.

For this reason we wanted to meet our colleagues from other countries to discuss their special interests and to hear about the work they had been doing. As the aim of the first Congress was exploratory, it was decided that there should be no central theme but that each contributor should be given complete freedom in his choice of subject. This led to a wide variety of papers. Though, for the most part, they have no formal relation to one another, it will be seen that they contain many common themes converging on the basic concepts of Analytical Psychology: the archetypal organization of the psyche and the process of individuation. All these themes were elaborated in the subsequent discussion; but, unfortunately, publication was not anticipated and these exchanges were not recorded. Even so, it was decided at the end of the Congress that the papers had been of sufficient merit to deserve collection in permanent form.

[1]There is one regrettable exception: Dr. Cahen, Paris, was unable, owing to the pressure of important work, to complete in time his paper on "Absentotherapie", which he had delivered from notes only.

## Preface

The aim of the present volume is to enable the reader to gain a picture of current trends in Analytical Psychology. For reasons of convenience, all papers have been published in English, but as an expression of the international character of the IAAP it has been decided to present the original text of those papers given in a language other than English as well as the English translation. The publication was made possible by the generosity of Mrs. Frances G. Wickes, who put the means of the Wickes Foundation at the disposal of the IAAP, and our special thanks are due to her. On the technical side I want to thank Tavistock Publications for the patient and efficient assistance given in the editorial preparation of this book.

It is hoped that this work will further the understanding and the development of Analytical Psychology. To its founder, C. G. Jung, we present these contributions of his pupils in gratitude and admiration.

GERHARD ADLER

# 1

## WHAT MAKES THE SYMBOL EFFECTIVE AS A HEALING AGENT?

M. ESTHER HARDING, *New York*

THERE have been many evidences in America, in recent years, of a desire to bring psychiatry and religion into closer relation. A number of societies have been formed with this end in view and Jungian lecturers have been asked to participate in their programmes. This new interest takes two forms. On the one side there is a real interest in searching out the psychological meaning of religious symbolism; on the other, various forms of "faith healing" as practised in some Churches are being discussed by psychiatrists and medical doctors. In this paper, I want to explore how it is that a symbol can affect the psychic condition of the individual.

The interpretation of religious symbols may range all the way from the Freudian "nothing but repressed sexuality" to the opposite extreme where they are taken as evidence of a transcendental reality, a more or less anthropomorphized deity, having a quite personal concern with the believer. The Freudian school considers that religious symbols are a substitute formation, an escape mechanism, whose purpose is to protect the immature ego from a task beyond its capacity; they are really wish-fulfilling fantasies, which keep the individual infantile. The theologians, in contrast, consider that the value and purpose of the symbols of religion are to implant in the individual faith in a divine being, a "person" who carries the burden of guilt or conflict and so brings healing for soul or body.

I have emphasized the extreme of these two positions intentionally, so as to bring into sharpest focus the irreconcilable conflict between them. Strangely enough, until quite recently, the clergy have preferred a Freudian approach to that of any other school. Freudian psychology is taught in their seminaries and their disturbed parishioners are referred to Freudian therapists, in complete disregard of the divergence of the basic principles on which the two points of view are founded, one mechanistic, the other metaphysical.

Neither of these schools has determined, however, just what it is makes a symbol effective as a healing agent, capable of resolving devastating conflicts and transforming the individual by producing a change in the not-personal part of the psyche. This understanding we owe to Professor C. G. Jung. What I have to say, in so far as it is true and of value, stems directly from his teaching. This is the area where he has done his most creative work. The subject is quite familiar to all of you, but it is so important that perhaps you will bear with me if I recapitulate it.

Many people regard symbols as merely picturesque expressions of well-known ideas, parables representing something one wished to convey to others. But real symbols, as we know, are not invented or made up, nor are they poetic or allegorical means to represent a known fact. On the contrary, they are numinous and autonomous products of the unconscious, expressions of unknown, that is unconscious, facts carrying an energy charge that can affect the psyche in drastic fashion.

No one would assume that dream images were under our personal control or were invented or imagined by ourselves, although some do hold that the symbols of religion may have been invented, perhaps by a priestly caste, as has been suggested by anthropologists. But just as dream symbols are autonomous, so, too, are all genuine religious symbols.

Not only is a symbol autonomous, but it remains unknown and inactive *in the unconscious* till at some particular moment it is activated by an access of energy and so rises above the threshold and assumes a form capable of being perceived by consciousness. Such symbols may have a peculiar fascination and awe-inspiring quality, i.e., they are numinous. All down the ages the religions have called such symbols *revelations*. They form the basis of dogma and religious mythologems. When an individual experiences such a symbol in his own dream he is compelled to recognize a powerful factor functioning, or intruding, within his own psyche and has to acknowledge that he is not the only master of his house, but that an unknown "other" also inhabits it and exerts a dominating influence in his psyche. As Jung has expressed it (Jung, 1942, *Coll. Wks.*, **11**, p. 150): "An archetypal dream . . . can so fascinate the dreamer that he is very apt to see in it some kind of illumination, warning, or supernatural help. Nowadays most people are afraid of surrendering to such experiences, and their fear proves the existence of a 'holy dread' of the numinous. Whatever the nature of these numinous experiences may be, they all have one thing in common: they relegate their source to a region outside consciousness. Psychology uses instead the concept of the unconscious, and specially that of the collective unconscious" to designate this region; the religious ascribe such experiences to the intervention of a divine personage.

Symbols having this kind of numinosity are, of course, expressions of the archetypes which exert such a powerful influence not only on the life of the individual but on that of society as well. But it is probable that the archetypes, in the form in which they exist in the unconscious, would not be recognizable by consciousness at all, for it lacks the categories of experience which would correspond to this totally "other" of the archetypes. Indeed, in deep dreams and especially in states of mental illness, such as schizophrenia, the experiences encountered may be quite indescribable in the terms of consciousness, and religious mystics, too, say that what they see and hear in the ecstasy of trance is ineffable and quite indescribable. But sometimes the experience of the "other side" comes through to consciousness in the form of a vision, a symbolic representation, which, although it may be strange and awe-inspiring, yet brings the unknown content closer to consciousness. For, as Jung has pointed out, a symbol has two sides or aspects. On one, it is related to man, to his conscious ego, it has a form that is comprehensible to him, or relatively so—the sky, the earth, man himself, or one of the animals, and even when the image represents something contrary to nature, such as a mythological beast, it still can be understood to some extent. But the symbol has also another side, which is not related to the categories of consciousness, instead it is turned towards the unknown facts of the unconscious psyche—a most incomprehensible statement, but one which it is important that we try to realize, especially when we come to consider the relation between psychic experience and the orthodox religions. The well-known progressive theologian, Paul Tillich, expresses this fact from the theological angle when he writes (Tillich, 1955, p.108): "Symbols of religious experience . . . are not God, but they point to God. . . . In these symbols there is expressed that which is the content of every religion, the basis of every religious experience and the foundation of every theology, the *divine-human encounter.*" And in another place he writes (Tillich, 1955, p.114): "The God of traditional theism is a symbol for the God beyond theism" [i.e. the God we know about is not God as He is in Himself. Our picture of God is an image of the unknowable Godhead and not that ineffable itself]. Tillich continues: "The true God is not a being existent beside others, but He is the symbolic expression of our encounter with the ultimate itself, with the ground of being. The God who is really God is the abyss of the symbolic material which we apply to Him."

By meditating on such a symbol some part of this obscure aspect comes gradually forward into the light of consciousness. By this means consciousness is enlarged so that it begins to include elements that are usually beyond its range of vision. Thus the personality is enriched, but in less favourable circumstances the ego consciousness, with its small light, can be engulfed in the darkness of the unconscious. If one catches a big fish there is a chance that one may land it. But if the fish is too huge the situation may be reversed and the fisher becomes the victim of his catch. It is most important, when one goes fishing in the waters of the unconscious, to have a firm anchorage in reality, otherwise one may be pulled overboard and swallowed by the whale-dragon, as Jonah was, or destroyed by a Moby-Dick, like Ahab.

In *Aion*, Jung discusses an old Patristic legend of the capture of the greatest of all fishes, Leviathan. There the Cross was said to be the hook and the Crucified the bait. Of this Jung says (Jung, 1951, *Coll. Wks.*, **9**, 2, p. 182): "A content (fish) of the unconscious (sea) has been caught and has attached itself to the Christ-figure." He goes on to show that Leviathan is a symbol of the self, and that it is caught because the figure or image of

Christ acts like a magnet, attracting to itself that which has a *secret affinity with it*. He points out that religious and mythological symbols have this power of bringing up the contents of the unconscious through their mutual attraction for each other.

Symbols of this kind have an arresting and numinous quality akin to the much rarer experiences of mystics and prophets. The dogmas of religions were undoubtedly founded upon such numinous experiences. But religious symbolism, as taught to the general congregation, rarely has this arresting quality. It has lost the ancient fire which it held for man of old. Dream symbols, however, or at least some dream symbols, do have this quality of awe and fascination because they are received hot, as it were, whereas religious symbols in their long passage from generation to generation have gradually cooled down. They have lost their *mana* through much repetition. But religious symbols were hot, exceedingly hot, when they first arose. Then they carried the amazement and power of true revelations. Today, they may merely be repeated as meaningless formulas, but unless they still have something of their old fire, for at least a minority of religious persons, they will gradually become petrified and the religion will die, while the spirit which informed these venerable symbols will depart, only to manifest itself somewhere else under some other form.

The question then confronts us as to how it happens that these dynamic symbols become activated once more or, more accurately, how do the archetypal motifs become activated so that they manifest themselves in the guise of symbols that can be grasped by the consciousness of this new age, or can take possession of consciousness without our even being aware of their intervention (Neumann, 1952, pp. 19 f. (trans.)). This question cannot be answered directly, for it is only by inference that we can get an idea of how the interaction between the conscious and the unconscious works. The symbol image that arises has always a complementary or compensatory relation to the conscious attitude of the moment. And if the conscious attitude is too one-sided, too much concerned with one aspect of life to the exclusion of another of immediate importance, then a compensatory energy is set free in the unconscious, and this manifests itself in the form of a symbol, or perhaps, a whole mythologem, a symbol series, which portrays the opposite or compensatory value that has been neglected by consciousness. This is why symbols have a curative or healing effect. Indeed, the great symbol dramas carry the whole story of redemption. It is these great, these fundamental, symbol myths, that form the basis of every religion, and their purpose is to bring to man the experience of wholeness.

Thus while the symbol is a means of representing something unknown, it is by no means only that, for it is also a psychic function, which performs a task. First, it serves to compensate for the one-sided, the lop-sided, development of consciousness; and second, it is the means by which the dynamic energy of the unconscious reality is carried over into consciousness. Without the symbol we could not come to terms at all with this dynamic energy, let alone comprehend it. For it would be like a force of nature, not only outside us, but inside as well—a hurricane, a blind emotion, rage, passion, desirousness, and fecundity and creativeness as well, in all their many aspects. For though the symbol brings us into contact with the unconscious, consciousness is needed if these blind and primitive emotions are to be humanized, transformed into love, friendship, and co-operation, or are to be submitted to law and order, by which cosmos can be created out of chaos.

In its beginnings this energy is attached to the instinctive processes of life. The life process in all its aspects, not excluding death, presses on with an inexhaustible dynamism. Freud, who first brought this fact to the attention of the modern world, spoke of the forms which it took as oral, anal, and oedipal, i.e. that they are related to the body functions—he also pointed out that the libido is dual, pulling in opposite directions, towards life and towards death. But he did not realize how the transformation of this same instinctive energy could be brought about by means of the very symbols which he took as merely showing from what lowly beginnings the life energy took its source. But Jung has demonstrated, what indeed the great religions also teach, that this energy may be freed from its instinctuality by means of a symbol, or mythologem.

How is it that this energy, so blind and potentially destructive in its unconsciousness, can possibly present itself in dreams and myths as a redeeming and life-giving force? The life energy is satisfied to fulfil itself in the instinctive processes in all nature, animal and vegetable alike, save only in *man*. But in him is found a striving towards psychic freedom and autonomy, in a word, towards consciousness. Is not this the meaning of the saying that God created man in his own image? In the struggle of man to transcend his bondage to the body and its functions, religion and religious symbolism have played the major, the determining, the indispensable role. Religion, and by this I do not mean the organized creeds, has consistently led the way by which man might develop consciousness, supplying not only the incentive, but the necessary energy as well. In his concern with "the gods" man has been enabled gradually to grow towards the restoration of the image of God that was imprinted in him at his creation.

This is a very meagre attempt to formulate the "why" of the change; we can be more definite when we come to the "how" of the process, and the question then becomes "In what way have the symbols of religion helped to free the libido from the hold of instinctive life? and what will guide it in the right path when it has been freed?" In his *Symbols of Transformation* Jung has explored this aspect of the problem extensively. He writes (Jung, 1912, *Coll. Wks.*, **5**, pp. 227 f.): "The libido has, as it were, a natural penchant: it is like water, which must have a gradient if it is to flow ... [This gradient is given by] the archetypes, ... [the] universal and inherited patterns which, taken together, constitute the structure of the unconscious."

The archetypal patterns govern, not only the structure of the unconscious psychic life, but the biological life with its instincts as well. There is, therefore, a correspondence between the life of the body and the unseen life of the psyche. The energy hidden in, inherent in, the very process of life itself, is made available to consciousness by means of the symbol, which is thus a sort of machine, a mechanism, which serves to transform the energy of the unconscious and carry it over into the conscious life, much as a turbine transforms the mighty energy of even a Niagara, so that it can serve the purposes of mankind. A very great importance, therefore, attaches to the nature of the symbol that performs this significant task. A symbol occurring in the dream of an individual has to be accepted for what it is, regardless of whether we think it "good" or "bad", but in the Church, redemptive symbols are taught or enacted with the intent of bringing healing to the worshipper. In these teachings analogies are freely used, and as Jung remarks (Jung, 1912, *Coll. Wks.*, 5, pp. 227 f.): "The nature of these analogies is . . . a serious problem because . . . they must be ideas which attract the libido. Their special character is . . . to be discerned in the fact that they are archetypes . . ."

Myths and legends telling of life and death, of rebirth and an after-life, of the beginnings of the world and of its ending, of its maker and redeemer, are universal and are to be found in all religions. These stories are not only told, as secular history might be, for educational purposes, but are regarded as the means by which a man's life can be directed and understood, and, frequently, their mere telling is thought to have power to heal, and in all mystery religions, of which Christianity is one, they form the core of rituals, which are performed in order to redeem man from his bondage to the body and transform him into a spiritual being.

The means by which this is accomplished is the *symbol*, which has the function of tapping the life-energy latent in the unconscious and transforming it. The symbols of religion are particularly apt for this work because they represent the way in which the libido has flowed for countless ages, resulting in its gradual transformation from instinctive drives to spiritual and cultural ends.

Take for example the symbols of rebirth. When an individual meets with some frustration in life, his libido retreats before the blow and regresses to the image of the mother with her warmth and tenderness. But, since he is an adult, his longing for protection and comfort may take the form of a sexual and incestuous wish in place of the more infantile longing for the womb. This wish will be expressed in some symbol which can be interpreted in two ways—and it makes all the difference which interpretation is chosen—for it could be taken quite concretely as a concealed wish for actual intercourse with the mother, an interpretation that leads only to carnality; or the symbol can be regarded as an attempt of the unconscious to lead the regressive libido over into a creative act of a different nature, that is, the symbol would point the way to a resolution of the conflict.

However, redemptive symbols do not usually arise unless there is a deep sense of need on the part of the individual, nor are they likely to occur unless he has concerned himself actively with the conflicting values whose claims he cannot reconcile by any device or conscious effort of his own. Neurotic suffering does not further the production of a reconciling symbol, for the neurotic individual is wrapped up in his personal distress and, as a rule, can spare little thought or attention to becoming aware of the nature of the forces that are at war in him, and still less is he inclined to take upon himself the difficult and painful task of enduring their opposition. But, as Jung has pointed out (Jung, 1921, trans. p. 607): "The living symbol cannot come to birth in an inert or poorly developed mind, for such a man will rest content with the already existing symbols offered by established tradition. Only the passionate yearning of a highly developed mind, for whom the dictated symbol no longer contains the highest reconciliation in one expression, can create a new symbol. But, inasmuch as the symbol proceeds from his highest and latest mental achievement and must also include the deepest roots of his being, it cannot be a one-sided product of the most highly differentiated mental functions, but must at least have an equal source in the lowest and most primitive motions of his psyche. ... Such a condition necessarily entails a violent disunion with oneself..." that is, it leads to the greatest conflict and inner division, which involves intense suffering. Religious "revivalists" seek to produce such a state by preaching the doctrine of man's guilt, believing that salvation can occur only in response to the most intense sense of need.

The analytical psychologist, too, is aware that this is a prerequisite for the coming of a reconciling or redeeming symbol. However, he does not have to resort to artificial means to produce a sense of need, for the individual who goes to an analyst is already aware of his inability to deal with his conflict, though its elements may not be very clear to him. The preliminary work of the analyst serves to clarify the conscious attitude and bring the opposing shadow side more fully into view. In this way the conflicting elements are brought into sharper focus and their irreconcilable nature is more clearly realized. Thus a general feeling of need or distress is replaced by a very clear recognition of the conflicting values whose warfare is disrupting the peace of mind of the patient and the normal flow of his life. These are the conditions in which a reconciling symbol is likely to arise.

It was in such a situation of conflict that a lawyer once came to consult me. He was a sensitive and rather artistic man, but was involved in a struggle for worldly success and prestige. His own innate desires would have led him to a less ambitious way of life, leaving time for intellectual interests and companionship, but his ambition forced him to a worldly social life and to competition with his more successful colleagues. During the early part of his analysis these two aims became increasingly clear, but always his choice led him, unwillingly, back into the worldly arena. Eventually he dreamed that he found himself in Egypt. A wise old priest led him into a pyramid and showed him many beautiful objects, which had been given to the dead Pharaoh to guide and help him on his after-death journey. When they emerged from the pyramid, the priest turned to him and, with a certain ceremony, presented him with one of the treasures from the tomb. He was delighted and started to thank the priest, but he had vanished. Now, from the dream it seems that this man's problem might be about to be resolved. In place of the treasures of this world he was given an emblem concerned with the spiritual journey, a treasure that would ensure success in the after-world, that is, in the eternal state. It was a big dream and one would expect that this man would find his conflict resolved in the direction of individuation. But there was a final statement of the dream, which put an end to all these optimistic anticipations. For he said, "When I saw that the priest had left, I looked again at my treasure, and thought 'I will take this to the museum in New York and sell it. It will bring a lot of money.'" And so, even when a reconciling symbol does make its appearance, the conflict is not always resolved by its means. Evidently another factor is involved before a successful outcome can occur.

Contrast this case with the next one. This was a man faced with such a devastating frustration that he had fallen into despair. He was utterly unable to summon sufficient energy to carry on his daily life. After some weeks of analysis in which his shadow problem has become clear to him, he dreamed that he was a small boy and was being bathed by his analyst in the bath-tub. Here, one might conclude, a regression is shown in full swing. The life problem was too hard, the man could not cope with it, and at least on a superficial view the dream seems to say "return to infancy and leave the problem to Mother". On this interpretation the analyst would be a mother-figure, and the bath a womb symbol. The patient is, as it were, in the womb again, bathed in the warm natal waters. So that on the surface we might conclude that his dream is an indisputable example of a wish-fulfilling fantasy. But the patient's associations carried the matter far beyond the banal bath-room situation depicted in the dream. For he said that the analyst was *not* his actual mother, but rather a sort of spiritual mother, who had opened a new dimension of life to him. To the bath he associated cleansing, and especially cleansing from the sin as in baptism, of which he felt greatly in need. This brought to his mind Jesus' conversation with Nicodemus, regarding the necessity of rebirth. Jung uses this story to illustrate the process of transformation of the libido from the instinctive to the psychic level. He writes (Jung, 1912, *Coll. Wks.*, **5**, p. 226): "The reason why Jesus' words have such great suggestive power is that they express the symbolical truths which are rooted in the very structure of the human psyche. The empirical truth never frees a man from his bondage to the senses; it only shows him that he was always so and cannot be otherwise. The symbolical truth . . . which puts water in the place of the mother and spirit or fire in the place of the father, frees the libido from the channel of the incest tendency, offers it a new gradient, and canalizes it into a spiritual form."

In another place Jung writes (Jung, 1942, *Coll. Wks.*, **11**, p. 183): "Spiritual transformation does not mean that one should remain a child, [compare 'The son stage is a transitory phenomenon and implies conflict'] but that the adult should summon up enough honest self-criticism admixed with humility to see where, and in relation to what, he must behave as a child—irrationally, and with unreflecting receptivity. Just as the transition from the first stage to the second [from child to son] demands the sacrifice of childish dependence, so, at the transition to the third stage [from son to father], an exclusive independence has to be relinquished."

That the interpretation of my patient's dream was correct was confirmed when, a few days later, he dreamed that he was standing in the street and saw a procession coming towards him. The procession was evidently to honour an important person and he had a strange feeling that he did not belong with these people and was unworthy to join in honouring this great man. So he stepped down into an area-way to watch unobserved. As the procession approached he suddenly realized that the central figure was the Christ. The dreamer was overwhelmed with awe and longing, but he drew still further back into the shadow so as not to be seen. But as the Christ passed the place where he was hiding, He turned and looked at him, beckoning him to follow. Naturally this dream was filled with deep emotion and made a powerful impression on this man, who because of his problem, had felt himself as an outcast from society.

My patient was not a religious man, he did not belong to any Church and although he had been brought up as a nominal Christian his knowledge of the Bible was pitifully inadequate. He could recall the conversation with Nicodemus, though he had never asked himself what it might mean, but he disclaimed any knowledge of the story of Zaccheus, who had actually had an experience very similar to that of my patient in the second dream. Indeed the two situations are surprisingly alike. Zaccheus, a Jew, was a taxgatherer for the Roman government, that is, he was a collaborator, and his confession at least suggests that he had used his position to feather his own nest. He, too, had not dared to approach the Rabbi Jesus directly, but had climbed into a tree hoping to see Him as he passed by. To his great surprise Jesus called him to come down so that He could dine at his house. Then, after dinner, Zaccheus confessed his wrong-doing and received acceptance and forgiveness.

The similarity with my patient's dream is remarkable. He, too, felt himself to be lost, a sinner, who could have no part even in doing honour to the Christ, and yet found that he was called and welcomed. And, in spite of the fact that he did not consciously know or remember them, the same symbols that form the language, not only of the Christian religion, but of others as well, appeared in his need to lead the libido from its fixation in carnality to a new and spiritual development.

Without these dreams, I do not think it would have done much good to have talked to this man in terms of Christian teaching: he would have heard the words, but they would not have touched him. It was only when a certain level of the unconscious was activated and the eternal, archetypal theme of rebirth was awakened in his own psyche, that his libido was able to be rechannelled into life on a different plane. Indeed, for him the symbol did not arise in the august form in which it is enshrined in the Church, rather it appeared in quite humble form, of a personalistic nature. And yet, perhaps for that very reason, it could speak to him as the sacred words of the ritual could not do.

Whenever the eternal truths are experienced anew they are apt to be couched in just such personalistic symbols, which may seem quite unacceptable to our conscious taste. But unless the symbol is living and is ever experienced anew in forms that speak directly to the individual heart, it will lose its efficacy and become hard like a fossil. It is the task of the analyst to take these symbols that arise spontaneously in the dreams of an individual who is in sore need, and so to elucidate them by using the associations of the dreamer and the relevant amplifications, that their hidden meaning may emerge with all its forward-looking implications. By an analysis of the unconscious material in this progressive spirit, the libido is led away from the carnal and concrete imagery to its real goal—the development of the personality.

The rituals and sacraments of the Christian Church contain in unsurpassed form the record of this process of transformation and, as we know, countless persons have been changed or "redeemed" by their means. But even in the days when faith in the teachings and rituals of the Church was much more universal than it is today, not *all* persons were transformed or experienced an inner redemption and enlightenment through participating in the offices of the Church. And, today, these truths, these "mysteries", are nothing more than a story—for many people, perhaps, they even seem like a stale and futile tale, whose manifest unreality, from the materialistic standpoint, is a source of incredulity and even of ridicule.

Why is it that what is life-giving to one is utterly meaningless to another? The answer the Churchman would give is that one man's heart is prepared to receive the message, another's is not. In one the grace of God is operative, whereas the other is not so moved. The analyst would say that to be effective the message and the ritual happening must correspond to the situation actually present in the man's own unconscious. It must speak to his condition, as the Friends say. For if the symbols portrayed really express the conditions already latent within him, then the life-energy can pass over into consciousness, and, in this way, life can really be renewed in him.

This leads to the next question, namely, how can one know whether an individual is in a state to profit by the symbol; is there any way by which he can be prepared to share in the life-giving process mediated by the symbol; and how can one discover which symbol will work with this particular man?

The experience of which we are speaking is called by the religious "conversion". This is a deeply-felt, emotional and personal experience, in which guilt and conflict are removed through a personal confrontation with a divine figure. In this respect "conversion" seems to have some kinship with the process of individuation, for each is concerned with the confrontation with a numinous "other", an experience that demands the displacement of the ego as centre of the psyche, expressed in religious terms as self-surrender. William James writes (James, 1901, p. 209): "that to exercise the personal will is still to live in the region where the imperfect self is the thing most emphasized", and adds (James, 1901, p. 210): "... self-surrender has been and always must be regarded as the vital turning-point of the religious life". And again, (James, 1901, p. 211): "Psychology and religion are thus in perfect harmony up to this point, since both admit that there are forces seemingly outside of the conscious individual that bring redemption to this life." Such a surrender of the ego feels like death, since all we know of our psyche, of ourselves, is that small part of it that is incorporated under the ego-complex. A confrontation with another of far greater power than the ego requires nothing less than self-surrender.

But a most fundamental problem remains, viz., who or what, is that "other", who is destined to replace the impotent ego and bring peace to the conflict-torn psyche? The Christian religion teaches that the sins and distresses of the individual are carried by Christ, a hypostatized, divine figure. The resolution of the conflict is achieved by identification with the good, through faith in the efficacy of Christ's sacrifice. In the analytic process the symbol of reconciliation points, not to perfection, but to wholeness, as the solution of the difficulty, and this must be achieved, not by faith, but by understanding and conscious work on the symbol in its relation to the life situation.

In the pursuance of his task of the cure of souls, the *minister or priest* has a long tradition of authority behind him. He preaches a general message, which, although it may not fit the particular individual, is generally valid. The analyst is seemingly at a disadvantage in comparison, for he cannot call on traditional ways of salvation nor expect his patient to exercise a faith which he obviously does not possess. He must confine himself to the actual facts, both conscious and unconscious, of the life situation with which he is confronted in order to discover where the life process is leading in this particular situation.

Although analysts and the clergy use different methods and seek different ends, they agree, as we have seen, that the first condition for success is the recognition of need. So important is this sense of need that Wesley used to say that unless the individual was aroused to a realization of sin nothing could be done for him. In an analysis, too, the story of difficulty and failure is confessed, and the individual comes to realize that he cannot remedy his situation by any conscious effort of his will. Indeed, the preliminary work leads to a clearer perception of the conflict and his need presses all the harder upon him, till he cannot see how he will ever be able to get out of the fix he is in or find sufficient energy or initiative to continue his life. At this point the analyst directs the patient's attention to the unknown part of his psyche to see what help can be found there, relying on the knowledge that every living organism contains within it an inner law or purpose, which leads towards the fulfilment of that particular life. This is an act of faith on the part of the analyst, who believes, or should one not say he *knows*, that the inner law of every being leads to the integration of that individual, and the achievement of this goal constitutes redemption from the state of division and unwholeness from which he is suffering.

When the dreams are approached in this way, symbols of regeneration presently begin to emerge in the vast majority of cases, indeed in all those persons in whom the conscious attitude is right, that is, in all who are really seeking for the truth and are not diverted from following their appointed path by selfish or false motives. The symbols that appear may take the form of some well-known religious teaching familiar to the dreamer, or they may utilize religious symbols that are strange to him, or they may be hidden under the guise of everyday, even perhaps banal, happenings having a personalistic slant. When these dream images are elaborated by the associations of the dreamer, or are compared with the symbols of other religions, their significance becomes clear.

The symbols that arise from the individual's own unconscious represent the actual state of his psyche, and demonstrate what is the natural way in which the healing energies of the unconscious could flow into his conscious life, and, since they are not static, but move within him and unfold their message from one dream to another, they map out a way that he must follow. At the same time they release the energy latent in the unconscious, which has power to produce a fundamental transformation of his personality, and of his life. But unless he allows himself to be moved by the inner happening, and unless he experiences the full affect connected with it, he will lose the blessing.

Whenever a numinous image is experienced it implies a confrontation with an "other" within the psyche. To the religious this "other" is interpreted as a divine being, who demands that the man surrender himself, give up his ego-will, and perform the will of God revealed in the vision. In the experience of a numinous "other" in the confrontation with the unconscious psyche, a similar demand is made, namely that the ego must renounce its hard-won supremacy in the psyche, and accept the fact that a stronger, though unknown, "other" rules from the unconscious. Only by the acceptance of this unknown potency can the true psychic centre of the individuality be found. Needless to say, this is not an easy recognition for the ego to make. It demands nothing less than a radical sacrifice of itself, but thereby the self is restored to its rightful place as centre of the psyche. Or, in religious terms, the image of God is restored to its original place within man (Jung, 1951, *Coll. Wks.*, **9**, 2, pp. 38 ff.).

There is, however, one further condition which must be fulfilled if this movement of the unconscious is to be effective. That is, the conscious personality must grasp the meaning of the symbolic happening and must begin to live by it. If he merely views his dreams, unfolding in the unconscious, as an interesting show, like a movie picture, nothing will be accomplished. The unconscious process will play itself out; the dreams may contain marvellous symbols, the whole drama of salvation may be enacted by the figures of the unconscious, but unless its meaning is seized by the conscious ego and used to direct the life, the whole process will subside once more, just as, when the waters of the pool at Bethesda were moved by the angel, unless someone stepped in, the waters subsided again and no one was healed. Here again, the part played by the affect is very important. Intellectual understanding and appreciation of the aptness, the beauty, the awe of the symbol process does not bring salvation. It is only emotional participation in the happening itself that effects any lasting change.

So it seems that for a reconciling or redemptive symbol to be fully effective four conditions must be fulfilled. *First*, the individual must be deeply concerned over his need; *second*, he must have struggled to the utmost of his ability to find a conscious way out of his dilemma; *third*, the symbol itself must express the life process of the unconscious, active in this particular individual; and *lastly*, he must grasp the meaning of the symbol that is presented to him, not only with his mind but with his heart also, and must act upon its teaching.

## REFERENCES

AMES, W. (1901). *Varieties of Religious Experience*. London and New York, Longmans, Green (quoted from 1922 ed.).

JUNG, C. G. (1912). *Wandlungen und Symbole der Libido*. Leipzig and Vienna, Deuticke. Trans. *Coll. Wks.*, **5**.

JUNG, C. G. (1921). *Psychologische Typen*. Zürich, Rascher. Trans. *Psychological Types*, by H. G. Baynes, London, Kegan Paul; New York, Harcourt Brace, 1923.

JUNG, C. G. (1942). "Zur Psychologie der Trinitätsidee". *Eranos-Jb.* **8**. Trans. *Coll. Wks.*, **11**.

JUNG, C. G. (1951). *Aion*. Zürich, Rascher. Trans. *Coll. Wks.*, **9**, 2.
NEUMANN, E. (1952). "Kunst und Zeit". *Eranos-Jb.* **20.** Trans. "Art and Time" in *Man and Time*, by R. Manheim. Bollingen Series 30, 3. New York, Pantheon, 1957; London, Routledge and Kegan Paul, 1957.
TILLICH, P. (1955). "Theology and Symbolism" in: *Religious Symbolism*, ed. by F. Ernest Johnson, New York, Harper.

# 2

## *DIE BEDEUTUNG DES GENETISCHEN ASPEKTS FÜR DIE ANALYTISCHE PSYCHOLOGIE*

ERICH NEUMANN, *Tel Aviv*

*"Das ferne Ziel, zu dem diese Forschungen führen, ist eine Phylogenie des Geistes."*
C. G. JUNG (1912)

WENN wir die Geschichte der Tiefenpsychologie betrachten, können wir ohne Zweifel feststellen, dass diese im ganzen, nicht nur in ihrer Entwicklung von der Psychoanalyse Freuds zur Analytischen Psychologie Jungs von der Betonung des personalen Aspekts zu der des transpersonalen Aspekts durchgedrungen ist. Die Psychoanalyse sieht den Menschen im wesentlichen als ein geschichtliches Wesen, das durch die personale Genese seines Lebens in einer bestimmten Umwelt und Zeitlichkeit zu verstehen ist. Die Einmaligkeit und Zufälligkeit des Geschehens zwischen Kind und Eltern ist nach ihr das schicksalbildende Element in der gesunden, besonders aber der kranken Entwicklung. Diese personalistischgenetische Auffassung hat dann dazu geführt, auf die Kindheit und ihre Analyse das entscheidende Gewicht zu legen. Der ergänzende transpersonale Aspekt kommt dann in der Entwicklung eines Modells der psychischen Struktur zum Ausdruck, das in den normativen Phasen der Libidoentwicklung einen allgemeinen Plan aufzeigt, in dem die personalistischen Ereignisse der Einzelentwicklung ihren Stellenwert bekommen, z.B. Fixierung auf der Analstufe durch falsche Reinlichkeitserziehung der Mutter, etc., etc.

Im Gegensatz zu dieser Betonung des Zeitlich-Personalen

entdeckte Jung die entscheidende Bedeutung der transpersonal-zeitlosen Faktoren der Psyche, der Archetypen, welche die Entwicklung des Menschen bestimmen. Diese Entdeckung und ihre Weiterverfolgung führte ihn dann fortschreitend zu einer Abwendung vom personalistisch-genetischen Aspekt der Psychoanalyse und ihrer Betonung der personalen Kindheit als dem eigentlichen Ursprungsort der menschlichen Entwicklung. Das seinen archetypischzeitlosen Aspekt ergänzende Zeit-Moment findet sich dann in der Betonung des Aktualkonfliktes und der von ihm skizzierten Psychologie der Lebensalter. Sowohl die Entdeckung der Archetypen wie die therapeutische Arbeit mit erwachsenen Menschen, welche die Psychoanalyse seinerzeit prinzipiell für "unheilbar" hielt, weil ihre Kindheit nicht mehr analytisch erreichbar war, verschob den Akzent der analytischen Psychologie von der Kindheit und dem zeitlich Personalen zum transpersonal-Zeitlosen als dem entscheidenden Schicksalsfaktor. In der Konsequenz dieser Auffassung und ohne die Tragweite seiner eigenen, im Laufe der Jahrzehnte immer reicher werdenden Entdeckungen voll zu realisieren, meinte Jung dann, die Therapie der ersten Lebenshälfte sei mit Hilfe reduktiver Methoden der Freud-Adlerschen Psychologie durchführbar.

Für uns, die wir, eine Generation später, auf den gesammelten Entdeckungen und Erfahrungen Jungs fussen, stellt sich, so scheint mir, die Aufgabe, die allzu stark auseinandergetretenen Aspekte des Personalen und des Transpersonalen, des Zeitlich-Genetischen und des Ewigen in einem veränderten Bild vom Menschen und seiner Entwicklung zu vereinigen. Dass wir dies tun müssen, ist nicht nur eine Notwendigkeit der Theorie, sondern mehr noch eine der Praxis. Die Ueberbetonung des Empirisch-Klinischen ist nur allzu oft damit identisch, seiner eigenen theoretischen Voraussetzungen unbewusst zu sein. Wenn Jung mit Recht betont, ein Empiriker zu sein, so ist sein Werk nicht zufälligerweise der grösstangelegte Versuch einer Theorie des Psychischen, den wir kennen. Gerade die überwältigende und fast nicht bewältigbare Fülle des empirischen Materials zwingt uns zur Theoriebildung, und in diesem Sinne ist auch mein Versuch zu verstehen, die archetypischen Stadien der Bewusstseinsentwicklung zu skizzieren.

Ich möchte als erstes betonen, dass die Ursprungsgeschichte

des Bewusstseins nicht identisch ist mit einer Ursprungsgeschichte der Psyche, die zu schreiben wir noch keineswegs imstande sind. D.h. wenn wir von archetypischen Stadien der Bewusstseinsentwicklung sprechen, meinen wir damit eine autonome Entfaltung der archetypischen Struktur der Psyche, innerhalb derer und an der die Ich- und Bewusstseinsentwicklung vor sich geht. So wie der Organismus sich in vorgegebener transpersonaler Weise entwickelt und das Zentralnervensystem in diese Entwicklung eingebaut ist, haben wir eine sich entfaltende archetypische Struktur der Psyche. In ihr wird die Dominanz des einen Archetyps von der eines anderen abgelöst und eine hierarchische archetypische Struktur aufgebaut. In dieser Entwicklung folgt mit Notwendigkeit die Entfaltung und Dominanz des einen Archetyps, z.B. des Vaterarchetyps, auf die des anderen, z.B. des Mutterarchetyps, so wie die Entwicklung des Bewusstseins auf die des Unbewussten und wie im Organischen die des zentralen Nervensystems auf die eines nicht zentrierten Nervensystems. D.h. aber das Transpersonal-Ewige, das jeder Archetyp darstellt und immer auch bleibt, begibt sich hier in ein zeitliches Nacheinander und bekommt damit einen genetisch-historischen Aspekt.

Wie wir für den Menschen eine transpersonale Entwicklung des Organischen kennen, die sich als Geburt, Pubertät, Lebensmitte, Klimakterium und Tod manifestiert, gibt es das Gleiche im Psychischen, und da der Mensch eine bio-psychische Einheit bildet, entsprechen diese Entwicklungsphasen des Organismus auch solchen der Psyche und der archetypischen Dominanz, wie Jung gerade an der Psychologie der Lebenswende und der Individuation in der zweiten Lebenshälfte nachgewiesen und dargestellt hat. Es handelt sich um eine transpersonale Entwicklung der psychischen Struktur, deren Nacheinander im Zeitlichen ebenso wie ihre strukturelle hierarchische Ordnung transpersonal artgemäss gegeben ist. So sprechen wir von einer verspäteten oder verfrühten, von einer verlängerten ebenso wie von einer verkürzten Pubertät.

D.h. es existiert eine transpersonal gegebene und sich entfaltende biopsychische Struktur, mit welcher das Individuum in Uebereinstimmung lebt, indem sie von ihm erfüllt wird, oder nicht in Uebereinstimmung lebt, wodurch es erkrankt. Dies Problem des "Uebereinstimmens" mit der artgemässen psychischen Struktur stellt den wesentlichen Konflikt dar zwischen dem Ich-Bewusstsein als dem Exponenten des Individuums und der artgemässen Kollektivstruktur der Psyche, wie sie durch die Instinkte repräsentierenden Archetypen gegeben ist. Diese artgemässe psychische Struktur aber enthält nicht nur ein Ewigkeits—sondern auch ein Zeitmoment, das man als transpersonal bezeichnen muss.

Aber nicht nur die Entfaltung der psychischen Struktur als einer Ganzheit ist archetypisch bedingt, sondern auch die des Bewusstseins, des Ich und der Beziehung des Ich zum Ganzen der Psyche. Dass die Phasen der Bewusstseins-Entwicklung transpersonal-archetypisch sind besagt, dass auch die Bewusstseins- und Ich-Entwicklung als artgemässe Entfaltung einer vorgegebenen psychischen Struktur anzusehen ist. Aber während die psychische Struktur, welche die Entwicklung der Lebensalter bestimmt, deutlich auf einem autonomen, d.h. in hohem Masse von der Unwelt unabhängigen, artgemässen und bio-psychischen Fundament fusst, haben wir es bei den archetypischen Stadien der Bewusstseinsentwicklung mit einem komplizierteren Phänomen zu tun. Es handelt sich nämlich nicht nur um das zeitliche Nacheinander einer spontan autonomen Entfaltung psychischer Dominanten, sondern dieser artgemäss angelegte und verlaufende Prozess ist gleichaeitig auf eine artgemässe Umwelt und deren Einwirkung angewiesen. D.h. das menschliche Kind in seiner Ich- und Bewusstseinsentwicklung ist seiner Art nach von Anfang an night nur ein psycho-biologisches, sondern ein soziales und kulturbedingtes Wesen. Wie die Geschichte der Wolfskinder lehrt, wird in einem nicht artgemässen Milieu, in welchem die menschliche Mutter fehlt, der Mutterarchetyp durch das kompensatorische Unbewusste nicht belebt, so dass sich das Kind nicht zu einem artgemässen menschlichen Wesen entwickeln kann. Nach den Forschungen Portmanns (1956) besteht eine der Besonderheiten der menschlichen Art darin, dass ein Teil der Embryonalentwicklung, nämlich das ganze erste Jahr, extrauterin in der Angewiesenheit des Säuglings auf die Mutter und die Prägung durch sie verläuft.

In der artgemäss archetypischen Strukturentwicklung der Psyche, folgt auf das anonym Enthaltende des Uroboros (vgl. Neumann, 1949) der Archetyp der Grossen Mutter und auf diesen der des Grossen Vaters. Da diese Reihenfolge ebensowenig umkehrbar ist, wie es unmöglich ist, ein Gebäude mit dem ersten Stockwerk zu beginnen, sprechen wir von einer hierarchischen psychischen Struktur. Die eine Phase ist strukturnotwendig die Grundlage der nächsten, die auf ihr aufbaut. D.h. die Aufeinanderfolge der archetypischen Stadien und Schichten konstituiert das transpersonale Zeit moment, nach dem artgemäss psychisches Nacheinander immer auch artgemässen Aufbau der psychischen Struktur bedeutet. So steht bei den Säugetieren, zu denen wir gehören, archetypisch immer das Enthaltensein im Uroborisch-Mütterlichen am Beginn, und immer folgt ihm als nächstes die Urbeziehung des Kindes zur Mutter. Dabei ist im Uroborischen das anonym Enthaltende der Intra-Uterin-Situation, in welcher das Ich-Bewusstsein des Kindes noch nicht erwacht ist, prägend, in der Urbeziehung dagegen der Bezogenheitscharakter eines von Mutter und Mutterarchetyp abhängig sich entwickelnden Ich und Bewusstseins. Wir sagen betontermassen "Mutter *und* Mutterarchetyp", denn bei den humanen, d.h. Menschengestalt besitzenden Archetypen ist immer die kompliziertere Konstellation gültig, die ich als die "personale Evokation des Archetyps" bezeichne. D.h. die in der Psyche des Kindes artgemäss angelegte und entwicklungsbereite transpersonale und zeitlose Struktur des Archetyps muss erst durch das personal-geschichtliche Ereignis der Begegnung mit einem Menschen ausgelöst und in Bewegung gesetzt werden. Diese Begegnung, z.B. die des Kindes mit der Mutter in der Urbeziehung, ist ebenfalls artgemäss, d.h. sie ereignet sich unter normalen menschlichen Bedingungen immer. Dieses Phänomen der Evokation des Archetyps ist individualgeschichtlich und personal, d.h. aber einer möglichen Störung ausgesetzt. Zwischen dem auszulösenden Archetyp in der kindlichen Psyche und der personalen auslösenden menschlichen Figur ist das Schlüssel-Schlüsselloch-Phänomen des Aufeinander-Zugepasstseins gültig, das uns aus der Instinktforschung bekannt ist. Aber während in der Tierwelt diese Prägungsstellen etwa im Sinne einer Stechuhr in der Entwicklung des Einzelwesens zeitlich genau festgelegt scheinen, muss im menschlichen Bereich die personale Auslösung des Archetyps zwar erfüllt werden, ist aber soweit wir wissen, nicht an einen genauen Termin gebunden. Gerade die Offenheit der psychischen Struktur des Kindes wird durch seine extrauterine Embryonalzeit, das erste Jahr nach der Geburt, gesteigert, in welcher es nicht mehr wie im Uterus von Ausseneinwirkungen fast abgeschlossen einer autonomen Entwicklung folgt, sondern in der Urbeziehung offen und ausgesetzt zugleich ist.

Damit wird aber die artgemässe Umwelt als Mutter und später als Eltern zu einem kulturbedingten und kulturbedingenden Einfluss, der neben die artgemässe Struktur der kindlichen Psyche tritt, und von Anfang an erweist sich das menschliche Schicksal als eine Synthese von archetypisch-zeitlosen und personalhistorischen Faktoren. Erst das artgemässe Einwirken der personalen Mutter in der Phase, in welcher der Mutterarchetyp dominant ist ebenso wie später erst das des personalen Vaters in der Phase, in welcher der Vaterarchetyp den Mutterarchetyp in seiner Dominanz abzulösen hat, garantiert eine artgemäss normative Entwicklung der psychischen Struktur des Kindes. So wie aber durch einen Schlüssel nicht nur das Schloss, sondern ein ganzer Raum eröffnet wird, wird durch die artgemässe personale Evokation des Archetyps eine ganze Welt und eine ganze Einheitsschicht der psychischen Struktur in Bewegung gesetzt. D.h. die personale Evokation ist schicksalsnotwendig, aber dann geschieht unendlich viel mehr, als was z.B. die Mutter oder der Vater tun oder intendieren. Ihr Tun setzt die angelegte Bereitschaft des transpersonalen Archetyps in der kindlichen Psyche in Bewegung, der deswegen in keiner Weise von der personalen Figur ableitbar, aber auf die personale Evokation artgemäss angewiesen ist.

Wenn diese Auffassung von der personalen Evokation der Archetypen richtig ist, hätten wir eine mittlere Stellung zwischen einer personalistisch genetischen und einer apersonal archetypischen Orientierung gefunden. Weder das Aufstöbern beliebiger personalistischer Daten in der Anamnese noch eine die Kindheit unberücksichtigt lassende und nur das Archetypische amplifizierende Methode wäre dann angemessen. Unser therapeutisches Augenmerk müsste sich besonders den Stellen der individuellen Entwicklung zuwenden, in welchen das Personale der Individualgeschichte sich nicht mit dem Transpersonalen der artgemässen archetypischen Stadienentwicklung in Uebereinstimmung befindet. So wissen wir z.B., dass der Ausfall der Mutter, falls sie nicht adäquat ersetzt wird, im ersten Lebensjahr zu Tod, Verblödung und psychotischer Gefährdung führen kann, wenn die Mutter dagegen erst nach einer normalen Urbeziehung der frühesten Entwicklungszeit ausfällt, sind die Entwicklungschancen des Kindes, selbst wenn es erkrankt, völlig andere geworden. Inzwischen ist der Mutterarchetyp in der psychischen Struktur des Kindes evoziert worden und kann damit auch unabhängig von ihrer personalen Realität z.B. im Sinne einer psychischen Kompensation wirken.

Das kompensatorische Verhältnis zwischen dem Ich-Bewusstsein und dem Unbewussten oder besser der psychischen Ganzheit wird, so scheint es, durch die Erfahrung der Urbeziehung konstelliert, in welcher die Mutter das Selbst, das Kind das Ich repräsentieren. Die durch die geglückte Urbeziehung gewonnene Sicherheit der Ich-Selbst-Beziehung kann nun auch beim Ausfall der Mutter als Person bestehen bleiben, sei es dadurch, dass der Mutterarchetyp nun projizierbar geworden ist, sei es dass er als schöpferisches Unbewusstes die Notsituation des Individuums auf andere Weise kompensiert.

Bevor wir aber diesen Gedanken weiterverfolgen, müssen wir einige prinzipielle Bemerkungen über das Wesen der psychischen Struktur in ihrer Beziehung zur geschichtlichen Entwicklung der Psyche einfügen. Denn nur so wird es möglich sein, den Einwänden zu begegnen, welche gegen die Ursprungsgeschichte (Neumann, 1949) und das in ihr dargestellte Prinzip der archetypischen Stadienentwicklung erhoben worden sind. Ich bin mir dabei dessen durchaus bewusst, dass es sich nur um einen Versuch handeln kann, denn in Wirklichkeit sind wir noch keineswegs voll imstande, die Tragweite dessen zu übersehen, was die Jungsche Konzeption des Archetyps bedeutet. Sie wird sich erst in Zukunft als das herausstellen, was sie ist, nämlich als eine neue Konzeption vom Menschen und von der Welt, welche in ihrer Tragweite bisher weder von den Geistes- und Kultur- noch von den sogenannten Naturwissenschaften geschweige denn von der Psychologie erfasst worden ist. Weder Einwände, die sich auf die heute herrschende Genetik noch solche, die sich auf die moderne unbewusst theologische Ethnologie des Pater Schmidt (1952) stützen, sind imstande, die auf einer ganz anderen, umfangreicheren und in ihrer Empirie viel eindeutigeren Konzeption des Archetyps fussenden Thesen der Tiefenpsychologie zu erschüttern. Umgekehrt wird sich möglicherweise gerade die Tiefenpsychologie mit ihrer Konzeption des Archetyps und der archetypischen Struktur des hierarchischen Aufbaus der Psyche als bahnbrechend und wegweisend für die anderen Wissenschaftsbezirke herausstellen.

Wenn wir davon sprechen, dass der Archetyp artgemäss sei, meint das, er konstitutiere allgemein menschliches Verhalten und existiere für das Individuum als eine Vorgegebenheit seiner psychischen Struktur. Wenn Jung deswegen sagt, der Archetyp sei Ahnenerfahrung, meint er natürlich nicht, er sei—wie bei Freud—Niederschlag sich wiederholenden historischen Geschehens z.B. als allmähliche Einprägung des im Zeitablauf offenbar unendliche Male sich wiederholenden Vatermordes. Wir finden nichts dergleichen Lamarckistisches bei Jung, müssen aber betonen, dass—worauf Portmann wiederholt aufmerksam gemacht hat—die heute moderne Vererbungstheorie der Auslese durch den Zufall nur die Varianten bestehender Ganzheiten erklären kann, aber sich ausserstande sieht, die Entstehung eines einzigen sinnvollen Organs auch nur wahrscheinlich zu machen. Wenn wir darüber hinaus wissen, dass die Erbbedeutung des Plasmas erst erforscht zu werden beginnt, scheint es berechtigt zu sagen, wir wissen nichts davon, wie die lebende Substanz Erfahrung macht und sich aus Systemen aufbaut die immer umfangreichere Erfahrung machen. Aber wir wissen, dass sie es tut und dass in jedem artgemässen Individuum eine Einheit von Erfahrung machender spezifisch aufgebauter lebendiger Substanz und einer diese Substanz prägenden und von ihr erfahrenen Welt vorhanden ist, auf welche diese Substanz bezogen ist.

Was bedeutet das artgemässe Funktionieren des Erbsenkäfers (Bruchus pisi), der für seine Brut in der noch weichen Erbse den Gang ausfrisst, da die später auskriechende Nachkommenschaft in der dann hart gewordenen Erbse sonst nicht auskriechen könnte? Ein derartiges Funktionieren kann niemals sukzessive durch wiederholte Erfahrungen, Einprägungen und Fortschritte erworben worden sein, da es keine Nachkommenschaft geben kann, wenn dieser Gang nicht da ist. Wir können keine Theorie des Geschehens geben, müssen aber darauf hinweisen, dass eine Konzeption unmöglich ist, in der ein Erfahrung machendes Subjekt von einer Welt als Objekt erst getrennt und danach aufeinander bezogen wird. Es handelt sich um ein Einheitsphänomen, wie z.B. auch in den sonst unerklärlichen Geschehen der Symbiose deutlich wird, in welcher die erfahrende lebendige Substanz des Lebewesens und die lebendige Substanz der Welt, in welcher sie existiert und auf die sie bezogen ist, in einem Einheitsfeld zusammengeschlossen sind.

Eine derartige Einheit aber ist der Archetyp, der immer zugleich Möglichkeit der Erfahrung der Psyche und eine durch diese Psyche erfahrene Welt in einem ist. So ist z.B. der Mutterarchetyp nicht nur eine Dominante der Psyche als eine archetypische Figur in ihr und eine Auffassung der Psyche von der Welt, sondern zugleich ein Sein der Einheitswirklichkeit, welches die Psyche enthält und hat entstehen Lassen. Dominanz des Mutterarchetyps in der archetypischen Stadienentwicklung bedeutet also nicht nur, dass hier dem Mutterarchetyp die führende Rolle in der Psyche zukommt, sondern dass der Mensch oder das Ich sich in einem spezifischen Abhängigkeitsverhältnis von einem umfassend ihn Nährendes und in einem Angewiesenheitsverhältnis auf dieses befindet—im Gegensatz z.B. zu einer späteren grösseren und selbständigeren Eigenaktivität.

Wenn ich deswegen von einer matriarchalen Phase als einer psycho-historischen Phase spreche, die nichts mit soziologischen und Macht-Verhältnissen zu tun hat, meint das diese Grundkonstellation, in welcher der Mensch und das Ich sich in der Welt vorfindet, wobei dieses sich so Vorfinden mit einer psychischen Konstellation identisch ist. Wenn mir daher z.B. vorgeworfen wurde (cf. Strech, 1958), nach der—mir übrigens theologisch verfärbt scheinenden—Erkenntnis der z.Zt. modernen Ethnologie stehe der "Urmonotheismus" und nicht das Matriarchat am Anfang der menschheitlichen Entwicklung, so verfehlt dieser Einwand das Entscheidende, nämlich den psychologisch-archetypischen Aspekt, um den es hier geht. Die in jedem populären Buch nachlesbaren Behauptungen oder auch Erkenntnisse der Ethnologie dürfen als bekannt vorausgesetzt werden. Aber die Urkulturen, in denen die Menschen, mit den Worten Pater Schmidts, "nur von dem leben, was die Natur in spontanem Wachstum hervorbringt und ihnen zur Nahrung darbietet", (1952, S.38 f.) sind psychologisch matriarchal, besonders im Gegensatz zu den charakteristischerweise produzierend genannten späteren Kulturstadien. In ihnen ist die Eigenaktivität des Menschen und des menschlichen Ich der Welt und der Natur gegenüber bewusst machtergreifend und soziologisch produzierend, d.h. aber psychologisch zu seiner neuen patriarchalen Selbständigkeit gekommen.

Aber die Frage, ob es sich psychologisch um eine matriarchale oder patriarchale Stufe handelt, ist in den Frühstadien auch keineswegs davon abzulesen, welches Geschlecht die Gottheit besitzt, wenn es in dieser Stufe eine gibt. Auch hier müssen wir lernen, psychologisch statt theologisch zu denken und zu verstehen suchen, welcher psychischen Situation des Menschen und einer Menschengruppe die spezifische Art und das Geschlecht einer Gottheit zuzuordnen ist. Eine gestaltlose männliche Geist-Gottheit, die erscheint oder gar nur zu erschliessen ist, kann wie wir wissen, durchaus zu einer matriarchalen Psychologie gehören, in der sie als patriarchaler Uroboros d.h. als gestaltlos Überwältigendes und Eindringendes erscheint. Wie leicht aber ist der Uebergang vom patriarchalen Uroboros, der deswegen diesen Namen erhalten hat, zu einer patriarchalen Gottheit, und wie schwer ist es zu entscheiden, was primär ist und was einer sekundären patriarchalen Umwertung entspricht.

Ich will dieses Thema hier nicht weiter verfolgen, sondern nur darauf hinweisen, dass es nicht die Aufgabe der Tiefenpsychologie ist, von Forschern, die psychologisch meist völlig unbewusst und einmal materialistisch-wissenschaftlich, einmal theologisch, fast immer aber patriarchal voreingenommen sind, Orientierungen entgegenzunehmen. Jeder, der in die Ergebnisse der gegenwärtigen Wissenschaft auch nur einen ungefähren Einblick hat, wird zugestehen müssen, dass die in der Tiefenpsychologie allmählich stärker werdende Bescheidenheit, welche aus der Bewusstwerdung der "persönlichen Gleichung" des Einzelnen stammt, in der Wissenschaft fast noch nirgends auch nur Problem geworden ist.

Im Rahmen dieser Auseinandersetzung, welche die Notwendigkeit betont, von den Erfahrungen der Tiefenpsychologie ausgehend zu allgemeinen verbindlichen Aussagen über den Menschen überhaupt zu gelangen, scheint es mir nötig, wenigstens den Versuch zu machen, einige Missverständnisse aufzuklären, welche sich an Inhalt und Begriff dessen geknüpft haben, was ich in der Ursprungsgeschichte in Uebereinstimmung mit Jung und seinem Satz: "Das ferne Ziel, zu dem diese Forschungen führen, ist eine Phylogenie des Geistes" (Jung, 1913, S.134) als "Psycho-Historie" bezeichnet habe. Es mag sein, dass ich diese Missverständnisse verursacht habe, obgleich ich mich ausserordentlich bemüht habe, sie zu verhindern. Fraglos sind aber dann durch die Interpretation Fordhams (cf. Fordham, 1957) weitere Missverständnisse entstanden. Erstens: Niemals habe ich von einem biogenetischen Gesetz gesprochen, niemals auch nur von einem Gesetz. Wenn man den grundlegenden Zusammenhang zwischen Phylogenese und Ontogenese als Gesetz ansprechen will, dann würde es sich um ein erst aufzustellendes psychogenetisches Gesetz handeln. Zweitens: Fordhams Erklärung, die Ontogenese entspreche nicht der Phylogenese und seine Polemik gegen die Anwendung des biogenetischen Grundgesetzes und des Evolutions-Gesichtspunktes in der Psychologie sind, wenigstens was meine Ausführungen betrifft, völlig fehl am Platze. Es wurde von mir immer und betont von der Entwicklungsgeschichte des *Bewusstseins* gesprochen, und die These der Ursprungsgeschichte sagt, die Phasen der Bewusstseinsentstehung der Menschheit, so wie sie sich meiner Auffassung nach z.B. im Mythos darstellt, seien mit der Bewusstseinsgeschichte des Einzelnen identisch. Drittens: Bei den Entwicklungsphasen, die nicht historisch nachweisbar oder jedenfalls bisher historisch unbewiesen sind, handelt es sich um Phasen der Psycho-Historie, d.h. um Phasen der psychischen Struktur, die deswegen in ihrem Nacheinander analog zu den S.D. Phasen (der "Sequence dating") der Archäologie sind, bei denen ebenfalls das Nach-und Aufeinanderfolgen der Phasen nichts über eine zeitliche und historische Datierung aussagt.

Ich will an einem einfachsten Beispiel das ausführen, was eine Selbstverständlichkeit zu sein scheint. Das Grundphänomen des kosmogonischen Mythos der Bewusstseinsentstehung ist die Geburt des Lichtes aus dem Dunkel. Dabei ist natürlich das Dunkel das Symbol des Unbewussten. Das Dunkel ist damit nicht nur das psychohistorische Frühere sondern auch die strukturelle Basis, die Grundlage des Späteren. Mit dem "Geburtssymbol" ist die ganze Vielfalt dessen, was wir ontogenetisch als "Urbeziehung" kennen, impliziert. Dass die Ontogenese der

Phylogenese entspricht besagt nicht nur, so wie im Individuum das Bewusstsein aus dem Unbewussten entspringt, ist auch in der Menschheitsgeschichte aus einer früheren Epoche des Unbewusstseins das Bewusstsein geboren worden, sondern die Struktur der Psyche ist so, dass immer Bewusstsein aus dem Unbewussten als dem Früheren und Grundlegenden entsteht. Das ist ein psychogenetisches, keineswegs aber ein biogenetisches Gesetz. Ganz gewiss handelt es sich hier nicht um die falsche Anwendung einer aus der Biologie entnommenen Theorie der Entwicklungsgeschichte auf die Psychologie.

Sogar wenn wir formulieren würden, es sei eine Anwendung des entwicklungsgeschichtlichen Gedankens auf die Psyche, hätten wir es falsch formuliert, denn es handelt sich um eine psychologische Aussage, welche die *Geburts- und Mutter-Kind Symbolik der Psyche* als das deutet und versteht, was diese meint, nämlich als eine Entwicklung.

Das der humane Archetyp im Bild einer zwischen-menschlichen Konstellation erscheint, z.B. als Urbeziehung von Mutter und Kind, oder als Beziehung von Mutter und Jünglings-Geliebtem, bedeutet einmal, dass hier ein für die menschliche Art Ewiges ausgesagt wird, bedeutet aber darüber hinaus, dass dieses Ewige von entscheidender und prägender Bedeutung für jeden Menschen ist. Im Bild der Urbeziehung offenbart sich nicht nur eine ewige Situation, sondern auch ein gleichermassen ewiges Entwicklungs-Schema, das für die psychische Struktur grundlegend ist : Uebergewicht des Ursprungs als Basis, Sicherheits- und Nahrungsgrundlage, Enthaltensein und Abhängigkeit des Entsprungenen und Späteren. Aber im Urbild der Mutter-Kindbeziehung ist gleichzeitig die Autonomie des Wachstums und die Notwendigkeit einer künftigen Befreiung vom Uebergewicht des Ursprungs zur späteren endgültigen Selbständigkeit "mitgegeben". Dabei ist das archetypisch-genetische Struktur-Moment mit der anscheinend banalen Tatsache identisch, dass Enthaltensein früher ist als Befreitsein. Dabei tritt das Enthaltende bei den Säugetieren, zu denen wir gehören, mit Selbstverständlichkeit als das Mütterliche auf, so dass Selbständigwerden zunächst Befreiung von der Mutter heisst.

Es ist wichtig zu erkennen, dass die Dominanz eines Archetyps, wie z.B. der Mutter der Urbeziehung, nicht so aufgefasst werden darf, als ob es sich nur um die Herrschaft eines bestimmten Archetyps in der menschlichen Psyche handle, die dem Menschen ein pattern of behaviour vorschreibt. Der Archetyp ist als Abbild einer Struktur viel mehr, er enthält in sich die Gesetzmässigkeit sowohl eines innerpsychischen wie eines zwischenmenschlichen und eines mensch-weltlichen Entwicklungsablaufs. Analog findet man schon beim tierischen Instinkt, dass er einen Ablauf im biopsychischen Organismus des Tieres, zwischen Tier und Nachwuchs und zwischen Tier und Umwelt bestimmt und ordnet.

Die *innerpsychische* entwicklungsbestimmende Struktur des Archetyps wird sofort deutlich, wenn wir uns bewusst machen, dass in der Urbeziehung die Mutter als dirigierender und schützend-ernährender Ursprung das Unbewusste und in der ersten Phase auch das Selbst bedeutet und das von ihr abhängige Kind das kindliche Ich und das Bewusstsein. Auch hier ist ein artgemässer Verlauf der innerpsychischen Entwicklung von Ich-Selbst-Abhängigkeit und Ich-Selbst-Konflikt, von Entstehung des Ich und des Bewusstseins aus dem Unbewussten und von mit dem Selbständigwerden mitgegebenem Konflikt zwischen Ich-Bewusstsein und Unbewusstem evident.

Aber der Archetyp der Urbeziehung bestimmt nicht nur eine inner-psychische sondern auch eine *zwischenmenschliche* Entwicklung. Gerade durch die personale Evokation des Archetyps würde die artgemässe Verflechtung des Innerpsychischen mit dem Zwischenmenschlichen deutlich. So bestimmt der Archetyp als zwischen-menschliches Phänomen nicht nur ein Verhalten des Kindes zur Mutter und der Mutter zum Kinde, sondern eine ganze Verhaltensreihe von Entwicklungen. Ambivalenz der Mutter und Ambivalenz der kindlichen Bezogenheit, Konfliktgenese durch Selbständigwerden des zunächst Abhängigen, damit zusammenhängend Uebergang von der positiv-enthaltend-nährenden zur festhaltend-verschlingenden Mutter etc. etc., alles diese Abwandlungen der zwischenmenschlichen Entwicklung sind als natur- und artgemässer Ablauf im archetypischen Bild der Urbeziehung mitgegeben.

Aber im Archetyp ist immer auch ein Weltaspekt enthalten. Deswegen sprechen wir von einer "matriarchalen Welt", von einer Welt des Jünglingsgeliebten, einer patriarchalen Welt usw.

Dabei ist das archetypische Bild z.B. der Urbeziehung nicht, wie wir früher annahmen, eine Reaktion der Psyche auf die Welt, sondern ebenso das Bild einer die Psyche konstituierenden Welt.

Wenn die Menschen "nur von dem leben, was die Natur in spontanem Wachstum hervorbringt und ihm zur Nahrung anbietet", handelt es sich um einen nicht-psychischen Tatbestand, aber wenn wir sagen, er sei Ausdruck einer "matriarchalen" Konstellation, besagt das, dass die Welt und Natur dem Menschen in der gleichen mütterlich-überlegenen Gestalt wie die Mutter dem Kind und das Unbewusste dem Ich gegenübertritt. Alles dies ist in dem Archetyp als einer Struktur enthalten. D.h. in dem Bild des Mutter-Kind-Archetyps der Urbeziehung ist die den Menschen konstituierende Einheit von welthafter, zwischenmenschlicher und innerpsychischer Bezogenheit fassbares Bild geworden. Deswegen können wir überall, wo dieser Archetyp auftaucht, gleichzeitig etwas über die Beziehung des Ich zum Unbewussten und Selbst, zur Mutter und allen ihren Vertretern und zur Welt als Natur aussagen.

Jetzt wird wohl evident geworden sein, was es bedeutet, dass psychologisch und psychohistorisch das Matriarchale und die matriarchale Welt primär ist, und dass diese Aussage sowohl ontogenetisch wie phylogenetisch gültig ist.

Der Archetyp ist immer auf eine Welt und Psyche umfassende Einheitswirklichkeit bezogen (vgl. Neumann, 1955a, 1956a, 1957). Der Uebergang von der Dominanz eines Archetyps zu der Dominanz eines anderen ist ein entwicklungsgeschichtlich kritischer Punkt, weil mit einem Dominanzwechsel immer eine innerpsychische, zwischenmenschliche und die Haltung zur Welt einschliessende Wandlung verbunden ist. Die Kindheit erweist sich uns jetzt als ein entscheidender Abschnitt der menschlichen Entwicklung, weil sich in ihr nicht nur die Psyche in ihren wesentlich archetypisch fixierten Stadien entfaltet, und strukturiert, sondern diese Struktur gleichzeitig die engere und weitere Beziehung zur Umwelt und die allgemeine Daseinshaltung als artgemäss oder als gestört einschliesst. So ist mit der Urbeziehung die Bezogenheit zum Selbst, zum Unbewussten, zum primären Du und zur Welt als Natur, mit der Dominanz des Vaterarchetyps die Möglichkeit der Ueber-Ich-Entwicklung, die Bewusstseinsentwicklung und Kulturierung mitgegeben, und keine Störung des einen verläuft ohne ein Mitgestörtsein des anderen Bezirks.

Leider können wir hier nur kurz auf einige genetisch bedingte Störungspunkte der artgemässen Entwicklung hinweisen. Wir tun es nur im Zusammenhang mit unseren prinzipiellen Ausführungen, aber jeder von Ihnen wird das Gemeinte mit seinem eigenen Material zu illustrieren imstande sein.

Die Ich-Selbst-Entwicklung verläuft von der uroborisch, mann-weiblich, väterlich-mütterlichen Vorfigur des matriarchalen Selbst zur matriarchalen Phase, in welcher der Mutterarchetyp dominant, das Väterlich-Männliche sekundär mit ihm verbunden ist. Das ist identisch mit einem Uebergewicht des dirigierenden Unbewussten, sei es dass dieses Dirigieren durch artgemässe Instinktformen oder spontane Manifestationen des Unbewussten erfolgt (Neumann, 1953a). Zugeordnet ist ein kindlich-unselbständiges aber sich zu relativer Autonomie entwickelndes Ich und Bewusstsein. Störungen können sowohl durch Ausfall oder Störung des personal-evozierenden Faktors, der personalen Mutter, eintreten, die in ihrer Persönlichkeit oder in Störungen der von ihr vertretenen Welt liegen. Auch "Umweltsstörungen" wie Hunger oder Krankheit sind Störungen der artgemäss normalen Entwicklung, die durch die Person der Mutter garantiert wird, und das Versagen der Mutter, die aus "äusseren" Gründen nicht nähren, schützen und kompensieren kann, führt zu einem Defekt in der personalen Evokation des Mutterarchetyps mit all den katastrophalen Folgen, die eine solche Störung mit sich bringt.

Die grundsätzlich andere Störungsform besteht in der Möglichkeit eines konstitutionellen Defektes des Kindes, in dem trotz artgemässer Evokation durch die Mutter und Normalität der von der Mutter vertretenen Welt das Evozierte, das archetypisch biopsychische Bereitschaftssystem, nicht ausgelöst wird. Einen solchen Fall stellen im Extrem z.B. die Kinder dar, die vom Moment der Geburt an keine Reaktion in der Urbeziehung zeigen und von ihren—normal-ungestörten—Müttern als "nicht antwortend" bezeichnet werden.

Entsprechende Störungszentren der Entwicklung sind alle "Uebergangsstellen" archetypischer Dominanz. Die Krisenpunkte Pubertät, Lebensmitte, Klimakterium sind keineswegs die einzigen. In der Kindheit sind derartige Krisenstellen aber gehäuft, weil in ihr der Aufbau der artgemäss psychischen Struktur mit dem Durchlaufen archetypisch artgemäss aufeinander folgender Phasen identisch ist. Die archetypischen Uebergänge, deren objektive Datierung in der Ontogenese wichtig wäre, sind Krisenstellen der Entwicklung. Wir wollen dies an einem Hinweis verdeutlichen, dem Wechsel der Geschlechtszuordnung zum Selbst. Wenn auch anfangs *immer* die umfassende und dirigierende Mutter das Selbst vertritt, kommt es später zu einer für Mädchen und Knaben verschiedenen Entwicklung, in der die Geschlechtszuordnung des Selbst für das Mädchen weiblich bleibt, für den Knaben aber von der Mutter abgelöst werden muss. Diese Krise der Selbstfindung steht natürlich im Zusammenhang mit der Loslösung des Kindes von der Urbeziehung. Selbstverständlich ist dieser Prozess bei dem Mädchen, für welches Mutter und Selbst geschlechtsverbunden bleiben, weniger problematisch als für den Knaben, der mit der Lösung von der Mutter seine bisherige Selbst-Zuordnung verändern muss. Viele Probleme der Geschlechsunsicherheit und Selbst-Unsicherheit hängen bei ihm mit diesem archetypischen Uebergang bei der Loslösung von der Mutter der Urbeziehung zusammen. Umgekehrt ist die Problematik bei der Begegnung des Kindes mit dem Vaterarchetyp, in welcher der Knabe zum "Eigenen", das Mädchen aber zum "Anderen" kommt.

Aber auch bestimmte Erkrankungsformen scheinen,—wir stehen hier ja erst am Anfang—mit den archetypischen Phasen und der für den Aufbau der Psyche artgemäss notwendigen archetypischen Erfahrung in dem Sinne zusammenzuhängen, dass eine ihrer Ursachen darin besteht, dass eine derartige Erfahrung fehlt oder nur ungenügend realisiert worden ist. So scheint die ungenügende Erfahrung der Urbeziehung, die dann in der Uebertragung nachgeholt werden muss, zu bestimmten Schizophrenieformen zu führen. Der Zusammenhang der gesetzmässigen magischen Stufe der Urbeziehung mit psychischen Erkrankungen ist von Whitmont (1957) verdeutlicht worden, auf die Zuordnung der Beziehung des Jünglingsgeliebten zur Grossen Mutter und der Homosexualität habe ich schon in der Ursprungsgeschichte (1949) aufmerksam gemacht. Dass in einer weiblichen Psychose eines Schwangerschaftswahnes einer Schizophrenen die Verfallsstadien der Psyche den nach meiner Ansicht (Neumann, 1952, 1953*b*) für die weibliche Psyche typischen Entwicklungsstadien folgen, hat Beyme (1957) wahrscheinlich gemacht, um nur einige Beispiele zu nennen. Kurz es besteht die Hoffnung, dass das Strukturgerüst der archetypischen Phasen sich als hilfreich erweist, genetische Störungen und Fixierungen mit Krankheitsgruppen in Zusammenhang zu bringen.

Psychohistorie heisst hier, den wesensmässigen Zusammenhang von Archetyp und Reaktion des Individuums zu verstehen und dem Strukturaufbau der Psyche zuzuordnen, z.B. zu erkennen, dass männliche Homosexualität immer vor-patriarchal ist, dass in ihr das Männliche vom Weiblichen nicht losgelöst ist und sich dauernd von ihm bedroht fühlt, weil bei ihm das Selbst noch nicht in der Eindeutigkeit als männlich erfahren wird, welche für die spätere patriarchale Männlichkeit selbstverständlich geworden ist. Diese psychohistorische Zuordnung hat nichts mit Geschichtlichkeit und soziologischen Zusammenhängen zu tun, macht es aber, was von entscheidender Wichtigkeit ist, möglich, die auftretende Symbolik in dem richtigen Zusammenhang zu sehen und zu erfassen.

Wir kommen damit zu einen letzten Punkt, der mit der Bedeutung der archetypischen Phasen als einer Entwicklungsreihe zu tun hat, nämlich mit der Bedeutung des Stellenwertes des Symbols in der S.D. Reihe der psychischen Entwicklung. Im allgemeinen haben wir das Verständnis des Symbols von seiner Amplifikation abhängig gemacht, d.h. von der Aufstellung einer horizontalen Reihe analoger Symbole, deren gegenseitige Erklärung im Sinne einer Anreicherung erfolgt. So macht z.B. die Zusammenstellung der Symbole der "Grossen Mutter" von "überall her" die Einheit und den Umfang des Archetyps sichtbar (vgl. Neumann, 1956).

Die Amplifikation ist aber für die Diagnose der psychischen Situation eines Menschen und für die Therapie unzureichend. Sie muss ergänzt werden durch den Stellenwert des Symbols, die vertikale Orientierung innerhalb der Psychohistorie, d.h. die Feststellung, zu welcher Entwicklungsphase das Symbol gehört. Erst dieser Stellenwert zusammen mit der Amplifikation ermöglicht die aktuelle Deutung des Symbols, so dass sich feststellen lässt, ob das Symbol progressive oder regressive Bedeutung hat, d.h. aber wie die Prognose der Situation ist. Ob z.B. die Grosse Mutter, die als Hexe erscheint, in der kindlichen Entwicklung die Progression zum Vaterarchetyp erleichtert, indem sie das kindliche Ich von der Mutter und der Bindung an sie abschreckt, ob sie in der Auseinandersetzung mit dem jugendlichen Ich des Jünglings oder des jungen Mädchens aufgesucht und besiegt wird, oder ob ihr, wie in der Individuation der zweiten Lebenshälfte, gedient werden muss, damit sie sich in der Wandlung als Sophia erweist, das lässt sich durch keine Amplifikation feststellen, sondern nur durch eine Orientierung und der Psychohistorie der menschlichen Entwicklungsstadien.

Erst die Einheit des Archetypisch-Ewigen mit seinem psychohistorischen Ort in der menschlichen Entwicklung ermöglicht uns, seine wahre Schickslasbedeutung für den Einzelnen zu erfassen. Auch diese Feststellung ist vielleicht eine Banalität, denn unbewusst haben wir wohl das Symbol immer in einen solchen Entwicklungszusammenhang gestellt. Meine Bemühung ging nur dahin zu zeigen, welchen Platz der genetische Aspekt deswegen auch in unserer Theorie einnehmen muss. Denn erst unsere fortlaufend zu erweiternde Theorie macht es uns möglich, das zu realisieren, was wir in unserer Praxis tun. Auch hier gilt das nicht genügend beherzigte Wort Goethes (1797): "Man erfährt wieder bei dieser Gelegenheit, dass eine vollständige Erfahrung die Theorie in sich enthalten muss".

## REFERENCES

Beyme, F. (1957). "Analyse eines schizophrenen Schwangerschaftswahnes im Lichte der Forschungen von J. J. Bachofen, C. G. Jung und E. Neumann", *Schweizer Archiv für Neurologie und Psychiatrie*, **80**, 1, 2.

Fordham, M. (1957). "Biological Theory and the Concept of Archetypes", *New Developments in Analytical Psychology*. London, Routledge & Kegan Paul.

Goethe, J. W. (1797). Brief an Schiller, 19 Oktober 1797.

Jung, C. G. (1913). *Versuch einer Darstellung der psychoanalytischen Theorie*. Leipzig and Vienna, Deuticke. Republished by Rascher, Zurich, 1955.

Neumann, E. (1953*a*). "Ueber den Mond und das matriarchale Bewusstsein" in *Zur Psychologie des Weiblichen*. Zürich, Rascher.

Neumann, E. (1953*b*). "Die psychologischen Stadien der weiblichen Entwicklung" in *Zur Psychologie des Weiblichen*. Zürich, Rascher.

Neumann, E. (1949). *Ursprungsgeschichte des Bewusstseins*. Zürich, Rascher.

NEUMANN, E. (1954). *The Origins and History of Consciousness.* Bollingen Series 42. New York, Pantheon; London, Routledge & Kegan Paul.
NEUMANN, E. (1955). *The Great Mother.* Bollingen Series 47. New York, Pantheon; London, Routledge & Kegan Paul.
NEUMANN, E. (1956). *Die Grosse Mutter.* Zürich, Rhein-Verlag.
NEUMANN, E. (1956*a*). "Die Erfahrung der Einheitswirklichkeit". *Eranos-Jb.* **24.** Also in: *Der schöpferische Mensch* (1959). Zürich, Rhein–Verlag.
NEUMANN, E. (1952). *Amor und Psyche.* Zürich, Rascher.
NEUMANN, E. (1956*b*). *Amor and Psyche.* Bollingen Series 54. New York, Pantheon; London, Routledge & Kegan Paul.
NEUMANN, E. (1957). "Der schöpferische Mensch und die 'Grosse Erfahrung' ". *Eranos-Jb.* **25.** Also in: *Der schöpferische Mensch* (1959). Zürich, Rhein–Verlag.
NEUMANN, E. (1955*a*). "Der schöpferische Mensch und die Wandlung". *Eranos-Jb.* **23.** Also in: *Der schöpferische Mensch* (1959). Zürich, Rhein–Verlag.
NEUMANN, E. (1959). "Creative Man and Transformation" in *Art and the Creative Unconscious.* Bollingen Series 61. New York, Pantheon; London, Routledge & Kegan Paul.
PORTMANN, A. (1956). *Zoologie und das neue Bild vom Menschen.* Hamburg, Rowohlt.
SCHMIDT, W. (1952). "Die Urkulturen" in "Frühe Menschheit", *Historia Mundi,* **1.**
STRECH, H. H. (1958). "Psycho-Historie oder Kulturhistorie?" *Psyche,* **11,** 12.
WHITMONT, E. (1957). "Magic and the Psychology of Compulsive States". *J. analyt. Psychol.,* **2,** 1.

# *THE SIGNIFICANCE OF THE GENETIC ASPECT FOR ANALYTICAL PSYCHOLOGY*

*The distant goal to which these researches lead is a phylogeny of the mind.*
C. G. JUNG (1912)

IF we survey the history of depth psychology, we shall be struck by the fact that not only as it developed from the psycho-analysis of Freud to the analytical psychology of Jung, but, in its whole general outlook, the emphasis laid on the personal has increasingly shifted to the transpersonal aspect. Psycho-analysis regards man essentially as a being who must be understood in terms of his personal history. The unique and accidental occurrences taking place between the child and its parents are, accordingly, the elements that determine the fate of the healthy, and especially the pathological, development of the individual. This personalistic genetic view led to decisive importance being attached to childhood and its analysis. The complementary transpersonal aspect finds expression in building up a model of the psychic structure revealing, in the normative phases of libido development, a general plan in which the personalistic events acquire their position and their value—for instance, fixation at the anal stage through the mother's wrong training of the child in regard to cleanliness, etc.

In contrast to this accentuation of the temporal and personal, Jung discovered the crucial importance of the timeless and transpersonal factors in the psyche—the archetypes—that determine man's development. This discovery and its implications led him to turn away more and more from the personalistic genetic aspect of psycho-analysis with its emphasis on childhood as the real source of human development. The time element that complements the timeless archetypal aspect is to be found in the emphasis Jung lays on actual conflicts, and in the psychology of the states of life sketched out by him. The discovery of the archetypes, and therapeutic work with adult patients whom psycho-analysts then regarded as "incurable" because their childhood was no longer accessible to analysis, shifted the accent of analytical psychology from childhood and the temporal and personal to the transpersonal and timeless as the fate-determining factor. In following up the logical consequence of this view, and without fully realizing the scope of his own discoveries, which grew steadily richer in the course of the years, Jung then believed that patients in the first half of life could be treated with the help of the reductive methods of Freudian and Adlerian psychology.

For us who, a generation later, can take our stand on the sum total of Jung's discoveries and experiences, the task must surely be to combine the aspects of the personal and the transpersonal, the temporal-genetic and the timeless, which have grown too far apart, in an altered picture of man and his development. To do this is a necessity not only in theory but even more so in practice.

The excessive emphasis laid on purely empirical and clinical factors is, only too often, identical with being unconscious of one's own theoretical preconceptions. Although Jung rightly stresses that he is an empiricist, it is nevertheless no accident that his work is the grandest attempt yet made to construct a theory of the psyche. It is just the overwhelming and almost unmanageable richness of the empirical material that forces us to build theories: and my own attempt to sketch out the archetypal stages of conscious development must also be understood in this sense.

I would like to emphasize, first, that the origins and history of consciousness are not identical with the origins and history of the psyche, of which we are in no position to write at present. When we speak of the archetypal stages of conscious development, we mean the autonomous unfolding of the archetypal structure of the psyche, within which and through which the development of the ego and of consciousness proceeds. Just as the organism develops in a transpersonal way laid down from the start with the central nervous system built into this development, so also we have an archetypal structure of the psyche that unfolds by itself. In it the dominance of one archetype is superseded by that of another and an hierarchical archetypal structure is built up: the unfolding of one archetype, say the father archetype, follows of necessity that of another, say the mother archetype. In the same way the development of consciousness follows that of the unconscious and, in the organism itself, the development of a central nervous system follows that of a non-centralized nervous system. This means that the transpersonal and timeless, which every archetype is and remains, enters into temporal succession and consequently acquires a genetic and historical aspect.

We know that in man the organism undergoes a transpersonal development that manifests itself as birth, puberty, middle age, climacteric, and death. The same thing happens in the psyche, and, since man is a bio-psychic unity, these phases of organic development correspond to phases of archetypal dominance within the psyche. Jung was able to demonstrate this in the psychology of the critical phase of middle life and the psychology of individuation. We can ascertain a transpersonal development of psychic structure, the sequence of which in time, like its hierarchal structural order, is determined transpersonally and fixed as a specific pattern. Thus we speak of a retarded or a precocious, a prolonged or a shortened, puberty. There is, in other words, a transpersonal, self-unfolding bio-psychic structure with which the individual lives in harmony when he fulfils it, or with which he does not live in harmony so that he becomes ill. This problem of living in harmony with the psychic structure of the species expresses the essential conflict between ego consciousness as the exponent of the individual and the specifically fixed, collective structure of the psyche as given by the archetypes which represent the instincts. This specific psychic structure contains a timeless as well as a time element that must be designated transpersonal.

Not only is the unfolding of the psychic structure as a whole determined archetypally, but also that of consciousness, of the ego, and of the ego's relation to the whole of the psyche and of the world. The fact that the phases of conscious development are transpersonal and archetypal means that the development of consciousness and of the ego must likewise be regarded as a specific unfolding of a pre-existent psychic structure. But whereas the psychic structure that determines the unfolding of the stages of life rests clearly on bio-psychic foundations peculiar to the species and largely independent of the environment, in the archetypal stages of conscious development we have to do with a more complicated phenomenon. Not only is there a temporal succession of psychic dominants unfolding autonomously, but this entire process, whose predisposed course is ingrained in the species, is at the same time dependent on the influence of a specific environment. The human child, with his development of an ego and consciousness, is by nature not only a psycho-biological being, but from the very beginning a social being conditioned by culture. As the history of the wolf children shows, in a non-human milieu in which the personal mother is lacking, the mother archetype is not activated by the compensatory unconscious, so that the child does not develop into a specifically human creature. According to the researches of Portmann (1956), one of the peculiarities of the human species is that part of the embryonic development, actually the whole first year, takes place outside the uterus, in the dependence of the infant on the mother and on her "imprinting".

In the archetypal development of psychic structure within the species the anonymous container, the uroboros (cf. Neumann, 1954), is succeeded by the archetype of the great mother, and this by the archetype of the great father. As this sequence cannot be reversed, any more than it would be possible to begin building a house from the roof downwards, we speak of the hierarchical structure of the psyche. The one phase is, by structural necessity, the foundation of the next. The sequence of archetypal stages and layers constitutes the transpersonal time element, in accordance with which a sequence of psychic events characteristic of the species is built up into an equally characteristic psychic structure. Thus among the mammals, to which class we belong, containment in the maternal uroboros always comes at the beginning, and this is always followed by the primary relationship of child to mother. In the uroboric phase the determining factor is the anonymously containing intra-uterine situation, in which the ego consciousness of the child is not yet awakened; in the primary relationship it is the development of an ego and consciousness in dependence of the mother archetype *and* the mother. We say emphatically "mother archetype *and* mother", because in the case of those archetypes which possess a human form the more complicated constellation I mentioned above becomes operative. I call this the "personal evocation of the archetype". That is to say the transpersonal and timeless structure of the archetype, ingrained in the specifically human psyche of the child and ready for development, must first be released and activated by the personal encounter with a human being. This encounter of the child with the mother in the primary relationship is also specifically human, and will always take place under normal human conditions. But the evocation of the archetype is a personal event in the individual's history and therefore subject to possible disturbance. Between the archetype to be released in the child's psyche and the human "releaser" figure a lock-and-key phenomenon comes into force: each must fit the other perfectly. This is comparable to the animal world in which the innate releasing mechanisms seem to function like clockwork at precise points of formative readiness for imprinting. But in the human realm the personal release of the archetype, though it must be fulfilled, is not, so far as we know, bound to any precise moment in time.

It is just the openness of the psychic structure of the child which is intensified by the embryonic period outside the uterus. Then it no longer follows an autonomous development practically cut off from all external influences, but is open and exposed at once in the primary relationship.

In this way the human environment—experienced as the mother and later as both parents—becomes a culture-conditioned and culture-conditioning influence appearing alongside the specifically human structure of the child's psyche, so that from the very beginning fate proves to be a synthesis of timeless archetypal and personal historical factors. It is only the specifically human influence of the personal mother in the phase when the mother archetype is dominant, and of the personal father in the phase when the father archetype has to replace it, that guarantees normal development of the child's psychic structure. But just as a key unlocks not only the door but a whole room, so the personal evocation of the archetype discloses a whole world and activates a unitary layer in the psychic structure. In other words, the personal evocation is necessitated by fate, so that infinitely more happens than what the mother or father does or intends. Their activity releases the ingrained propensities of the transpersonal archetype in the child's psyche, which cannot be derived in any sense from the personal figure though it is specifically dependent on personal evocation.

If this view of the personal evocation of archetypes is correct, then we would have found a position midway between a personalistic, genetic orientation and a transpersonal, archetypal one. Neither ferreting out personal data during the anamnesis nor amplifying only the archetypal material leaving childhood unconsidered could be appropriate. We have to turn our attention more particularly to those critical places where the personal factors in the individual's history have to be in harmony with the transpersonal stages of archetypal development, characteristic of the species, or where their disharmony has a pathogenic effect. Thus we know that the loss of the mother (without adequate substitute) during the first year of the child's life can lead to death, severe deterioration, and psychotic disturbances, whereas if the loss occurs after a normal primary relationship in the earliest developmental period the chances of the child's healthy development are much more promising even if he becomes ill. For in the meantime the mother archetype in the psychic structure of the child has been evoked and can function independently of the mother's reality, for instance as a compensating psychic factor.

The compensatory relationship between ego consciousness and the psychic totality seems to be constellated by the experience of the primary relationship in which the mother represents the self and the child the ego. The security of the ego-self relationship achieved in a successful primary relationship can now survive even the loss of the mother as a person, whether it be that the mother archetype can now be projected or, functioning as the creative unconscious, compensate the plight of the individual in some other way.

Before we pursue these thoughts further, we must make a few remarks on the nature of psychic structure in relation to the historical development of the psyche. For only then will it be possible to counter the objections that have been raised against the archetypal stages of development depicted in my book, *The Origins and History of Consciousness*. I am fully aware that this can be no more than an attempt, for it seems to me that in reality we are still very far from being able to survey the full scope of Jung's conception of the archetype. The future will show that this is really a new conception of man and the world, whose implications have been grasped neither by the human nor by the so-called natural sciences, let alone by psychologists. No objections based on present-day genetics, nor those supported by the unconsciously theological ethnology of Father Schmidt (1952), are in my opinion capable of shaking the theses of depth psychology, because they are grounded in a quite different, more comprehensive, and from the empirical point of view much clearer conception of the archetype. Conversely, it is very likely that depth psychology, with its conception of the archetypal and hierarchical structure of the psyche, will prove to have broken new ground and pointed the way for the other sciences.

When we speak of an archetype as "specifically human", we mean that it constitutes a general mode of human behaviour which exists as an *a priori* datum of psychic structure in the individual. When Jung therefore says that the archetype is ancestral experience, he naturally does not mean that it is the deposit of a self-repeating historical event, in the Freudian sense of the gradual imprinting of an endlessly repeated father-murder. We do not find any such Lamarckian ideas in Jung's writings, though in the beginning his formulations are somewhat ambiguous. Here we want to emphasize a point to which Portmann has repeatedly drawn attention: that the modern theory of heredity based on chance variation can explain only the changes in existing wholes, but is incapable of giving a plausible explanation of the origin of a single meaningful organ. And when, on top of that, we consider that the plasma's significance for heredity is only now beginning to be investigated, we would seem justified in saying that we know nothing about how living substance accumulates experience and builds itself up out of systems that accumulate ever greater experience. All we know is that it does do this, and that "specific structure" means the unity of a specific substance which accumulates experience and of a world which in its turn imprints this substance and is experienced by it, and to which this substance is related.

What are we to make of the behaviour of the pea-weevil (*Bruchus pisi*), which eats out a passage for its young in the still-soft pea, because otherwise, when they hatched out later, they would not be able to crawl out of the pea that in the meantime had grown hard? This kind of functioning can never have been acquired successively, by repeated experience, imprinting, and progress, for the simple reason that there can be no progeny unless this passage is there. We can offer no theory about it, but must point out that any conception is untenable in which an experiencing subject and a world as object are first separated and then related to each other afterwards. We are concerned here with a unitary phenomenon, similar to those otherwise inexplicable symbiotic relationships in which the experiencing, living substance of the organism and the living substance of the world it lives in and to which it is related are joined together in a unitary field.

The archetype is such a unit, for it is always at one and the same time the possibility of the psyche's experience and the world experienced by this psyche. The mother archetype, for example, is not only a dominant of the psyche, an archetypal figure in it, and the psyche's view of the world, but is at the same time a being *in* the world that contains the psyche and originally produced it. Dominance of the mother archetype in the archetypal stages of development therefore means not only that the mother archetype has acquired the leading role in the psyche, but that the individual or the ego is in a specific relationship of dependence on an encompassing and nourishing "mother"-world, in contradistinction to the greater degree of independent activity that will ensue later.

When, therefore, I speak of a matriarchal phase as a psychohistorical phase which has nothing to do with sociological and power conditions generally, I mean this fundamental constellation in which individual and ego find themselves in the world. The very fact of their finding themselves there is identical with a psychic constellation. One of my critics (cf. Strech, 1958), basing his position on the views of certain modern ethnologists—which it seems to me, have a strong theological colouring—points out that "primitive monotheism" and not the matriarchate stands at the beginning of human development. In this he misses the crucial point, namely that we are concerned with the psychological archetypal aspect. The statements that can be read in any popular book on ethnology may be taken as known, but the primitive cultures in which human beings, in the words of Father Schmidt, "lived only from what Nature produced by spontaneous growth and offered for nourishment" (1952, pp. 38 f.) are, in the psychological sense, matriarchal, and contrast essentially with the later stages of culture characteristically named "productive". In them the activity of man and of the human ego is consciously bent on conquering the world and nature and is sociologically productive, which in a psychological sense means that a new, patriarchal independence has been reached.

Nor can the question as to whether we are dealing psychologically with a matriarchal or a patriarchal stage be decided, in the early stages, by the sex of the deity, if there is one. Here too we must learn to think psychologically instead of theologically and try to understand to what particular psychic situation of a human being or human group the specific kind and the sex of a deity are to be correlated. When, for instance, a formless masculine spirit-deity appears or is merely to be inferred, it can, as we know, quite well pertain to a matriarchal psychology, appearing then as the patriarchal uroboros, that is, as the formless overpowering, penetrating masculine principle. But how easy is the transition from the patriarchal uroboros to patriarchal divinity, and how difficult it is to decide which is primary and which is the result of secondary patriarchal revaluation.

I will not pursue this theme any further but will only point out that it is not the task of depth psychology to take its orientation from investigators who for the most part are entirely unconscious psychologically, and in addition are afflicted now with materialistic, now with theological, but almost always with patriarchal, prejudices. Anyone who has the least insight into the conclusions of present-day science will have to admit that the increasing modesty apparent in depth psychology, which springs from the awareness of the "personal equation" of the investigator, has still not become anything of a problem for most scientists.

In this discussion, which stresses the need to formulate valid statements about man in general on the basis of depth psychology, it seems to me necessary to make at least an attempt to clear up some of the misunderstandings that have attached themselves to my conception of what, in accordance with Jung's dictum: "The distant goal to which these researches lead is a phylogeny of the mind" (Jung, 1913, repub. p. 194), I have called "psycho-history". It may be that I myself have been the cause of these misunderstandings, though I have taken extraordinary pains to forestall them. First, I have never at any time spoken of a biogenetic law, or of any other law (cf. Fordham, 1957). If one wants to speak of the fundamental connection between phylogeny and ontogeny as a law, it would be a question of a *psycho*genetic law that would first have to be established. Second, a declaration that ontogeny does not correspond to phylogeny and a polemic against the application of biogenetic law and the evolutionary viewpoint in psychology are, at least so far as my remarks are concerned, completely out of place. I have always spoken, with the utmost emphasis, of the evolutionary history of *consciousness*, and the thesis of my book is that the phases in the development of mankind's consciousness, so far as they are depicted in mythology, are identical with the history of consciousness in the individual. Third, in phases of development that cannot be demonstrated historically, or at any rate have not yet been historically proven, we are dealing with phases of psycho-history, that is, of psychic structure, which for that reason are analogous to the "sequence-dating" phases in archaeology, where the sequence of phases likewise says nothing about their historical dating.

I will show by means of the simplest example what, in a sense, seems to be perfectly obvious. The fundamental phenomenon in the cosmogonic myth of the origin of consciousness is the birth of light from darkness, darkness being naturally the symbol of the unconscious. The darkness not only is psycho-historically earlier but is also the structural basis for what comes later. In the "birth symbol" the whole multiplicity of what we know ontogenetically as the "primary relationship" is implicit. That ontogeny corresponds to phylogeny means not only that, as in the individual, consciousness develops out of the unconscious, so in the history of mankind consciousness was born from an earlier epoch of unconsciousness, but that the structure of the psyche is such that consciousness always evolves out of the unconscious as the earlier and more fundamental stage. This is, if you like, a psychogenetic law, but it is by no means a biogenetic one. It is certainly not a question of the false application of a biological theory of evolution to psychology.

Even if we were to formulate it as an application of evolutionary thinking to the psyche, it would be a false formulation, because the above proposition is a statement which interprets and understands the *birth and mother-child symbolism of the psyche* for what it means, namely a psychic development.

The fact that a human archetype appears in the image of an "inter-human" constellation, for instance the primary relationship of mother and child, or the relationship of mother and youthful lover, means firstly that a timeless statement is being made about the human species, but over and above that it means that this timeless statement is of crucial importance for every human being. In the image of the primary relationship there is revealed not only a timeless situation but a timeless pattern of development which is fundamental to the psychic structure: dominance of the origin as the basis of security and nourishment, containment and dependence of its progeny. But in the image of the mother-child relationship the autonomy of growth and the necessity of later liberation from the dominance of the origin for the purpose of achieving final independence are "given" at the same time. Here the archetypal-genetic structural element is identical with the seemingly banal fact that containment is earlier than liberation. But among our congeners the mammals the container naturally appears as the mother, so that independence primarily means liberation from her.

It is important to realize that the dominance of an archetype, say that of the mother in the primary relationship, should not be understood as though it were merely the dominance of a definite archetype in the human psyche, which prescribes a definite pattern of behaviour. The archetype, as the reflection of a structure, is much more than that. It contains within itself the laws *regulating a course of development* on three levels: within the psyche, between man and man, and between man and world. Similarly, in the case of the animal instincts, we find that it determines and regulates a course of development in the bio-psychic organism of the animal, between the animal and its young, and between the animal and its environment.

The *intrapsychic* structure of the archetype, which determines this development, becomes immediately apparent when we realize that in the primary relationship the mother as the directing, protecting, and nourishing source represents the unconscious and, in the first phase, also the self, and that the dependent child represents the childish ego and consciousness. Here again a specifically human process of intrapsychic development is evident: interdependence of ego and self, conflict between ego and self, growth of ego and consciousness out of the unconscious, conflict between ego consciousness and the unconscious as a result of increasing independence.

The archetype of the primary relationship, however, determines not only an intrapsychic but also an *interhuman* development. It is just the personal evocation of the archetype that makes the interweaving of the intrapsychic and the interhuman apparent. As an interhuman phenomenon, the archetype determines not only the behaviour between mother and child but a whole series of behavioural developments. Ambivalence of the mother and ambivalence of the child's relationship to her, conflicts caused by its growing independence, and the consequent transition from the positive, sustaining, nourishing mother to the clutching and devouring mother—all these modulations of interhuman development are by nature implicit in the archetypal image of the primary relationship.

But the archetype always contains an *aspect of the world* as well. That is why we speak of a "matriarchal world", a world of the youthful lover, a patriarchal world, and so on. At the same time the archetypal image—of the primary relationship, for example—is not merely, as we previously supposed, a reaction of the psyche to the world, it is just as much the image of a world constituting the psyche.

If human beings "lived only from what Nature produces by spontaneous growth and offers for nourishment", this would be a non-psychic fact, but when we say that it is the expression of a "matriarchal" constellation we mean that the world and nature confront man in the same maternal guise as that in which the mother confronts the child and the unconscious the ego. All this is contained in the structure of the archetype, so that in the archetype of the primary relationship the unity of man's relationships to the world, to other men, and to his own psyche, has become a concrete image. That is why, whenever this archetype appears, we can say something simultaneously about the ego's relation to the unconscious and the self, to the mother and all her representatives, and to the world as nature.

It will now have become clear what is meant when we say that, psychologically and psycho-historically, the matriarchate and the matriarchal world are primary, and that this statement is valid ontogenetically as well as phylogenetically.

The archetype always refers to a unitary reality embracing world and psyche (cf. Neumann, 1956*a*, 1957, 1959). The transition from the dominance of one archetype to that of another is therefore a critical point, because a change of dominance is always bound up with a transformation on all three of the above-mentioned levels. Childhood now appears to us as a crucial segment of human development, not only because the psyche then unfolds in fixed, archetypal stages and becomes structured, but because this structure includes at the same time the child's relation to the environment and his general attitude to the world, which may be specifically determined or else disturbed. Thus, while the primary relationship involves relationship to the self, the unconscious, and the world as nature, the dominance of the father archetype brings with it the possibility of developing the superego, extension of consciousness, acquisition of culture, and every disturbance of the one sphere involves disturbance of the others.

Unfortunately, we can cast only a quick glance here at some of the genetically conditioned points of disturbance in the child's "specific" development. We do so only in conjunction with our statements of principle, but the reader will be able to use his own material to illustrate what is meant.

The course of ego-self development runs from the uroboric, male-female, paternal-female figure of the matriarchal self to the matriarchal phase in which the mother archetype is dominant and the masculine, paternal element is associated with it secondarily. This is identical with a predominance of the directing unconscious, no matter whether its influence is mediated through spontaneous manifestations or through specific forms of instinct (cf. Neumann, 1953*a*). Correlated with it is a childishly dependent ego consciousness, gradually acquiring relative autonomy. Disturbances can supervene through loss or disturbance of the "evoking" factor, the personal mother, which lie in her personality or in disturbances of the world she represents. Disturbances like hunger or illness are likewise disturbances of the normal development guaranteed by the person of the mother, and the failure of the mother, for so-called external reasons, to feed, protect, and compensate leads to a defect in the personal evocation of the mother archetype, with all the disastrous consequences this entails.

The other, fundamentally different, form of disturbance is the possibility of there being a constitutional defect in the child, in whom, despite specific evocation through the mother and the normality of the world she represents, that which is evoked, the archetypal and biopsychic system of reactivity, is not released. We find an extreme instance of this in those children who, from the moment of birth, show no reaction in the primary relationship and are described by their normally undisturbed mothers as "unresponsive".

Similar centres of disturbance are all the "transition phases" of archetypal dominance. Puberty, middle life, and the climacteric are by no means the only critical points. These points accumulate in childhood because the building up of a specifically human psychic structure involves passing through a sequence of archetypal phases. The archetypal points of transition, whose objective dating in ontogeny would be important, are the critical places of development. We shall make this clear by a reference to the change of sex-correlation to the self. Even though at the beginning the all-embracing and directing mother always represents the self, later there is a different development for girls and for boys. The sex-correlation of the self remains feminine for a girl, while for the boy it must be detached from the mother. This crisis of self-discovery is naturally connected with the detachment of the child from the primary relationship. Obviously the process is less problematical for a girl, for whom mother and self remain sex-linked, than it is for a boy, who must alter his previous correlation to the "maternal "aspect of the self with his detachment from the mother. Many problems of sexual insecurity and self-uncertainty are connected with the boy's detachment from the mother at this archetypal point of transition. The problem is reversed in the case of the male and the female child's encounter with the father archetype.

Definite forms of illness, too—though here we are only at the beginning—seem to be connected with the archetypal phases and the archetypal experience needed by the species to build up the psyche. One of their causes is the fact that this experience is lacking or is realized insufficiently. Thus, insufficient experience of the primary relationship, which then has to be made up for in the transference, seems to lead to certain forms of schizophrenia. The connection of the "magical" stage of the primary relationship with psychic illnesses have been clarified by Edward Whitmont (1957), and I myself have already drawn attention to the correlation between homosexuality and the youthful lover's relationship to the great mother (Neumann, 1954). Beyme (1957) has shown that the stages of psychic degeneration in a case of pregnancy psychosis follow in descending order the stages of development which in my view are typical of the feminine psyche (Neumann, 1953*b*, 1956*b*). These are only a few examples. In short, there is reason to hope that the structural framework of the archetypal phases will prove helpful in bringing genetic disturbances and fixations into relation with various groups of illness.

Psycho-history, in this context, means understanding the essential connection between the archetype and the reaction of the individual and coordinating it with the structure of the psyche. We must recognize, for instance, that male homosexuality is always pre-patriarchal, and that in it the masculine is not detached from the feminine and feels constantly threatened by it, because the self is not yet experienced in the unequivocally masculine form which is self-evident for a later patriarchal masculinity. This psycho-historical coordination has nothing to do with history or with sociological conditions, but—what is of decisive importance—it enables us to see and understand the symbolism in correct perspective.

We come now to a final point which has to do with the significance of the archetypal phases as an evolutionary sequence; we have to ask what is the positional value of the symbol in the "sequence-dating" phases of psychic development. In general we have made our understanding of the symbol dependent on its amplification, i.e. on the drawing up of a horizontal series of analogous symbols whose explanation of one another acts as an enrichment. Thus the mustering of symbols of the great mother "from all over the place" enables us to see the unity and scope of this archetype (cf. Neumann, 1955).

But amplification is not sufficient for diagnosing the psychic situation of a person and for therapy. It must be supplemented by the positional value of the symbol, its vertical orientation in psycho-history, and this means discovering to what phase of development the symbol belongs. It is only this positional value, together with amplification, that enables us to undertake the actual interpretation of the symbol, and to find out whether it has a progressive or a regressive significance, and what the prognosis of the situation is. Whether the great mother, appearing as a witch, facilitates progression to the father archetype in the child's development by frightening the childish ego away from the mother and fixation to her, or whether, in her encounter with the adolescent ego of the young man or young girl, she must be sought out and conquered, or served as in the individuation process during the second half of life, so that she may transform herself into Sophia—none of this can be ascertained by amplification, but only be orientation about the position of the individual in the psycho-history of the stages of human development.

Only when we see the unity of the archetypally timeless with its psycho-historical place in human development can we grasp its significance for the fate of the individual. But this is perhaps a banal statement, for unconsciously we have always connected the symbol with a place in our psychic development. I have merely endeavoured to show what place the genetic aspect must therefore occupy in our theory. For it is only the continual broadening of theory that enables us to understand what we do in practice. We should take to heart the insufficiently appreciated saying of Goethe (1797): "In this matter one discovers again that any complete experience must contain its own theory."

(*For References see pp. 36–37*)

# 3

## DE QUELQUES COUPLES D'OPPOSÉS OU D'UNE PHILOSOPHIE IMPLICITE

CHARLES BAUDOUIN, *Geneva*

L'INVESTIGATION analytique, décantant les conflits du sujet, place sous une lumière singulière certains *couples d'opposés*. Or lorsqu'on veut désigner ceux-ci par la formule la plus simple, il arrive communément que l'on tombe sur des termes qui appartiennent au registre de la *Weltanschauung*.

Ceci nous permet d'élucider le malentendu en vertu duquel on a souvent reproché à C. G. Jung de présenter, sous le nom de science psychologique, une philosophie camouflée. Il s'en est toujours fortement et justement défendu, mais le malentendu renaît sans cesse, du fait que cette investigation psychologique explore la région de la psyché où naissent les philosophies, où existe chez les sujets, à titre de fait d'expérience, une sorte de *philosophie implicite*, que le psychologue dégage, mais n'invente pas. L'erreur commune revient en somme à confondre l'explorateur avec l'objet exploré, en bref, comme je le disais un jour avec humour, à prendre Lévy-Bruhl pour un nègre du Zambèze.

Nous nous sommes attaché ici à certains de ces couples d'opposés dont l'examen nous a paru propre à redresser les perspectives. Nous en avons échelonné la série, à partir de ceux qui ont un caractère d'évidence presque banale, pour aboutir à ceux qui surprennent davantage et donnent enfin le sentiment de la découverte. Chacun de ces couples est illustré par un ou deux cas concrets où il nous est apparu sous une forme particulièrement typique.

Nous considérerons ainsi successivement les couples suivants: I) l'intellect et la vie, II) l'esprit et la nature, III) la fantaisie et la réalité, IV) le mérite et la grâce, V) l'irréparable et le renouvellement, VI) le moi et le soi, VII) chercher et trouver.

### I. L'INTELLECT ET LA VIE

Cette polarité, qui est loin d'être rare, s'est présentée à nous avec une force singulière dès les premières séances de l'analyse d'un jeune homme, Christophe N., étudiant épris de sciences exactes.

La résistance à l'analyse s'exprime d'emblée (3e séance) par un rêve où il s'agit de visiter un château, qu'on peut en bref assimiler à l'inconscient, mais où "le propriétaire du château, qui nous conduisait, nous dit que nous sommes prisonniers" et une bagarre s'engage. Il s'avère bientôt que cette *peur d'être pris* est, chez Christophe, une conduite fondamentale, qui se répète sur tous les plans et rend compte d'une certaine angoisse, patente ou latente, dont il souffre.

Dans un rêve de la 5e séance, il se trouve avec une troupe d'enfants; il regrette de leur avoir dit de venir tous ensemble chez lui, non sans avoir essayé d'ailleurs de leur donner une fausse adresse; il craint leur tumulte, ce qui s'avère en rapport avec une crainte du collectif irrationnel (inconscient collectif). Les associations le conduisent à l'opposition de la "science-fiction" à la littérature, puis à un roman dont le héros séduit une jeune fille, se fiance avec elle, voudrait la quitter, se demande "comment il en sortira"—expression typique, qui renvoie d'une part aux prisonniers du château, et d'autre part au thème connu de la "femme-trappe", ou de la "femme-gouffre" (au "vagin denté" du registre freudien), thème que nous avons reconnu assez fort chez ce sujet, en liaison avec des difficultés effectives dans la réalisation sexuelle. Dans un second rêve de la même séance, et qui complète bien le premier, il achète des crevettes, mais celles-ci s'organisent en un "groupe autonome", comme un animal composé d'une quantité de crevettes, qui s'approche du rêveur et lui inspire dégoût et terreur—terreur qui provient surtout de "l'incompréhensible du phénomène". Le monstre marin, familier aux connaisseurs du mythe, est lié au thème précédemment évoqué, aux angoisses du gouffre, et nous ramène explicitement, dans le cas particulier, à l'angoisse du collectif irrationnel. En ce qui concerne le collectif, il faut dire que ce sujet souffre aussi de difficultés sociales; il n'a "pas le contact facile". Et commentant ce point, il arrive très vite, par association, à sa "crainte de l'engagement" (15e séance) que nous retrouvons en effet sur tous les plans. Dans la région des images, l'engagement est toujours engagement trés concret dans quelque chose où l'on pourrait "être pris", de sorte que l'on ne saurait pas "s'en tirer". Dans une région plus consciente, il se traduit par *l'indécision*, car toute décision comporte aux yeux de ce sujet un irrationnel: "Quand je me décide, j'ai l'impression de me lancer à l'eau sans beaucoup de raisons. J'essaie de me représenter comme fait quelqu'un qui n'est pas indécis et je n'y arrive pas. Je ne comprends pas qu'on puisse se décider" (56e séance). C'est, en somme, le refus du "pari", du "nous sommes embarqués" pour parler en termes pascaliens. Il ajoute: "Entre 16 et 22 ans, je n'étais pas du tout dans la vie" comprenant bien que toute cette disposition aboutit à une *peur de la vie*, cette vie qui a "des raisons que la raison ne comprend pas".

La vie, ou "le cœur". En termes de "fonctions" jungiennes, Christophe est nettement un type *pensée*, qui refuse le *sentiment*. Dès la 2e séance, il rêve de deux camarades qui sont à ses yeux respectivement des images typiques de l'intellect et de la vie; il parle de camarades qu'il a trouvés "superficiels, car ils voulaient jouir trop tôt de la vie", et qui "lui reprochaient de se perdre dans les idées".

On a ici un exemple de ce que nous avons appelé autrefois la "polarisation des conflits". Et les deux pôles peuvent bien être désignés, le plus simplement peut-être, comme l'intellect et la vie. Quant aux résonances philosophiques de cette opposition, nous avons déjà rencontré Pascal au passage; nous pourrions aussi évoquer Bergson, qui a construit toute une partie de sa philosophie sur cette opposition, en relevant que "l'intelligence se caractérise par une incompréhension naturelle de la vie".

## II. L'ESPRIT ET LA NATURE

On peut dire des couples d'opposés que nous considérons ici, ce que nous avons dit ailleurs des complexes, des symboles, des archétypes classiques. On passe de l'un à l'autre, par transition, par une sorte de glissement; les limites ne sont pas tranchées, mais tout à coup on s'aperçoit que l'un a passé la main et qu'on est sous la juridiction de l'autre. Ainsi, on conçoit aisément un glissement entre le couple de l'intellect et de la vie, et celui de l'*esprit* et de la *nature*—la nature conçue comme une ambiance vivante, aux résonances cosmiques.

Nous sommes au point de transition avec le cas de Simon E., dont le tableau rappelle fort, à certains égards, celui de Christophe N. C'est lui aussi un indécis typique, évitant les risques du monde, replié sur lui-même; il présente des tendances obsessionnelles et, aux approches de la trentaine, il n'a pu encore se décider à aborder la vie sexuelle. Ses intérêts philosophiques d'ailleurs valables, sa lecture des philosophes de *l'esprit*, comme Emerson, lui servent trop souvent d'alibi et de défense contre la vie. La femme est pour lui l'image de l'inconnu, de l'étranger, du lointain. (Son plus ancien souvenir d'enfance, c'est, à l'école enfantine, la présence d'une petite fille *japonaise*.) Lorsque, au cours de l' évolution analytique, il commence à sortir de lui-même, il a ce joli symbole: il rêve qu'il pénètre dans un dancing, où il rencontre des femmes, et qui s'appelle. . . *l'Univers*—ce qui introduit, d'une manière imprévue, le thème d'un contact "cosmique".

C'est ici le lieu de rappeler un cas que nous avons présenté ailleurs (Baudouin, 1957a, III, 3, p. 193), celui de Nine. Son conflit conscient est de se sentir partagée entre "l'école et la vie". Elle rêve d'un repas de famille. Mais sur la table de ce repas, elle est occupée à ranger dans des cartons des papiers concernant l'école du dimanche, qui lui sont passés par son père, tandis qu'il y a d'autre part une belle rose rouge, qu'elle doit, croit-elle, donner à sa mère. Les associations développent tout un conflit polarisé: ce sont les papiers contre la rose rouge—l'école contre la vie—mais du même coup le père contre la mère, et au-delà, c'est le conflit de deux conceptions religieuses: d'un côté, une religion conforme à l'éducation protestante et fidèle au Dieu-père, mais qui lui apparaît à ce moment comme sèche et livresque; de l'autre, une aspiration plus chaleureuse à la communion avec la maternelle nature, et qu'elle désigne elle-même du nom de "panthéisme", nouvelle allusion au "cosmique". Or il n'est pas rare de voir, comme dans ce cas, la dualité esprit-nature polariser avec la dualité père-mère, ce qui la situe dans le prolongement des complexes fondamentaux du sujet.

On a pu étudier sous cet angle ce cas que représente Kierkegaard, chez qui une tension particulièrement forte entre les images de la mère et du père se répercute, dans la doctrine et dans la vie spirituelle, en une tension également extrême entre les notions de nature et d'esprit (cf. Künzli, 1948).

Partant du thème esprit-nature, il y aurait lieu d'en étudier une importante variation, celle que figure le couple *esprit-matière*. Matière est certes autre chose que nature, mais on passe de l'une à l'autre notion par un glissement facile. Notons seulement que toutes deux se fondent sur des complexes sous-jacents assez proches, car ici et là, c'est la mère qui se retrouve. L'étymologie suffit à l'indiquer; puisque *nature* renvoie à *naître*, et *matière* directement à *mère*. Etudier à cette lumière les grandes philosophies dualistes, et au premier chef celle de Descartes, apporterait sans nul doute des vues rafraîchissantes.

### III. LA FANTAISIE ET LA RÉALITÉ

Des transitions encore, et nous voici au couple *fantaisie-réalité*. Parfois le premier terme se présente sous le nom d'*idéal*, et le couple paraît alors très voisin de celui de l'esprit et de la matière, mais dès que l'idéal se confond avec l'*illusion*, le *rêve*, la *fantaisie*, nous nous apercevons que nous sommes passés dans un tout autre climat.

Edmond G. se plaint d'un certain *flottement* dans sa vie, d'un certain manque de mordant dans ses activités. Au cours d'une séance (la 37[e]), il développe, dans ses tenants et aboutissants, le thème *fantaisie et réalité*.

Un curieux souvenir d'enfance est présenté: celui d'un cambriolage du poulailler. Mais dans son souvenir, Edmond ne parvient pas à revoir le poulailler du jardin familial; il lui a substitué l'*image* qu'il se faisait du poulailler en écoutant une histoire de renard voleur de poules: bref, la fantaisie plus forte que la réalité. Un autre souvenir du même âge (8 ans) est celui d'un camelot qui vendait des plumes brillantes comme de l'or; le lendemain, il ne restait plus dans la main que des plumes, de cuivre quelconque: thème des illusions perdues, de la fantaisie qui, en s'envolant, ne laisse, comme une sorte de résidu, qu'une réalité ordinaire et décevante.

C'est là un thème fréquent, et d'une large signification humaine. Nous l'avons relaté, au cours des souvenirs d'enfance réunis sous le titre de *L'Éveil de Psyché* (1948): les jouets merveilleux apportés par Saint-Nicolas, découverts à la lumière singulière de la lampe inaccoutumée, et qui ne sont plus ensuite, sous l'éclairement cru du jour ordinaire, que des jouets quelconques, que l'enfant est presque déçu de pouvoir manier. Dans la même ligne se situeraient bien des exemples littéraires: ainsi, chez Baudelaire:

*Ah! que le monde est grand a la clarté des lampes*[1]
*Aux yeux du souvenir, que le monde est petit.*

Ainsi, chez Hugo, le titre *L'Écu changé en feuille sèche*, qui est celui d'un chapitre (VIII 1) de *Notre-Dame de Paris*.

Pour en revenir à notre sujet Edmond G., il apporte, lors de cette même séance, deux rêves—qui mettent l'un et l'autre en scène des déceptions analogues. Dans l'un, il voit un homme de sa connaissance—en fait jeune, svelte et de caractère idéaliste—qui s'est transformé en une sorte d' "homme d'affaires très gros, avec une chaîne d'or à son gilet", ce qui marque bien l'alourdissement et la chute dans le réel. L'autre rêve commence par une scène qui est une reproduction du vol au poulailler, et continue par une scène de marché ou de foire. (C'est un vendeur de cette foire qui appela comme association le camelot aux plumes d'or); mais tout à coup, toute cette scène vivante disparaît et il reste seulement "un lampion avec des papiers poissés par terre"—une sorte de piteux lendemain de fête. D'autres associations conduisent aux bateleurs, aux trapézistes, et le sujet lui-même répète qu'il se sent "flottant", comme sur un trapèze. Ainsi se dessine une fois de plus la polarité bien connue du léger et de l'alourdi, de la fantaisie aérienne et de la réalité terre à terre; mais l'aérien est aussi le flottant.

Cette opposition se rattache, par un côté, à la situation infantile qui oppose le moment bienheureux où l'enfant *est porté* sur des bras, et celui où il doit s'efforcer de *marcher à terre*; ce qui, en dernière analyse, ramène au complexe classique du *sevrage*. Et lors de la description que nous avons donnée de ce complexe dans

[1] BAUDELAIRE, *Les Fleurs du Mal:* le Voyage.

*A'Lme et l'Action* (1944), nous avons rencontré, en belle place, précisément, le thème du "flottement".

C'est l'occasion de le remarquer: en perspective strictement "réductive", il ne fait aucun doute que le pôle "aérien" est régressif et que le sujet progresse en acceptant le "terre à terre". Mais les choses sont plus complexes, et une telle simplification est dangereuse. S'il faut, d'une part, décrire honnêtement les structures, leurs tenants et aboutissants, leurs oppositions, cette description de faits ou de "fonctions" biologiques doit réserver le registre des "valeurs", comme l'a bien marqué Charles Odier. L'accent de valeur est à placer différemment selon les cas. Et la valeur que peut présenter le pôle "fantaisie", sous ses aspects d'"idéal" et d'imagination créatrice, ne saurait être méconnue sans de lourdes fautes.

### IV. LE MÉRITE ET LA GRÂCE

Il convient peut-être de nous excuser de faire ici, à titre indicatif, un emprunt au vocabulaire théologique. Ces notions: mérite et grâce, ne sauraient marquer certes, dans leur sens propre, que le terme extrême d'une série que le psychologue considérera dans ses manifestations, aussi, les plus profanes et les plus humbles, voire les plus aberrantes. Mais ils ont l'avantage de faire image pour orienter l'esprit sur deux attitudes psychologiques qui se retrouvent à tous les niveaux, l'une qui ne compte que sur l'effort propre, l'autre qui s'abandonne à quelque puissance auxiliatrice; celle-ci pourra s'appeler parfois "Providence", mais elle pourra aussi, d'autres fois, s'appeler "chance" ou plus noblement "étoile" ou plus familièrement "veine": ce sera toujours alors, et plus ou moins enrobée de superstition et de magie, une sorte de divinité maternelle. Dans cette région, où se meuvent avec désinvolture, avec insolence, avec angoisse, le joueur, le spéculateur, nous reconnaissons que nous sommes en continuité avec le couple précédemment envisagé. La chance est une mère de la petite enfance, une mère d'où l'on reçoit tout et dans les bras de laquelle il n'y a qu'à s'abandonner. Ce pôle est à celui de l'effort, ou du mérite, comme sont entre elles les deux situations d'avant et d'après le sevrage, de l'enfant porté et de l'enfant qui marche. Nous voyons cela clairement en étudiant ces sujets mous, à l'optimisme facile, que nous avons présentés dans *L'Ame enfantine et la Psychanalyse* (1951) au chapitre des *Conduites élusives;* ils sont de ceux qui, selon le dicton, "attendent que les alouettes leur tombent toutes rôties"; mais nous avons retrouvé, à un tout autre niveau, les mêmes structures en étudiant un mystique authentique, tel que saint Jean de la Croix (dans Baudouin, 1957*a*). Il devient plus visible encore que tout à l'heure, que la description des structures est une chose, l'appréciation des valeurs une autre.

Il arrive qu'un sujet, à un moment de son analyse, croie découvrir qu'il serait bon de se tendre moins vers l'effort, de s'abandonner davantage, et il n'est pas rare que cette découverte rende quelque résonance religieuse. Ainsi Sigmund N. voit dans un rêve (53e séance) son ancien directeur "type soucieux, consciencieux" (pôle du mérite) venir vers lui "reposé et dêtendu" et il le reçoit avec émotion "comme un sauveur" (pôle de la grâce); à la fin du rêve, un bateau (flottement, être porté) conduit la compagnie à une fête champêtre dans des jardins pleins de roses, qui évoquent explicitement "le paradis sur la terre". Devant un déferlement d'images de cette sorte, on doit demeurer perplexe. Marquent-elles un mouvement tout régressif vers le règne du moindre effort, vers le paradis d'avant le sevrage? Ou signifient-elles l'accès nouveau à une attitude détendue et confiante, qui doit être tenue pour valable et réjouissante? Le contexte éclaire. Dans le cas particulier, la séance suivante apport, de la part de ce sujet, chrétien convaincu, des réflexions comme celles-ci: "Je voulais tout contrôler; j'accepte de laisser une marge que je ne contrôle pas. Acceptation d'un risque, d'un irrationnel. Je sème, mais ce n'est pas moi qui fais pousser. J'étais enfermé dans mon moi hypertrophié; maintenant, un dialogue peut s'établir, alors qu'avant c'était un monologue... Comme si la chose devait m'être donnée, que je ne doive pas la prendre. Une conception plus nette de la grâce au lieu des œuvres". Ce n'est pas nous qui le lui faisons dire.

Quoi qu'il en soit, chacun des deux pôles n'a son sens qu'en fonction de l'autre. Ce que souligne, de sa manière narquoise, la sagesse des nations, lorsqu'elle énonce: "Aide-toi, le Ciel t'aidera".

## V. L'IRRÉPARABLE ET LE RENOUVELLEMENT

Le pôle que nous avons convenu de désigner comme celui de la "grâce" peut se présenter, à tous les niveaux, comme celui du don *gratuit*, qui ne se mesure pas, qui coule de source (comme le lait maternel), avec une surabondance inépuisable—la fontaine de Jouvence, l'eau qui ne tarira point—, et par cette ligne, nous rejoignons un autre couple, celui qui oppose la perte irréparable au *renouvellement* inespéré.

Les enfants nous offrent volontiers le spectacle de ces désespoirs et de ces colères sans mesure provoqués par un petit objet détruit, un jouet cassé, ou qui a seulement perdu, surtout si c'est par la faute d'autrui, le lustre parfait du neuf. Ces colères tournent aisément en une attitude butée, d'où l'on ne voit pas comment on sortirait, car l'enfant exige d'une part que la chose soit restituée dans son état antérieur, sans qu'il y manque un iota, et d'autre part il sait que cette restitution est impossible, et que, quoi qu'on fasse pour le satisfaire, il le refusera parce que ce ne sera "pas ça"; et même si on lui rachète un jouet semblable, ce ne sera pas le même, ce ne sera encore "pas ça". Il semble qu'on doive rattacher ces attitudes à la psychologie du *narcisme*, exigeant d'intégrité—cette exigeance étant ici transférée du corps propre aux possessions. Pourtant, on sort bel et bien de cette impasse; mais c'est comme on sort d'une bouderie; par une sorte de conversion de l'attitude, par l'acceptation d'une ouverture, qui est aussi ouverture à autrui, et par laquelle s'engouffre à nouveau le flot inépuisable de la vie. Rien n'est perdu, pour peu qu'on cesse de se cramponner. Cette conversion du *fermé* à l'*ouvert* ne va guère, semble-t-il—pour user du vocabulaire de l'école—, sans un passage de l'attitude *captative* à l'attitude *oblative*, de celle de la prise à celle du don, deux pôles encore, dont nous avons marqué ailleurs le rapport avec l'opposition philosophique de l'*avoir* et de l'*être*, au sens de Gabriel Marcel (1957).

Kurt E. nous apporte (69e séance) une mise en pages saisissante de ce système; elle est particulièrement exemplaire, parce que dépouillée, et réduite fort joliment à ses lignes essentielles. Il s'agit d'un rêve, composé de deux scènes successives: dans la première, le sujet voit deux vases à fleurs qu'il aimait pour leur forme, et qui sont cassés, ébréchés; il éprouve devant cet accident un cruel sentiment "d'irréversibilité". Mais dans la seconde, comme en réplique, à ces vases ébréchés sont substitués d'autres très beaux. Cependant que, dans un autre rêve de la même séance, il a d'abord un sentiment de *frustration*, à l'idée que les plantes qu'on va lui apporter ne seront peut-être pas celles qu'il a achetées; mais tout s'arrange; le syndic a tout pris à son compte et tout payé. Dans une autre scène du même rêve, il est question de deux églises, l'ancienne et la nouvelle, que l'on inaugure; celle-ci est *ouverte* de part en part; c'est une sorte de passage, comme si la route la traversait. A l'inauguration, il veut avoir sa place; il songe d'abord à s'installer égoïstement au milieu d'un banc, pour n'etre pas dérangé; mais enfin il s'assied au bout du banc, et peut-être a-t-il gracieusement donné sa place à une femme (passage à l'oblativité).

Cet exemple simple nous suffira, parmi beaucoup d'autres plus orchestrés, et qui nous conduiraient bientôt—on l'a peut-être entrevu déjà—à un mythe fondamental et fort étudié, celui de la *mort* et de la *nouvelle naissance.*

## VI. LE MOI ET LE SOI

Nous nous excusions tout à l'heure de désigner un de nos couples d'opposés par des termes du vocabulaire théologique. C'est par un raccourci semblable, et qui pourra sembler prématuré, que nous recourons cette fois d'emblée à deux termes techniques de la psychologie de C. G. Jung, le *moi* et le *soi.* Aussi bien est-ce l'occasion de remarquer, une fois de plus, comme les notions et les termes proposés par ce psychologue comportent, en définitive, un faible coefficient d'abstraction, combien au contraire ils sont "*phénologiques*", c'est-à-dire combien ils collent à l'expérience psychologique et clinique, par laquelle ils lui sont immédiatement dictés, et qu'ils résument plus qu'ils ne l'interprètent. D'une part, certes, la polarité du moi et du soi rejoint certaines oppositions philosophiques célèbres, ainsi celle de *phénomène* et de *noumène* chez Kant (comme Jung lui-même l'a marqué), mais c'est que ces oppositions sont bel at bien enracinées, ici encore, dans une *philosophie implicite* qui procède directement de l'expérience intime. Et c'est bien celle-ci qui nous met sans cesse en présence de la perception, par nos sujets, d'une dualité intérieure, d'une tension entre un moi infirme et contingent, qui existe dans la vie quotidienne, et d'un "vrai moi" auquel il aspire, qui devrait être, et qui se présente parfois avec un caractère "numineux", participant à l'expérience du "sacré".

Le couple du *moi* et du *soi* se suite bien dans le prolongement de celui du mérite et de la grâce. Le moi progresse pas à pas, avec effort; le soi se présente plutôt comme une découverte, un don reçu. Ce peut être la découverte du "trésor", de "l'or". Dans le même rêve, que nous présentions tout à l'heure, où notre sujet Sigmund N. accueille "comme un sauveur" son directeur détendu, il découvre peu après, avec un compagnon, sur la crête d'une colline, un "amas de pièces d'or et d'argenterie"—et ils se mettent à "ramasser ce trésor", qui d'ailleurs "résultait d'un vol". Il n'est pas exceptionnel en effet que le moi hésite devant le soi comme devant quelque chose qui justement n'est pas "à moi", qui est "trop beau pour moi". Ainsi Igor N. (obs. 1619) se trouve en rêve (138e séance) chez un horloger (analyste) pour y rechercher sa montre. "Elle est en pièces détachées. . . Je ramasse le tout mais au milieu il y a *une perle assez grosse*; je ne sais pas *si cette perle m'appartient*, et cela m'ennuie de la prendre, vu sa grosseur, si elle ne m'appartient pas. Je la ramasse, me proposant de voir ce que je dois en faire".[1]

C'est ainsi que se présente volontiers une véritable dialectique du moi et du soi. Chez Henri E., médecin en analyse didactique, l'opposition de ces deux pôles s'affirme très joliment à travers celle de la *maison* et du *temple* (dans lequel Jung a su nous montrer un symbole du soi dans son aspect "numineux"). "L'idée du temple, dit Henri E., m'est venue par cette vielle maison de bois. *On passe de l'une a l'autre.*" Puis le temple lui évoque la Grèce, la perfection, laquelle est bien, selon lui, le terme vers lequel tend l'analyse. Au reste le "passage" n'est pas si aisé. "Celui qui pénètre dans le temple n'en est peut-être pas digne." C'est bien le *non sum dignus intrare.*

## VII. CHERCHER ET TROUVER

Nous abordons ici un thème qui peut apparaître comme une simple variation sur le précédent. Nous avons déjà parlé de la découverte du trésor; en somme, le moi *cherche*, alors que le soi

[1] Igor N. était d'ailleurs sensibilisé, en général, à cette difficulté de tracer les limites du *mien* et du *tien*, et surtout d'attribuer à son moi des possessions et des pouvoirs qu'une éducation dépréciative lui avait trop montrés comme "n'étant pas pour lui". Il a déjà en certaines difficultés à constituer son moi, à conquérir son autonomie. Il nous a fourni (dans *Y a-t-il une science de l'âme?* 1957*b*, p. 94) une belle imagerie du moi se constituant. Or les mêmes difficultés se répètent au niveau du soi.

*est trouvé*. Mais en désignant les deux termes par ces deux verbes, nous écoutons surtout les résonances de la parole inépuisable de Pascal: "Tu ne me chercherais pas si tu ne m'avais trouvé". C'est elle peut-être qu'il faudrait mettre en exergue à ce dernier paragraphe; la situation paradoxale qu'elle désigne est assez particulière, assez digne d'intérêt, pour mériter d'être considérée isolément.

Aussi bien, les deux sujets qui viennent de nous instruire sur la tension du moi et du soi, nous présenteront aussi des exemples typiques de ce nouveau couple.

Sigmund N., au cours de la même série de séances où nous avons déjà puisé, apporte un rêve (52e séance) où, "apres une *longue déambulation* pour *chercher* la clef dans la ville" (thème de la *circumambulatio* bien dégagé par Jung), il aboutit à un couloir où est étendue une femme malade qui lui "indique où cette clef *se trouve*". On remarquera que le précieux objet cherché n'est pas directement trouvé, mais que seulement est obtenue, concernant cet objet absent, une garantie—l'indication du lieu où il "se trouve". De même, peu après, dans un autre rêve (54e séance), Sigmund s'intéresse à un groupe d'enfants qui accomplissent un exploit sportif, qui le tente lui-même; ensuite "je ne *retrouve* pas les enfants, mais une enveloppe contenant toutes les indications nécessaires".

La garantie sur l'objet cherché et absent apparaît parfois sous la forme d'un souvenir incomplet, d'une *réminiscence*. Nous avons rapporté ailleurs le rêve typique de cet homme de 78 ans qui errait à travers la campagne (*circumambulatio*), cherchant une ville qui était "le *centre* du pays" (le centre, symbole classique du soi)[1] où il avait été jadis, mais dont il avait oublié le nom (Baudouin, 1950, p. 188).

Ce theme de la réminiscence se présente chez Igor N. dans un contexte qui n'est pas sans analogie avec celui des exemples précédents. Au cours d'un rêve mouvementé (113e séance) il est question d'Amérique, d'un nègre, d'un hôtel où le rêveur s'installe, puis "nous *circulons*". Dans la rue, on lui vole son portefeuille; sa femme disparaît. Le voilà "seul, sans argent, dans une ville inconnue, ignorant même le nom de mon hôtel.

[1]Et auquel Mircea Eliade a consacré une étude attentive à travers les mythologies et es rites (1952, cap. I, notamment p. 65).

Cependant *je me doute de ce nom*, j'arriverai bien à le retrouver. .. *en circulant*".

Si l'on interroge les prolongements philosophiques d'une telle situation, il est difficile de ne pas rencontrer, d'une part, le mot de Pascal que nous rappelions tout à l'heure, d'autre part, la "reminiscence" platonicienne.

## CONCLUSION

Nous avons voulu nous borner à la description de situations psychologiques typiques. Mais les systèmes que nous avons ainsi repérés s'étendent dans toutes les régions de la psyché. Par un côté (biologique) ils rejoignent les notions freudiennes (l'"irréparable" rejoindrait la "castration"), certains complexes de base (le "sevrage" auquel nous avons dû plusieurs fois nous référer); ils touchent d'autre part aux fonctions (cf. p. 56) et aux archétypes de a psychologie de Jung; ils rencontrent les mythes en maint endroit; et enfin, nous n'avons pu nous dissimuler leurs implications philosophiques qui sont, comme le reste, une donnée "phénologique"; c'est comme si nous saisissions là, en certains moments de l'expérience, l'existence d'une philosophie *in statu nascendi*, dont le rapprochement avec les philosophies constituées ne peut manquer d'être suggéré.

Nous devons maintenir ce que nous rappelions au début: que notre psychologie n'est pas une philosophie camouflée: elle décrit du vécu humain, purement et simplement, et une certaine philosophie, exprimée ou non, fait partie de ce vécu. Mais d'autre part, il est bien permis d'espérer que nos explorations, en se poursuivant, permettront de dégager toujours mieux la physionomie de cette *philosophie implicite* qui se dessine spontanément au tréfonds de l'esprit humain.

La connaissance de la philosophie implicite ne permettrait-elle pas de cerner, avec des armes dont ni Kant, ni Husserl ne disposaient, les "formes a priori" et les "prolégomènes" de toute philosophie explicitée, et, à la limite, de dégager peut-être la perspective d'une "philosophie comme science"? Dès maintenant, la prédominance, dans ces explorations, des "couples d'opposés" soulignerait, semble-t-il, le caractère *dialectique* de toute philosophie implicite.

On voit dans quel sens, strictement délimité, et cependant riche de promesses, il est permis d'assigner à notre psychologie une tâche philosophique.

## REFERENCES

BAUDOUIN, C. (1944). *L'Ame et L'Action*. Geneva, Mont-Blanc.

BAUDOUIN, C. (1948). *L'Éveil de Psyche*. (13th ed.) Paris, L'Arche.

BAUDOUIN, C. (1950). *De l'instinct a l'esprit*. Bruges-Paris, Desclée de Brouwer.

BAUDOUIN, C. (1951). *L'Ame enfantine et la Psychanalyse*. (2nd ed.). Neuchâtel. et Paris, Delachaux et Niestlé.

BAUDOUIN, C. (1957*a*). *Psychanalyse du symbole religieux*. Paris, Arthème Fayard.

BAUDOUIN, C. (1957*b*). *Y a-t-il une science de l'âme?* Paris, Arthème Fayard.

ELIADE, MIRCEA (1952). *Images et symboles*. Paris, Gallimard.

KÜNZLI, ARNOLD (1948). *Die Angst als abendländische Krankheit*. Zürich, Rascher.

MARCEL, G. (1957). *Avoir et être, faire et créer*. Communication au Congrès de philosophie d'Aix-en-Provence.

# *SOME PAIRS OF OPPOSITES: OR REFLECTIONS ON AN IMPLICIT PHILOSOPHY*

AMIDST all the conflicts brought to light by analytic investigation, certain pairs of opposites attract particular attention. In order to arrive at a simple formula by which to classify them, we find ourselves choosing terms that are normally employed to define a philosophy or *Weltanschauung*.

This may help to explain the misunderstanding that has led to the frequent reproach that C. G. Jung is really presenting a philosophy camouflaged as scientific psychology. Jung himself has always firmly and justifiably denied this charge, but the misunderstanding persists, since psychological investigations expose that layer of the psyche in which philosophies are born, a region where a kind of *implicit philosophy* arises in the patient, as a fact of experience, to be disentangled, but not invented, by the psychologist. The common error is, in fact, to confound the explorer with the object explored, in brief, as I remarked jokingly the other day, to equate Lévy-Bruhl with an African from the Zambesi.

We shall now consider certain pairs of opposites which seem most likely, on examination, to restore the perspective. The series is graded, ranging from those which are self-evident almost to the point of banality, to those which are sufficiently surprising to arouse a sense of discovery. Each of these pairs will be illustrated by one or two practical examples that seem to show them in their most typical form.

The pairs to be considered are as follows: I. Intellect and Life; II. Mind and Nature; III. Fantasy and Reality; IV. Merit and Grace; V. the Irreparable and Renewal; VI. the Ego and the Self; VII. Seeking and Finding.

### I. INTELLECT AND LIFE

This polarity, by no means unusual, appeared with remarkable intensity early in the analysis of a young man, Christopher N., a student of the exact sciences.

Even at the beginning of analysis (third session), his resistance was expressed by a dream in which he had to visit a castle which can, in brief, be equated with the unconscious, but "the owner of the castle, who was our guide, told us we were prisoners". A scuffle then ensued. It soon appeared that *this fear of being captured* was a fundamental attitude in Christopher, repeated at all levels, and betraying a certain obvious or latent anxiety from which he suffered.

In a dream reported during the fifth session, he finds himself with a group of children; he regrets having invited them all to his house, though he had, incidentally, tried to give them a false address; he is afraid of the noise they make, which turns out to be associated with a fear of the irrational collective (collective unconscious). Associations lead him to the contrast between science fiction and literature, then to a novel in which the hero seduces a girl, becomes engaged to her, would like to leave her, and asks himself "how he can get out of it"—a typical expression, referring on the one hand to the prisoners in the castle and on the other to the "trap-woman" or the "gulf-woman" (the *vagina dentata* of the Freudians), a theme that was strongly accentuated in this patient in connection with practical difficulties of sexual achievement. In a second and complementary dream of the same session, he is buying some shrimps, but they organize themselves into "an autonomous group", like an animal made up of a number of shrimps, which approaches the dreamer and fills him with disgust and horror—the terror being mainly due to the "incomprehensibility of the phenomenon". The sea monster, familiar to students of mythology, is related to the preceding theme, to the fear of the abyss, and is an explicit reference, in this particular case, to the fear of the irrational collective. In so far as the collective is concerned, it must be added that the patient also suffered from social difficulties; he had no "ease of contact". In his comment the patient quickly produced the association of a "fear of commitment" (fifteenth session), which we meet again at every level. In his imagery the fear of commitment is always the fear of being committed to something concrete, in which he might "get caught" so that he "couldn't get out of it". At a more conscious level this fear was expressed by *indecision* since, to his mind, every decision contained an element of the irrational: "When I do decide, I feel as if I were jumping into the water without any good reason. I try to form a picture of myself as a resolute person, but I can't do it. I can't understand how anyone decides things." It is, in fact, the refusal to "wager", the refusal to "embark", to use Pascal's words. He adds, "From 16 to 22 I just wasn't in life at all," realizing quite well that this frame of mind leads to a *fear of life*, of life that "has reasons that the reason does not understand".

Life, or "heart". In terms of Jung's functions, Christopher is distinctly a *thinking* type, who denies *feeling*. After the second session he dreamed of two friends who were, to him, typical images of intellect and life respectively: he spoke of friends whom he found "superficial because they wanted to enjoy life too soon", and who "reproached him for getting lost in ideas".

This is an example of what I have called elsewhere the "polarization of conflict". And the two poles may perhaps be most simply described as intellect and life. As for their philosophical overtones, we have already encountered Pascal; one might also mention Bergson, who built up a large portion of his philosophy on this pair of opposites, by pointing out that "intelligence is characterized by a natural incomprehension of life".

## II. MIND AND NATURE

What we have said elsewhere about complexes, symbols, and classical archetypes is also true of the pairs of opposites we are considering here. There is a transition from one to the other by an imperceptible gradient: the boundaries are not fixed, but we suddenly perceive that the outlines of one have faded and that we have moved into the orbit of another. Thus it is easy to perceive the transition between the pair intellect and life and the pair mind and nature—nature conceived as a living environment with cosmic significance.

We reach the transitional point in the case of Simon E., a patient whose clinical picture strongly resembles, in certain aspects, that of Christopher N. He also is a markedly irresolute type, avoiding the dangers of the world by withdrawing into himself; he has obsessional tendencies and, although approaching the thirties, has not yet been able to bring himself to attempt any sexual experience. His alibi, his defence against life, is all too often his interest in philosophy, for which he was, incidentally, gifted, and a study of the more "spiritual" philosophers, such as Emerson. Woman is to him all that is unknown, alien, or remote (his earliest childhood recollection is of a little *Japanese* girl at his kindergarten). When, in the course of analysis, he begins to come out of his shell, this engaging symbol appears: he dreams that he is entering a dance-hall, where he meets some women: the hall is called . . . The Universe, which introduces, unexpectedly, the theme of a cosmic relationship.

It is appropriate to refer here to the case of Nina which has been reported elsewhere (Baudouin, 1957a, III, 3 p. 193). Her conscious conflict is the sense of the incompatible demands of "school and life". She dreams of a family meal. But on the dining-table there are boxes into which she is putting papers dealing with the Sunday School, as they are passed to her by her father. There is also a red rose which she feels she must give to her mother. Associations bring out the polarity of the conflict: the papers in opposition to the red rose—school against life—but also father against mother; and behind these, the conflict between two conceptions of religion: on the one hand religion on the Protestant model, centred on God-the-Father, which seems to her at that moment, dry and bookish; on the other hand, an ardent longing for communion with maternal nature, which she herself describes as "pantheism", a further allusion to the cosmic element. It is not uncommon to find, as in this case, the duality of mind-nature linked in polar opposition with the duality of father-mother, which establishes its connection with the patient's basic complexes.

We can look at the case of Kierkegaard from the same angle. In him we find a particularly high tension between the father and mother images, expressing itself, both in his doctrine and in his spiritual life, in a corresponding tension between the concept of nature and mind (see Künzli, 1948).

Following the theme of the duality mind-nature, we might study one of its important variations, the pair mind-matter. Matter is, admittedly, something other than nature, but one passes almost imperceptibly from the one to the other. It should be noted in passing that both are based on closely associated underlying complexes, for the mother-figure reappears in both. The etymological indication is sufficient in itself. "Nature" leads to "nativity" and "matter" to "mater". If we were to study the great dualistic philosophies, in particular the Cartesian, from this angle, we should no doubt make some interesting discoveries.

## III. FANTASY AND REALITY

Some further transitions and we come to the pair *fantasy-reality*. The first term sometimes occurs under the guise of the *ideal*, and the pair then seems to be closely related to that of mind and matter, but as soon as the ideal is confused with *illusion*, *dream*, and *fantasy*, we perceive that we have moved into a different climate.

Edmond G., complained of the "floating" quality of his life, and of a lack of incisiveness in his activities. During his thirty-seventh session he developed the theme of fantasy and reality in extraordinary detail.

An odd childhood memory had reappeared: the robbery of a hen-run. But Edmund was not able to visualize the hen-run in the family garden: he provided as substitute the *image* he had formed of the hen-run whilst listening to a story about a fox stealing chickens: in short, the fantasy was stronger than the reality. Another memory from the period (his eighth year) was that of a pedlar selling feathers as bright as gold; on the following day he found nothing but feathers of ordinary copper: the theme of lost illusions, of the fantasy which, as it vanishes, leaves behind only traces of a disappointing and ordinary reality.

It is a common theme, and one of much human significance. In a collection of childhood memories entitled *L'Éveil de Psyché* (Baudouin, 1948), we recounted the story of the toys brought by Santa Claus, so entrancing when examined under the unfamiliar lamplight, which by the crude light of day turn out to be ordinary playthings that, to one's disappointment, one can even play with. There are many examples of this same theme in literature, for instance, Baudelaire's lines:

*Ah, in the light of the lamp how large the world!*
*In the eye of memory, how small it is!*[1]

To return to our patient Edmond G.; during the same session he produced two dreams, both dealing with similar disappointments. In the first he saw a man he knew, who was in fact young, slim, and of idealistic temperament, and who had been transformed into a kind of "fat businessman, with a gold watch and chain", which clearly showed a coarsening and a descent into reality. The second dream started with a scene that was a reproduction of the hen-run robbery, and led into a scene in a market or at a fair. (It was one of the salesmen at the fair which brought up the association to the pedlar with the golden feathers.) But suddenly the lively scene disappeared and all that remained was "a lamp-post and some litter on the ground"—a sort of pathetic aftermath. Other associations led to jugglers and trapezists, and the patient himself repeated that he was "floating" as if on a trapeze. This was yet another indication of the well-known polarity of the light and the heavy, of aerial fantasy and down-to-earth reality; but the aerial was also the floating.

[1] *Ah! que le monde est grand à la clarté des lampes!*
*Aux yeux du souvenir, que le monde est petit!*
BAUDELAIRE, *Les Fleurs du Mal:* "Le Voyage".

Similarly in Hugo, one of the chapters in *Notre Dame de Paris* is entitled "The gold piece turned into a dry leaf".

This apposition is, on the one hand, related to the infantile situation, in which the happy time, when the child is *carried* in someone's arms, is contrasted with the moment when he has to try *to walk on the ground.* In the last analysis, this brings us back to the classic complex of *weaning.* When we described this complex in *L'Ame et l'Action* (1944), we encountered the concept of "floating" as one of its major themes.

It is worth while pointing out that in strictly reductive terms there is no doubt that the "aerial" pole is regressive and the patient is progressing when he accepts the "down-to-earth". But the matter is more complex and such a simplification is dangerous. Though we must, on the one hand, describe every detail of structure as carefully as possible, this description of facts should eschew any attribution of value, as Charles Odier has rightly remarked. The value judgement will vary according to the circumstances. And the value represented by the pole of fantasy, in its aspect of the ideal or of creative imagination, can be neglected only at grave risk.

### IV. MERIT AND GRACE

We must, perhaps, apologize for borrowing terms from the vocabulary of theology for our title. These concepts, merit and grace, are, of course, in their true meaning only the extreme limits of a series which the psychologist has to consider in all its manifestations, however humble or profane or even perverted. But they provide images that are useful in drawing attention to two psychological attitudes to be found at every level, one of which relies solely on personal effort, whereas the other abandons itself to an exclusive reliance on some beneficent power: sometimes this is called "providence", but it may also be "chance" or, more elegantly, "my stars" or, more popularly "luck", but it is always, however, enfolded in superstition and magic, a sort of maternal divinity. In this domain, in which the gambler and speculator move with such carelessness, insolence, or anxiety, we recognize that we are still dealing with the pair of opposites already described. Chance is the mother of early childhood, the mother-figure that gives everything, whose arms invite total abandonment. This pole is to effort or merit what the situation before weaning is to that after weaning, the child in arms to the child that walks. We see this clearly when studying the weak-willed, over-optimistic patients, whom we described in *L'Ame enfantine et la Psychanalyse* (1951) in the chapter on "Elusive Behaviour": they are those who wait, as the popular saying goes, for everything to fall into their laps, but we have also found the same structure, at an entirely different level, when studying an authentic mystic, such as St. John of the Cross (Baudouin, 1957*a*).

It may happen that a patient, at some period of his analysis, may feel that it would be better to make less effort, to abandon himself more, and it is not unusual for this decision to have some religious flavour. Thus Sigmund N. reported a dream during his fifty-third session, in which he saw his former director, "a worried, conscientious type", coming towards him "relaxed and carefree". He welcomes him with emotion, "as a saviour" (pole of grace); at the end of his dream a ship (floating, being carried) takes the company to a picnic in gardens full of roses, which explicitly recall "the earthly paradise". When a succession of images such as these unfold before one's eyes, what is one to do? Should one consider them a totally regressive movement towards the pole of least effort, towards the paradise before weaning? Or do they represent the achievement of a new attitude of confidence and relaxation which can be considered valuable and encouraging? The context will show. In this particular case the patient, a convinced Christian, advanced the following remarks: "I used to want to control everything. Now I accept an area which I cannot control. Acceptance of risk, of the irrational. I sow, but I do not make it grow. I was shut up in a hypertrophied ego: now there can be a dialogue where previously there was only a monologue . . . It's as if something has to be given me. I must not try to take. A much clearer concept of grace instead of works." It is the patient speaking, not us.

However, neither pole has any meaning without the other. Popular wisdom, in its sardonic manner, underlines the point: "Heaven helps him who helps himself."

## V. THE IRREPARABLE AND RENEWAL

The pole we agreed to call that of grace can appear, at every level, in the guise of a *free gift*, which cannot be measured, which flows from a spring (like mother's milk) in inexhaustible abundance—the Fountain of Youth, the well that never dries up—and, pursuing this sequence, we find another pair of opposites in irreparable loss and unexpected *renewal.*

It is quite normal to find children giving way to inordinate despair or rage over some small object, some broken plaything, or a toy which has lost its pristine freshness, particularly if someone else is to be blamed for it. After such rages, a child frequently falls into a fit of stubbornness, and it is difficult to see how he can get out of it, for he requires the object to be reconstituted in all its former glory but knows that this is impossible. Whatever may be done to satisfy him, he will refuse it, because "that's not it"; even if one buys him a similar toy, it still will not be the same, it is still "not it". It seems that such attitudes are explicable by the psychology of *narcissism,* which insists on integrity—the integrity, in this case, being transferred from one's own body to one's possessions. However, one does emerge from this *impasse,* but one does so in the same way that one recovers from a fit of sulking, by a sort of conversion of attitude, by the acceptance of an opening, which is at the same time an opening towards others, through which the life-stream can flow once more. Nothing is lost, the moment one ceases to hang on. This conversion from the *closed* to the *open* seems never to occur—to use rather formal terminology—without a transition from the *captative* to the *oblative* attitude, from taking to giving, another pair of opposites, which are closely related, as we have shown, to the philosophic opposition between *having* and *being,* as expressed by Gabriel Marcel (1957).

Kurt E. provided, during his sixty-ninth session, a striking illustration of this system; a particularly good one, because it was beautifully simple and reduced to its bare essentials. It was a dream in two successive scenes: in the first he saw two flower vases which he liked for their shape, and which were now cracked and broken; this accident provoked a bitter sense of "irreversibility". But in the second scene, as if in answer to the first, they were replaced by two new and beautiful vases. Whereas, in another dream reported in the same session, he had at first felt frustrated by the belief that the plants that were to be delivered to him would not be those he had purchased; but everything turns out all right; the public trustee is seeing to it, and has paid for everything. In another scene of the same dream there were two churches, an old one, and a new one that was being consecrated: the later is *open* from one end to the other, as if it were a passage, with the road running through it. He is trying to find a seat for the ceremony of consecration; first of all he thinks of sitting egoistically in the middle of a bench, in order not to be disturbed, but finally he sits down at one end—and may even have offered his seat courteously to a lady (transition to oblation).

This simple example should suffice, although there are many others, more detailed, which would soon lead us, as may have already been suspected, to the basic and well-known myth of *death* and *rebirth*.

### VI. THE EGO AND THE SELF

We apologized a little earlier for employing theological terms to describe our pairs of opposites. By a similar perhaps rather premature short cut, we are now borrowing two technical terms from analytical psychology, the *ego* and the *self*. It is opportune to point out once again what a relatively low coefficient of abstraction is to be found in the concepts and terminology of C. G. Jung: they are, however, markedly *phenological*, that is to say, they adhere strictly to the immediate dictates of psychological and clinical experience, of which they are a summary rather than an interpretation. It is, admittedly, true that on the one hand the polarity of the ego and the self is akin to certain well-known opposities in philosophy, such as the *phenomenon* and the *noumenon* of Kant (as Jung has himself pointed out) but this is because, once again, these opposites are deeply rooted in an *implicit philosophy* which proceeds directly from inner experience. Thus we are constantly confronted with the fact that our patients are aware of an inner duality, a tension between a weak and dependent ego, which exists in ordinary life, and the "true ego" to which they aspire, the "ego" as it should be, which sometimes appears to have a numinous aspect, partaking of the experience of the "holy".

The pair ego-self appears as a confirmation of the pair merit and grace. The ego progresses with difficulty, step by step: the self appears more as a discovery, a gift. It may be the discovery of the "treasure", or of "gold". In the dream we have just mentioned, in which Sigmund N. welcomes his relaxed director "as a saviour", he discovers later at the top of a hill, which he climbs with a friend, a heap of gold coins and silver plate—and they begin to pick up the treasure, which was, incidentally, "the fruit of a robbery". Not uncommonly, in fact, the ego is hesitant before the self, as though it were "not mine" or "too beautiful for me". Thus Igor N. had a dream (one hundred and thirty-eighth session) in which he had come to the watchmaker (the analyst) to collect his watch. "The watch was in pieces . . . I pick up the pieces, but in the middle there is a *pearl of considerable size*: I don't know *whether the pearl belongs to me*, and I feel rather embarrassed at taking such a big pearl, in case it does not belong to me. I pick it up, with the idea of seeing what should be done about it".[1]

This is the way a true dialectic of the ego and the self usually presents itself. In a dream reported by Henry F., a doctor undergoing a professional analysis, the same opposites were beautifully portrayed by the theme of *house* and *temple* (which Jung has shown to be the symbol of the self in its numinous aspect). "The idea of the temple", said Henry F., "came to me from the old wooden house. *One passes from one to the other.*" Then the temple evoked the idea of Greece, which is perfection, and the goal, according to him, of analysis. However, the "passage" is not so easy. "Those who penetrate into the temple are perhaps not worthy of it." Truly, *non sum dignus entrare.*

## VII. SEEKING AND FINDING

We are now about to consider a theme that may appear to be a simple variation on the preceding one. We have already mentioned the discovery of the treasure: in short, the ego *seeks*, whereas the self is *found*. But when we describe these two aspects by these two verbs, we cannot escape the association to Pascal's timeless words: "Thou wouldst not seek Me, if thou hadst not

[1]Igor N. found it, incidentally, very difficult to draw the line between mine and thine and particularly to attribute any qualities or capacities to the ego, owing to the disparaging attitude of his family expressed in terms of "such things are not for you". He had considerable difficulty in ego formation and in achieving independence. He has already provided some remarkable imagery of ego formation (see Baudouin, 1957b, p. 94). The same difficulties are now repeated at the level of the self.

already found Me." This is perhaps the key to the whole paragraph, illustrating as it does the peculiar paradox of the situation, which is sufficiently interesting to deserve separate consideration.

The two patients who furnished such typical examples of the tension between the ego and the self provide equally striking examples of this new pair of opposites.

Sigmund N., during the period of treatment we have already mentioned, produced in the fifty-second session a dream in which, after a *long perambulation looking* for the key in the town (Jung has pointed out the significance of the *circumambulatio*), he reaches a corridor in which a sick woman is lying. She "shows him where the key *is to be found*". It will be noticed that the precious object of the search is not directly found, only a guarantee as to the presence of the missing object is given—the indication of the place where "it is to be found". Similarly, in another dream, a little later (fifty-fourth session), Sigmund N. is taking an interest in a group of children who are performing some athletic feat, which attracts him; then "I don't find the children again, only an envelope containing the necessary instructions."

The guarantee as to the missing object sometimes appears as an incomplete recollection, a *reminiscence*. We have quoted elsewhere a typical dream of this nature, from a man of 78, who was wandering about the countryside (*circumambulatio*) looking for a town which was "the *centre* of the country" (the centre is the classic symbol of the self)[1] where he had once been, but whose name he had forgotten (Baudouin, 1950, p. 188).

The theme of reminiscence appeared in Igor N.'s dreams in a somewhat similar context. During a very lively dream (one hundred and thirteenth session) there appeared in succession America, a negro, a hotel in which the dreamer takes a room, then "we walk around". In the street his wallet is stolen; his wife disappears. There he is, "alone, without money, in an unknown city, not even knowing the name of my hotel. However, I have a vague idea where it is, and I shall hit on it . . . *by walking around*."

If one looks more deeply into the philosophical development of such a situation, it is difficult not to be aware, on the one

[1]Mircea Eliade (1952, Ch. I, particularly p. 65) has made a careful study of this symbol as it appears in mythology and ritual.

hand, of Pascal's words, and, on the other, of Plato's theory of "remembering".

## CONCLUSION

We have tried to limit this paper to the description of certain typical psychological situations. But the systems we have noted extend to every region of the psyche. From the biological angle, they relate to certain Freudian concepts (the "irreparable" would relate to "castration") and certain basic complexes (weaning, for instance, to which we have often referred); from another angle, they link up with the functions (cf. p. 69) and the archetypes of Jung's psychology; frequently they are associated with myths; and, finally, it is not possible to evade their philosophical implications, which are, like everything else, "phenological" data; it is as if, at certain moments of experience, we were able to apprehend the existence of a philosophy *in statu nascendi*, suggesting a connection with the established philosophies.

We must insist on the point mentioned at the beginning of this paper: our psychology is not a disguised philosophy: it describes purely and simply a human experience, and a certain philosophy, explicit or not, is part of this experience. But on the other hand we may be allowed to hope that further investigation may permit us to become better acquainted with the physiognomy of this *implicit philosophy* which arises spontaneously from the recesses of the human soul.

A better acquaintance with this implicit philosophy would surely allow us, who have advantages denied to both Kant and Husserl, to delimit the *a priori* forms and the *prolegomena* of explicit philosophy, and even perhaps one day to lay down the outlines of philosophy as science. Even now, we may say that the predominance of the pairs of opposites in our examples would suggest the *dialectic* nature of all implicit philosophy.

It is therefore clear how, within certain narrow limits, yet with infinite possibilities of development, it is possible to ascribe a philosophical task to our psychology.

(*For References see p. 67*)

# 4

## *DIE KLINISCHE BEDEUTUNG VON EXTRAVERSION UND INTROVERSION*

H. K. FIERZ, *Kreuzlingen, Schweiz*

Extraversion und Introversion sind konstitutionelle, typische Einstellungen. Das primäre Interesse des Extravertierten ist beim Objekt, dasjenige des Introvertierten beim Subjekt.

Um zu untersuchen, welche medizinischen Auswirkungen diese beiden Einstellungsmöglichkeiten haben, müssen wir zunächst jenen Augenblick erfassen, in welchem Objekt und Subjekt entstehen.

Objekt und Subjekt zeigen sich immer dann, wenn die Beziehungen, die in einer participation mystique herrschen (*Lévy-Bruhl*), der Kritik unterstellt werden, sei es der eigenen Kritik des Subjektes, sei es der Kritik eines anderen. Jetzt entsteht Bewusstsein, und Objekt und Subjekt werden geboren. Ein solches Ereignis kann die Gesamtpersönlichkeit betreffen, z.B. beim Kleinkind, oder bei weitgehend unbewussten, primitiven Menschen. Aber auch bei differenzierten Erwachsenen ist immer noch ein Sektor in Entwicklung, immer noch Unbewusstheit vorhanden, und dann kann es zu Konflikten kommen, die die Kritik wachrufen und eine participation mystique auflösen.

Konflikt heisst, dass Zwei, die aufeinander bezogen sind, sich nicht völlig harmonisch zueinanderfügen. Erlebt ein Individuum diese Störung der Harmonie, so ist es als erlebender Mensch Subjekt. Der Konfliktpartner, zu welchem Disharmonie herrscht, wird ihm Objekt.

Am Individuum lässt sich in diesem Moment der Störung beobachten: im Individuum entsteht ein Affekt; hier zeigt sich das Animus/Anima-Problem. Und zur nun objektiv gewordenen Umgebung besteht eine Anpassungsstörung, die Affekte schafft; denn hier zeigt sich das Schatten-Problem. Klassisch das Beispiel der heranwachsenden Kinder: Es wird entdeckt, dass die Eltern nicht immer so vollkommen sind, wie erwartet wurde. Dies führt zum Aerger über die Eltern, dem Affekt. Und zur Anpassungsstörung, dem flegelhaften Verhalten. Jetzt ist dem Kinde die Türe offen zur Frage: Wer bin ich? Und zur anderen Frage: Wer sind meine Eltern? Weiter: Was ist das, "Ich"? Was ist das, "Vater", "Mutter"? Und so wird Subjekt und Objekt geboren. Wie bald dann der Archetypus (eben z.B. Vater und Mutter) sichtbar wird, erkennen wir; daher das oft erhebliche Ausmass des Affektes.

Wo eine participation mystique aufgelöst wird, steht jeder vor demselben Problem. Das Problem ist ein allgemeines. Die Bearbeitung des Problems ist jedoch verschieden, je nachdem das Primär-Interesse sich dem Subjekte zuwendet oder dem Objekte. Die Form der Bearbeitung zeigt den Einstellungs-Typus.

Der Introvertierte beachtet primär das Subjekt. Hier wird ihm das bewusst, was im Subjekt störend wirkt. Das ist der Affekt. Sein Anliegen ist, diesen zu beschwichtigen, und eifrig gibt er sich dieser Aufgabe hin, indem er eine neue, beruhigendere Einstellung sucht. Nicht—oder weniger—beachtet wird die Anpassungsstörung nach aussen, zum Objekt. Leicht wirkt der Introvertierte deshalb schattenhaft-negativ, z.B. sonderlich, schrullig, hochmütig oder gar böse. Dieser Schwierigkeit wird nicht durch fortschreitende Bewusstheit, also Erkenntnis, begegnet, sondern durch Ausweichen. Ein Introvertierter kann deshalb seinen Freundeskreis systematisch beschränken, auslesen, ungefährlich wählen. Oft aber stösst er an der realen Aussenwelt, die ihm ja überall entgegentritt, an. Die "Tücke des Objekts" kann seine Crux sein, er kann Pechvogel sein. Auch ein noch jugendlicher Introvertierter kann sich auf einer Treppe das Bein brechen . . . er konnte ja nicht die Treppe beachten, sondern musste seinen Aerger darüber, dass der Treppenläufer so hässlich rot ist, bearbeiten (mit dem Ziel, zu sagen: "Es ist gleichgültig, wie Treppenläufer gefärbt sind", oder vielleicht: "Dieses Rot gefällt mir nicht, weil es mir nicht liegt"). Natürlich tut ihm die Bearbeitung des Affektes gut. Die Emotion legt sich wieder, und so bleibt er z.B. von nervös gesteuerten Stoffwechselstörungen verschont. Der Chirurg hat wohl eher mit ihm zu tun, jedoch meist nur im Gebiete der kleinen und mittleren Chirurgie. In diesem Stadium der Entwicklung scheint es, wie wenn der Geist befriedigt würde, aber der Instinkt vernachlässigt. Gleichsam geistig hochstehend, aber weltfremd stösst der Introvertierte mit der Welt zusammen; eine Lebensgefahr besteht aber in der Regel nicht. Eine besondere Frage wäre vielleicht, ob der Introvertierte—um sich ruhig zu halten und der Welt auszuweichen—ungenügend und gehemmt atmet, sodass er verhältnismässig anfällig ist für Lungentuberkulose.

Der Extravertierte beachtet primär das Objekt. Er will seine Beziehung zum Objekt ordnen. Er gibt sich ihm hin und wirkt gar nicht schattenhaft. Dass etwas in ihm vorgeht, dass etwas in ihm in Bewegung geraten ist, übersieht er. Trotz der guten Objektanpassung des Extravertierten lässt sich dies ab und zu äusserlich feststellen. Denn der missachtete Affekt zeigt sich in gelegentlichen Stimmungsschwankungen, die noch recht bald animösen Charakter haben. Der unberücksichtigte Affekt kann sich auch auf den Stoffwechsel auswirken; Leberleiden sind kennzeichnend. Auch das Herz kann angeschlagen werden. In diesem Stadium der Entwicklung begegnet er viel eher dem Internisten als dem Chirurgen. In der Regel besteht aber keine Lebensgefahr, wenn der Extravertierte gleichsam dem Instinkt folgt, aber den Geist vernachlässigt.

Auf das erste Stadium der Entwicklung folgt jedoch ein nächstes. Die äussere Unangepasstheit des Introvertierten kann zunehmen. Trotz allen Strebens nach "innerlichem Ausweichen" und trotz des Versuchs, die Objektzahl durch Auslese zu beschränken, kann ein Zusammenstoss mit der Welt eintreten, der die Wirklichkeit des Objekts zwingend sichtbar macht. Und nun lässt sich eben der Affekt nicht mehr befriedigen, er wird deutlich sichbar, und der Introvertierte wird animös, und zwar meistens deutlich giftiger als ein harmloser Extravertierter.

Der Extravertierte hingegen wird einen Punkt erreichen, wo sein Affekt dringlich nach Befriedigung ruft. Dann bricht der Affekt heftig nach aussen durch, die Anpassung an die Aussenwelt wird zerschlagen, und es zeigt sich ein sehr dunkler Schatten. Der Extravertierte aber wird vor die Frage nach dem

Subjekt, nach der Wirklichkeit seiner eigenen Person, gestellt.

In dieser Lage sollte der Introvertierte extravertieren, sich mit Interesse dem Objekt zuwenden. Und der Extravertierte sollte introvertieren und sich seiner eigenen Wenigkeit, dem Subjekt, zuwenden. Wird die Gegeneinstellung nicht als Aufgabe angenommen, so zeigen sich klinische Folgen.

Dann wird nämlich einseitig und krampfhaft am ursprünglichen Einstellungstypus festgehalten. Dieser aber ist bereits überaltert, hat Energie an die Gegen-Einstellung abgegeben und befindet sich in einem *abaissement* (P. Janet). Die ursprünglich hochwertige Einstellung funktioniert nicht mehr zuverlässig. Sie ist minderwertig geworden. Der Zusammenbruch des alten Systems zeigt sich bis in den Körper.

Der Introvertierte wird anfällig gegen plötzliche Infektionen, die gefährlich sind. Der übergrosse Affekt kann seinen Stoffwechsel so stören, dass lebensgefährliche (perniziöse) Lagen entstehen. Die Gefahr kommt nun von innen, der Introvertierte braucht den Internisten; das Leben ist in Gefahr.

Auch für den Extravertierten besteht grosse Gefahr, wenn er seine überalterte Primär-Einstellung einseitig aufrecht erhalten will. Seine Anpassung ans Aussen funktioniert nicht mehr zuverlässig. Nun kann er verunfallen, und nun braucht er den Chirurgen. Der aber ist oft zu grosser Chirurgie aufgerufen, denn die Unfälle des "dekompensierenden Extravertierten" sind häufig sehr schwer (Auto-Unfälle, Absturz in den Bergen). Nicht immer aber ist is der Chirurg, der helfen sollte. Oft erhält das Problem auch ein juristisches Kleid. Die Blindheit für die subjektive Seite und den schwarzen Schatten kann zu Konkursen, Betrügereien und anderen forensischen Tatbeständen führen. So kann der Extravertierte durch Unfall oder törichtes Delikt sein Leben gefährden . . . um ein Leben durch Straffälligkeit zu zerstören, braucht es ja nicht Todesstrafe; auch Gefängnis und Zuchthaus können ein Leben brechen.

Dieses Stadium der Entwicklung ist eine Krise. Der Introvertierte kann der Krise ausweichen durch Suicid. Dieser geschieht in plötzlichem Affekt, als Panik vor eben diesem gehassten Affekt, der die subjektive Ruhe vernichtet. Auch der Extravertierte kann dem Problem ausweichen durch Suicid. Er plant ihn in schattenhaft-schwarzer Ueberlegung und kann so erreichen, dass er den Verlust der geliebten Objekt-Sicherheit nicht bearbeiten muss.

In der Krise zeigt der Introvertierte demnach die Symptome des Extravertierten, aber in bedeutend bedrohlicherem Ausmass. Gerade dann, wenn er die Extraversion nicht annehmen will, zeigt sie sich automatisch, archaisch und mit viel bösartigerer Problematik. Die gefährlichen Störungen können allerdings heute bedeutend erfolgreicher behandelt werden als noch vor 20 Jahren. Die gefährliche Infektion lässt sich durch Antibiotika bekämpfen. Die lebensgefährliche Stoffwechselstörung lässt sich durch Pharmaka, wie z.B. Serpasil, Largactil u.a. mildern. Es besteht aber doch die Gefahr des geistigen Todes, wenn der übergrosse Affekt den Stoffwechsel so stört, dass eine Verblödung eintritt. Und eine Gefahr des körperlichen Todes, wenn unter dem grossen Affekt die Infektionsabwehr zusammenbricht. Die Gefahr kommt von innen.

Der Extravertierte seinerseits zeigt, wenn er in der Krise steht, die übersteigerten Symptome des Introvertierten. Denn eine nicht realisierte Introversion setzt sich in gefährlich-archaischer Form durch. Ist der Extravertierte durch Unfall mit der Welt zusammengestossen und schwer verletzt, so kann immerhin die moderne Chirurgie mit ihrer verbesserten Technik, auch der ausgefeilten Narkosetechnik, viel helfen; die wiederherstellende orthopaedische Chirurgie kann Manchem, der zum Krüppel wurde, wieder zur Tätigkeit verhelfen. Wenn der schattenhafte Zusammenstoss mit der Welt forensische Folgen hatte, so darf man bedenken, dass immerhin die Todesstrafe zunehmend abgeschafft wird, und dass Bestrebungen sich durchsetzen, den Strafvollzug nicht zur Vernichtung, sondern zur Erziehung des Sträflings zu verwenden. Dennoch besteht Lebensgefahr. Sie kommt, als Unfall oder als Strafe, von aussen, Sie kann durch Unfall töten, oder durch soziale Vernichtung das geistige Leben brechen.

Beim Introvertierten lässt sich die Minderwertigkeit seiner Extraversion auch formal beobachten, z.B. in der Perception: es kann intuiert werden, fasciniert vom Aussen. Es wird aber minderwertig intuiert. Es werden deshalb nicht Möglichkeiten gesehen, wie dies einer entwickelten Intuition entspricht, sondern es werden die "unmöglichsten Möglichkeiten" gesehen. Von hier zum Verfolgungswahn mit Wahnideen ist nur noch ein kleiner Schritt.—Wird mit der Empfindung percipiert, so wird die Aussenwelt nicht geordnet erfasst, sondern zerfahren. Auch hier ist der Befund oft erheblich pathologisch.

Die minderwertige Introversion des Extravertierten zeigt sich darin, dass sich zwar eine reflektierende Betrachtung des Subjekts aufdrängt, dass sich diese Betrachtung aber oft zu einem hilflosen Abquälen entwickelt. Dies vor allem, weil ungenügend unterschieden wird. Im Nachdenken über sich selbst wird "pars pro toto" genommen. Wegen eines einzigen Fehlers wird der ganze Mensch verworfen. Schuld-Gedanken, ja ein Versündigungswahn, können so entstehen. Es wird weiter die Autonomie der persönlichen Entwicklung sehr deutlich wahrgenommen, sie wird aber als Katastrophe empfunden. Als Ganzes ergibt dies ein depressives Bild. Gelegentlich erlahmt eventuell die Fascination durch das Subjekt, und dann wird nur noch die bereits minderwertig gewordene ursprüngliche Extraversion sichtbar, als Manie.

Es lässt sich demnach feststellen, dass die minderwertige Gegeneinstellung beim Introvertierten eine eher schizophrene Symptomatik bewirkt, während sie beim Extravertierten manisch-depressive Symptome verursacht. Sind die psychotischen Symptome deutlich, dann lässt sich die Konstellierung der minderwertigen Gegeneinstellung besonders eindrücklich beobachten. Man muss nur zuhören, was der Mensch sagt. Ein Introvertierter kann, wenn er sich dem Aussen auwendet, paranoisch reagieren. Es zeigt sich dann eine abwegige Fascination durch das Objekt, und der Mensch sagt: "Er hat getan, er darf, er darf nicht, er sollte, er will". Dabei wird die Minderwertigkeit der Extraversion ins Objekt projiziert. Das Gegenüber ist deshalb böse, töricht oder verwerflich. Wird umgekehrt ein Extravertierter, der introvertieren sollte, melancholisch, so sehen wir ein ausschliessliches Kreisen der Gedanken um das Subjekt. Der Mensch sagt: "Ich habe getan, ich sollte, ich bin". Und die Minderwertigkeit der Introversion wird dem Subjekt zugeschoben. So hält sich der Depressive für schuldig, für unwürdig, für schlecht und für verarmt.

Bemerkenswert ist im Hinblick auf den Einstellungstypus auch eine psychiatrische Erfahrung. Bekanntlich empfiehlt der Psychiater bei Schizophrenen eine möglichst frühe Entlassung aus der Klinik, die sogenannte Frühentlassung. Bei Manisch-Depressiven ist anderseits eine Spätentlassung angezeigt. Im

Hinblick auf das Problem der minderwertigen Gegeneinstellung könnte man hier sagen: Der Schizophrene, der primär introvertiert ist, in dessen Krankheit sich eine minderwertige Extraversion zeigt, soll möglichst früh ins Leben hinaus, um seine Extraversion zu üben. Der Manisch-Depressive aber, der extravertiert veranlagt ist, soll lange genug in der Klinik bleiben, denn er sollte dort seine unentwickelte Introversion üben.

So deutlich nun aber der psychopathologische Fall gewisse Einzelprobleme aufzeigt, so ist er selbstverständlich nicht der Normalfall. Normalerweise dürfte sich die Frage nach der minderwertigen Gegeneinstellung als Auftakt zur zweiten Lebenshälft stellen. Gerade bei den pathologischen Fällen stellt sie sich aber oft bedeutend früher. Eine der Ursachen hiefür dürfte sein, dass familiäre oder Milieu-Einflüsse den Menschen schon früh verfälscht haben. Es kann dann vorkommen, dass einem konstitutionell Extravertierten eine introvertierte Einstellung eingeflösst wird, die ihm gar nicht liegt und aus der die in ihm vorhandene Entwicklungstendenz ihm verhältnismässig bald befreien möchte. Dass Zusammentreffen einer gesunden, jedoch unentwickelten Extraversion mit einem verfälschten, dem Menschen nicht angemessenen habituellen Bewusstsein, das introvertiert ist, kann dann zu sehr komplexen, eben pathologischen Befunden führen. Einem Introvertierten kann die analoge Verfälschung widerfahren. Im Einzelnen ist diese Frage noch ungenügend untersucht. Ich glaube aber, dass die Verfälschung des konstitutionellen Einstellungstypus durch das Milieu eine der wichtigen Ursachen von psychotischen Symptomen und von sogenannten Psychopathien ist.

Der ideale Normalfall wäre nun der, bei dem sich die Entwicklung der Gegenstellung störungsfrei vollzieht. Wie immer in der Medizin, und insbesondere in der Psychologie, ist dieser Fall aber gar nicht leicht zu beobachten, da zur Beobachtung eben auch kein Anlass besteht. Kommt es zu Störungen, so können im Ausmass natürlich alle Abschattierungen auftreten. Als Einzelheiten wären vielleicht noch anzuführen: Der Introvertierte, der seine Extraversion entwickeln sollte, ist relativ anfällig für ein Magengeschwür. Beim Extravertierten, der introvertieren sollte, besteht nach meiner Erfahrung die Gefahr einer vorzeitigen Arteriosklerose. Dass das Magengeschwür psychotherapeutisch angehbar ist, dürfte bekannt sein. Weniger bekannt ist vielleicht, dass auch relativ schwere arteriosklerotische Befunde unter geeigneter Psychotherapie oft erstaunlich aufhellen, ganz im Gegensatz zur defaitistischen psychiatrischen Prognose, wie sie in allen Lehrbüchern steht. Insbesondere dort also, wo ein Extravertierter die Gegeneinstellung bearbeiten sollte und allenfalls depressiv ist, sollen arteriosklerotische Symptome in Bezug auf die Prognose keinesfalls überwertet werden; man darf ihretwegen auch nicht eine Psychotherapie unterlassen.

Im Ueberblick ergibt sich nach dem Gesagten die folgende Auswirkung der Einstellungs-Typen auf medizinischem Gebiet: Der Introvertierte befriedigt primär den Affekt und stösst mit der Welt zusammen. Er ist durch leichte bis mittelschwere Unfälle gefährdet. Der Extravertierte passt sich der Welt an und übersieht den Affekt. Bei ihm sind Stoffwechsel und Herz gefährdet. Beide Einstellungstypen stehen dann früher oder später vor dem Problem, auch die minderwertige Gegeneinstellung zu entwickeln. Gelingt dies ungenügend, so können Störungen auftreten, die schwer sind, ja sogar vital gefährlich. Beim Introvertierten können Infektionen einbrechen oder perniziöse Stoffwechselstörungen auftreten. Der Extravertierte ist durch schwersten Unfall gefährdet, eventuell auch forensisch. Weiter ist der Introvertierte für ulcus ventriculi, der Extravertierte für Arteriosklerose anfällig. Die Fascination des Introvertierten durch das Aussen kann sich dann auch in einer paranoiden Symptomatik zeigen, während die Fascination des Extravertierten durch das Innen die minderwertige Introversion in der Melancholie zeigt.

Im Hinblick auf den zuletzt angeführten psychiatrischen Aspekt sei noch hervorgehoben: Auch in der Krise bleibt (neben der von Kretschmer meisterhaft dargestellten körperlichen Konstitution) die spontane, ursprüngliche Primärbeziehung sichtbar. Wenn sich der asthenische Schizophrene wahnhaft dem Aussen zuwendet, so gilt doch seine Spontanneigung dem Subjekt. Entsprechend ist der affektive Rapport, der ihn mit dem Aussen verbindet, schlecht. Und wenn sich der pyknische Melancholiker dem Innen zuwendet, so gilt doch seine Spontanneigung dem Objekt. So ist sein affektiver Rapport gut. Es ist auch eindrücklich, wie—gegen alle Widerstände des habituellen Bewusstseins—

die Psychose der minderwertigen Gegeneinstellung zum Durchbruch verhilft. Der introvertierte Schizophrene wird durch eine hervorbrechende Aggressivität zum Kontakt mit dem Aussen geführt. Und der extravertierte Melancholiker schliesst sich von der Aussenwelt ab, indem er die Idee entwickelt, es könne ihn niemand verstehen, es wolle ihn auch niemand verstehen, und niemand könne ihm helfen; so wird er auf sich selbst zurückgeworfen.

Wir müssen nun noch fragen, welche Anforderungen an eine moderne medizinische Auffassung des Problems der Einstellungstypen gestellt werden müssen. Ganz allgemein ist es ja selbstverständlich, dass internistische, chirurgische und psychiatrische Komplikationen, die im Verlauf der Entwicklung auftreten, nach den Regeln der ärztlichen Erfahrung und der ärztlichen Kunst zu behandeln sind. Darüber hinaus ist aber die Diagnose nicht unwesentlich, dass der Kranke ein Mensch ist, welcher in einer Krise seine minderwertige Gegeneinstellung realisieren sollte. Denn diese kritische Lage schafft erhöhte Gefahren. In solcher Lage ist deshalb eine ganz besonders sorgfältige und wache Aufmerksamkeit erforderlich. Wenn z.B. die innere Stabilität des Introvertierten zusammenbricht, so kann eine Infektion überaus plötzlich hereinbrechen. Antibiotika müssen unbedingt zeitig gegeben werden, sonst ist es zu spät. Im Zweifelsfalle sind deshalb die Leukozyten regelmässig zu zählen—Puls—und Temperaturkontrolle allein genügen nicht. Steigen sie über 10,000, so ist allenfalls mit der antibiotischen Therapie zu beginnen. Bricht hingegen die äussere Anpassung des Extravertierten zusammen, so ist die erhöhte Unfallgefahr sehr zu beachten. Gewagte Bergtouren z.B. sind zu untersagen, eventuell auch das Lenken eines Motorfahrzeugs.

Neben einer solchen wachen ärztlichen Einstellung ist aber auch ein Verständnis für den psychologischen Gehalt der Symptomatik zu fordern, seien die Symptome physisch oder psychisch. Krankhafte Symptome sind abwegig und minderwertig. In dieser Abwegigkeit und Minderwertigkeit muss jenes Unternehmen des Menschen erkannt werden, das das Problem der minderwertigen Gegeneinstellung bearbeiten will. In diesem Sinne ist die medizinische Symptomatik positiv aufzufassen, d.h. nicht als krankhafte Abirrung, sondern als ein Weg zu einem ganzen Menschen.

ZUSAMMENFASSUNG

Wenn die "participation mystique" sich auflöst, wird Bewusstsein geboren.

Dann ist das Interesse des Introvertierten auf der subjektiven Seite der Objekt-Subjekt-Beziehung. Deshalb beachtet er den Affekt und vernachlässigt die Anpassung an die äussere Welt; die Folge ist eine typische medizinische Problematik (z.B. Unfälle, die aber nicht lebensgefährlich sind). Dass Interesse des Extravertierten ist in diesem Moment auf der objektiven Seite. Er beachtet die Anpassung an die Welt und vernachlässigt den Affekt. Das medizinische Problem zeigt sich dann in Störungen des Stoffwechsels (z.B. Leberleiden, ohne Lebensgefahr).

Im Verlaufe der Entwicklung begegnet der Introvertierte seiner minderwertigen Extraversion, und der Extravertierte seiner minderwertigen Introversion. Gleichzeitig verliert jedoch die Introversion des Introvertierten ihre alte Sicherheit ("abaissement du niveau mental"); beim Extravertierten geschieht das Umgekehrte. Deshalb sind beide in (oft vitaler) Gefahr durch eine minderwertige Introversion und eine minderwertige Extraversion, mit chirurgischer Probelmatik (Unfälle), intern-medizinischer Problematik (lebensgefährliche körperliche Krankheit) und psychiatrischen Symptomen (Psychose, Suicid).

Die ursprünglichen Tendenzen des Introvertierten und des Extravertierten—denen körperlich die Konstitution entspricht, wie dies Kretschmer beschrieben hat—führen jedoch in dieser Krise zu von einander unterschiedenen Zustandsbildern. In Bezug auf die kritische Situation des Introvertierten und diejenige des Extravertierten wird eine kurze Uebersicht betreffend die medizinischen Symptome und die medizinische Therapie gegeben.


## *THE CLINICAL SIGNIFICANCE OF EXTRAVERSION AND INTROVERSION*

EXTRAVERSION and introversion are typical, constitutional attitudes. The primary interest of the extravert lies in the object, that of the introvert in the subject.

If we wish to study the possible medical consequences of these two basic attitudes, we must first understand the moment at which subject and object arise.

Subject and object always appear when relationships which have hitherto been governed by a *participation mystique* (Lévy-Bruhl), are exposed to criticism, whether from the subject himself or from someone else. Such an event may affect the whole personality, for instance, in the young child, or in largely unconscious, undifferentiated people. But even in differentiated adults we still find unconscious areas in need of development. This situation is conducive to conflicts that may provoke criticism and thus lead to the dissolution of a *participation mystique*.

By conflict we understand that two persons in a given relationship find that they are not in complete harmony. The individual who experiences this disturbance of harmony is the subject and the partner to the conflict, with whom he feels in disharmony, is his object.

We can observe how this disturbance manifests itself in the individual: an affect is created, involving an animus-anima problem. There is also a disturbance of adjustment to the now objectivated environment, which creates further effects, constellating the problem of the shadow. A classic example can be found in young children: they discover that the parents are not always as perfect as they had expected. The affect created is anger with the parents: the ensuing churlishness leads to a problem of adjustment. The child is now exposed to doubts such as: "Who am I?", or "Who are my parents?" And further, "What is this I?", "What is 'father', 'mother'?" In this way subject and object are born. This situation soon constellates the parental archetypes, hence the often considerable energy of the affect.

The same problem arises for everyone when a *participation mystique* is dissolved. Although the problem is a general one, the way it is worked through varies according to whether the primary interest is directed towards the subject or object. The individual way in which the problem is solved indicates the basic attitude.

The introvert is primarily concerned with the subject, and so he becomes aware of the disturbing factors in the subject. At this point the affect arises. He has a tendency to damp down this affect, and devotes himself to this task with alacrity by seeking a new and reassuring orientation. His difficulty in external adjustment to the object is less—or not at all—important to him. For this reason the introvert frequently appears as negative, "shadowy", showing himself as odd, whimsical, haughty, or even malicious. This difficulty will not be dealt with by greater awareness, and realization, but by evasion. An introvert may thus systematically reduce his circle of acquaintances by selection of the most "harmless". But he often comes up against the reality of the external world. The "malice of the object" can be his stumbling-block: he will always have "bad luck". Even a young introvert may break his leg on the stairs. He could not pay attention to the stairs, but had to express his anger at the horrible red colour of the stair carpet (with the object of being able to say later "I don't mind what the colour is" or perhaps "I don't like this red because it doesn't suit me"). Naturally it does him good to let out his affect. The emotion subsides and he is thus, for instance, protected against metabolic disturbance. It is more likely that the surgeon will be called in, although mainly for minor or only moderately serious interventions. At this stage of development it would seem that the spirit is satisfied but the instinct neglected. Mentally "superior", but alienated from his surroundings, the introvert comes into perpetual collision with the world, though usually without endangering his life. It is perhaps possible that the introvert—in order to remain calm and aloof from the world—breathes in an inadequate and inhibited way, and thus may become relatively easily susceptible to pulmonary tuberculosis.

The extravert is primarily concerned with the object. He likes to organize his object relationships. He gives himself up to them, and has anything but a 'shadowy' appearance. He overlooks the fact that something is happening inside him, that something has been set in motion. In spite of the extravert's successful adaptation to the object, this oversight becomes apparent from time to time when the underestimated affect manifests itself in occasional changes of mood that soon develop into animosity. The unrealized affect can also influence the metabolism: liver troubles are typical and even the heart may be affected. At this stage of development he is more likely to need the physician than the surgeon. Generally speaking there is no danger to life when the extravert follows his instinct and neglects the spiritual side.

This first stage of development is, however, followed by another. In the case of the introvert, the lack of external adaptation increases. In spite of all attempts at "escaping inwards", and in spite of his endeavour to restrict the number of objects by selection, he may come into such a collision with the world that the reality of the object is forced upon him. And now the affect can no longer be pacified: it manifests itself clearly, and the introvert shows his animosity usually much more bitterly than the harmless extravert.

The extravert, on the other hand, reaches a point where his affect clamours for satisfaction. The affect breaks through with violence, the adjustment to the external world is shattered and a dark shadow side becomes evident. The extravert is faced with the question of the subject, of the reality of his own person.

In such a situation the introvert should become more extraverted and direct his interests towards the object. And the extravert should become more introverted and turn towards his own humble person, the subject. When the task of reversal of attitudes is not accepted, clinical developments will follow.

For there follows a stubborn and one-sided attempt to cling to the original attitude type. But this is now outmoded, has lost energy to the opposite attitude, and the struggle ends with an *abaissement du niveau mental* (P. Janet). The originally superior attitude no longer functions reliably and has become inferior. The break-up of the old system has its physical consequences.

The introvert becomes liable to sudden and dangerous infections. The excessive affect can disturb his metabolism so seriously that a highly dangerous, even pernicious, condition may arise. The danger comes from within: the introvert needs the physician, for his life may be in danger.

For the extravert also there is grave danger if he tries to maintain his one-sided, outmoded, primary attitude. His adaptation to external reality is no longer reliable. Now he can have accidents and be in need of the surgeon. The surgical intervention needed will be serious, for the accidents that occur to a "decompensating extravert" are usually severe (car or mountaineering accidents). However it is not always the surgeon who has to help, as the problem often impinges on the legal sphere. Blindness to the subjective side and to the black shadow often lead him into bankruptcy, swindling, and other delinquencies. Thus the extravert may endanger his life through an accident or stupid misdemeanour. . . it does not need capital punishment to destroy a life: prison or Borstal may do it equally well.

This stage of development is critical. The introvert can evade the crisis by suicide. This occurs under pressure of a sudden affect, panic at the power of the hated affect which ruins his subjective tranquillity. The extravert may also evade the problem by suicide. He plans his suicide with the deliberation of the dark shadow, and can thus avoid having to deal with the loss of the beloved object—security.

In this crisis the introvert develops all the symptoms of the extravert, but to a much more menacing degree. Precisely because he will not accept his extraverted side, it appears as automatism, in archaic form, and with more intractable problems. However, these dangerous disorders can nowadays be handled much more successfully than 20 years ago. Dangerous infections respond to treatment by antibiotics. Disturbances formerly fatal to the metabolism yield to drugs such as Serpasil and Largactil. There is, however, a danger of mental death when the excessive affect disturbs the metabolism to such an extent that mental deterioration occurs; there is also a danger of physical death when the force of the affect destroys the resistance to infection. Again, the danger comes from within.

The extravert, in his crisis, develops in exaggerated form, the symptoms of the introvert, as his not realized introversion takes over in dangerously archaic form. If the extravert has come into collision with the world through an accident and been badly injured, the technical improvements in modern surgery, particularly in the highly developed technique of anaesthetics, can help a good deal: rehabilitation by orthopaedic surgery can restore to active life many who would otherwise have been permanently crippled. When the shadow has brought the extravert into conflict with the world with legal consequences, we must bear in mind that capital punishment is falling increasingly into disuse, and that it is becoming more customary to use a penal sentence for education and not for destructive purposes. Yet there is still danger to life coming, whether from accident or punishment, from without. The accident may kill, or social annihilation may destroy, spiritual life.

There are also formal manifestations of the inferiority of the introvert's extraversion, for instance, in perception. He may intuit, fascinated by the outer world, but the intuition is of poor quality. Thus he does not perceive possibilities as they present themselves to a differentiated intuition, but only "impossible possibilities". From this to paranoia is only a short step. If perception takes place through sensation, the outer world is not understood in an organized manner, but in a disordered way. Here too the condition is often pathological.

The inferior introversion of the extravert manifests itself in the fact that although he is compelled to consideration of, and reflection on, the subject, this often turns into a helpless state of anxiety, largely owing to the lack of discrimination. In reflecting upon himself he takes *pars pro toto*, and rejects himself completely for a single shortcoming. A sense of guilt and sin amounting to mania may then arise. Further, although perfectly aware of the autonomy of personal development, he looks upon it as a catastrophe. The overall picture is one of depression. Sometimes the fascination of the subject gives way again to the original extraversion, which now, however, has become inferior and manifests itself as mania.

It therefore becomes clear that the inferior attitude in the introvert tends to the development of schizophrenic states, whereas in the extravert they may induce manic-depressive ones. If psychotic symptoms are manifest, then the constellation of the inferior attitude becomes particularly impressive. One need only listen to what they say. When an introvert directs his attention outwards, he may show paranoid reactions. His morbid fascination by the object shows itself in such ruminations as: "He did it, he may, he must not, he should, he will." In this way the inferiority of the extraversion is projected on to the object: the other side is therefore bad, stupid or contemptible. On the other hand, if the extravert, who ought to introvert, becomes depressed, we find his thoughts revolving interminably around the subject. He says: "I did it, I should, I am." And the inferiority of the extraversion is thrust on to the subject. So the depressive patient considers himself guilty, unworthy, miserable and impoverished.

Psychiatric experience also sheds a useful light on the two types. It is well known that in schizophrenic cases the psychiatrist orders the earliest possible discharge from the clinic, the so-called "early release", whereas with manic-depressive cases a retardation of the discharge is indicated. Relating this to the problem of the inferior attitude, we could say: the schizophrenic, who is primarily introverted and is displaying an inferior extraversion in his illness, should be sent out into the world to exercise his extraversion. But the manic-depressive, of extraverted disposition, should stay long enough in the clinic to have an opportunity of practising his still undeveloped introversion.

But however clearly the psychopathological case may demonstrate certain problems, it is, of course, abnormal. In normal cases the problem of the inferior attitude becomes constellated with the second half of life. But in pathological cases it often presents itself very much earlier. One of the reasons for this may be that family or environmental influences may have led to an early distortion of the original character. It may be that a constitutional extravert has had an introverted attitude that is quite alien to him forced on him, and the opposite tendency of development aims at restoring the genuine attitude as soon as possible. This clash between a healthy, yet undeveloped extraversion and a distorted, basically alien introverted consciousness, can lead to a very complex, even pathological state. An introvert can be subjected to a corresponding distortion. The details of this problem have not yet been sufficiently studied. I believe, however, that the distortion of the constitutional attitude by environmental factors is one of the principal sources of psychotic symptoms and of the so-called psychopathic pattern.

It would, of course, be ideal if the normal development of the opposite tendency were to take place without disturbance. But, in medicine and particularly in psychology, we seldom observe such cases, as a normal development leaves little to be observed. Where there are disturbances, naturally every shade and variety is forthcoming. One might add a few further details: the introvert, who has to develop his extraversion, is relatively liable to peptic ulcers. In extraverts, who should introvert, there is, in my experience, a danger of premature arterio-sclerosis. It is well known that sufferers from peptic ulcers may derive relief of symptoms from psychotherapy. But it is perhaps less well known that even relatively serious arterio-sclerotic conditions can be helped considerably by suitable psychotherapy, despite the defeatist psychiatric prognoses to be found in all text books. So that in the case of an extravert who has to work out his introversion, and has become depressive, arterio-sclerotic symptoms should not be allowed to influence the prognosis too seriously, and psychotherapy should by no means be neglected.

Let me sum up the effect of the two basic attitude types from the medical aspect. The introvert lives primarily in his affect and comes into conflict with the world. He is liable to slight or moderately serious accidents. The extravert adapts himself to the world and neglects the affect. For him the danger lies in the heart and metabolic system. Both attitude types are then, sooner or later, faced with the same problem, to develop the opposite, inferior attitude within themselves. If this development is inadequate, serious, even fatal disorders may ensue. The introvert may be affected by infections or by pernicious disturbances of the metabolism. The extravert is liable to dangerous accidents and to conflicts with the law. Further, the introvert is liable to peptic ulcers and the extravert to arterio-sclerosis. The introvert's fascinated absorption in the outer world may lead to paranoid symptoms, that of the extravert with the inner world may lead to a manifestation of his inferior introversion in melancholia.

With regard to the psychiatric aspects, we should also stress that the spontaneous, original, primary relationship remains apparent even in crisis (as well as the constitutional types so ably described by Kretschmer). When the asthenic schizophrenic turns outwards in a hallucinatory way, his spontaneous inclination is towards the subject, and his affective rapport with the external world is correspondingly poor. And when the pyknic melancholic directs his attention inwards, he still remains spontaneously directed towards the object, and his affective rapport is good. It is impressive to note how—in spite of the resistance set up by the established consciousness—the psychosis helps the inferior attitude to break through. The introverted schizophrenic is brought into contact with the outer world through outbursts of aggression. And the extraverted melancholic shuts himself away from the world in order to develop the idea that no one can understand him, no one wants to understand him, and no one can help him: so he is thrust back upon himself.

We should now ask what treatment is to be expected from a modern medical understanding of the problems of the two attitude types. Generally speaking, it goes without saying that internal, surgical and psychiatric complications appearing in the course of development, are to be treated according to the general rules of medical science and experience. But, in addition, it is important in diagnosis to think of the patient as a human being who has to achieve, through his crisis, an acceptance of his inferior other side. This critical situation creates special dangers requiring particular care and close attention. If, for instance, the inner stability of the introvert breaks down, his whole system may be invaded by infection with unexpected suddenness. Antibiotics must be administered in good time, or it may be too late. In doubtful cases there must therefore be a regular count of leucocytes—records of pulse and temperature are not enough. If the count exceeds 10,000, antibiotic therapy must begin at once. If, on the other hand, the external adaptation of the extravert breaks down, the increased risk of accidents must be guarded against. Mountaineering, for instance, should be forbidden and perhaps even driving a car.

But apart from such special medical care, an understanding of the psychological meaning of the symptomatology is also required, whether the symptoms be physical or psychological. Illness is symptomatic of something aberrant and inferior. In this aberration and inferiority we must recognize the struggle of a human being trying to work out the problems of his opposite attitude. So, in this sense, the medical symptoms are to be interpreted positively, that is, not as morbid aberrations but as a path to wholeness.

# 5

## *THE EMERGENCE OF A SYMBOL IN A FIVE-YEAR-OLD CHILD*

MICHAEL FORDHAM, *London*

THIS paper about a child called John has two main purposes: first to study the relation between image and symbol, and second to demonstrate how inner symbolic activity leads to ego growth.

### PRE-SYMBOLIC BEHAVIOUR

John had exhibited states of violent and often manic excitement for about one year before he was seen at the clinic; in them his sense of reality was so defective that ordinary methods of control, such as restraint and punishment, were not effective away from home; in the end a good nursery school, after many attempts to help him, was compelled to exclude him and refer him for analytic treatment. As a first step before this was begun, he was placed in a small group of children who needed special educational care.

John's mother, a warm-hearted woman, tended to become too permissive in her handling of him because of her guilt at having produced such a child. His father, on the other hand, resented his son's behaviour and being a mixture of bombast and sentimentality was ineffectual when he tried to exert control; his punishments were often violently resented. In spite of these defects the home was good, because both parents loved their child and wanted to keep him at home. They proved to be helpful and reliable in bringing John for treatment, and the preliminary assessment of them was amply confirmed by several years' knowledge of them.

John was four years old when I first saw him and had already been in analytic treatment for about one year before the symbolic process developed, which therefore happened in his fifth year.

Before describing the rather dramatic changes which came about later, it will be valuable to sketch a few events in the child's first year of analysis so that the later ego development can be described against this background experience. The material will also place the synthetic events in their context and contribute to their understanding. John's behaviour will be considered under three headings: aggression, hearing, and speech.

(*a*) *Aggression*

At first he showed little overt sign of the aggression for which he came, though its presence was suggested by his anxieties. They were so intense that he could not enter my room without his mother and she remained with him during the interview. It is my practice to give the child virtual control over his mother when he needs her, so I made no effort to prevent her being present (cf. Fordham, 1957*a*).

Soon his aggression began to reveal itself and a repetitive drama started. First a pathetic look of fear would come into his eyes and he stood rooted to the spot transfixed before an apparently innocent object as if he were hallucinated, as indeed I believe he was. Then he would creep towards the object and abandon himself maniacally to its destruction.

The necessity for physical intervention on my part led to the aggression being directed on to my body. He was very alarmed when he emptied water over me for the first time and rushed out of the room after he had done it. Only when I interpreted the situation as follows did he return to the playroom: "There is a good John and a good Dr. Fordham who are together, but in the playroom there is a bad John and a bad Dr. Fordham who are destroying each other."

As he became less afraid of what I would do, he started behaving as if he wanted to force his way into my body by attacking it with his head. He held a theory that adults had a special hole down below that he could get into, and he was trying to test whether that was true or false. This idea was also reflected in his play and linked with his anal aggression, which he demonstrated by bending forward and making gestures with his hands to indicate that faeces were shooting out of his anus, saying at the same time that he was exploding "bombs". These activities varied and were elaborated from interview to interview within wide limits. The impulse that occurred regularly was to bite various parts of my body; soon it became apparent that my genital organ was the ultimate object of his aggression.

### (*b*) *Hearing*

When he started making pictures I noticed that ears were a prominent feature in them. He always drew them in the same way, which I can best describe as follows: they resembled the two cotyledons on a seedling; the two side leaves, corresponding to the ears, were spread out horizontally on a single stem, which would correspond to the head, body, and legs of a person who was not pictured. There were in fact no real head, body, or legs; indeed the picture was scarcely more than a diagram suggesting an auditory schema, split off from the more integrated parts of his body ego. If this were so it would follow that the ears did not convey noise into anybody and this correlated in my mind with his apparent failure to hear what was said to him, and with the negligible notice he took of the noise he made himself.

### (*c*) *Speech*

At first he hardly spoke at all and only started to talk freely when I was able to interpret his silences, which were most marked early on in the interview. I told him that his words had got separated from his body, like the ears, and perhaps he had left them outside the clinic. He then told me that the words were indeed in the house opposite the clinic; they got put there, though he did not explain how.

These examples show some of the many signs of his disintegration; they illustrate how primitive was his sadism and how his body image was split. I may add here that I had concluded that his sadistic acts resulted from a counter-phobic identification with a demonic part of his psyche, the cause of his anxieties. The rest of his behaviour could be understood as defensive projection and splitting: when the archetypal energy was felt inside him it was immediately projected into toys and my body or it was split off from his ego in the form of hallucinated objects, ears, or speech.

## THE SYMBOLIC IMAGE AND ACTS

One day he came into the playroom with his mother and planted several pieces of paper down on the table, saying, "For frighten people," and his mother explained what had happened. It will be remembered that, as he was too uncontrolled in his relation to other children for an ordinary nursery school, he was being educated in a small special group for difficult children. There he had been unnaturally compliant to the control exerted by his teacher, in very marked contrast to his behaviour at the clinic and to his regular habit of attacking other children when the teacher was absent. Because of his aggression the children teased him and this made him more violent; thus a vicious circle was set up which disrupted his relationships with children in his own age group. Today when his teacher attempted to control him so as to break the vicious circle, he behaved quite differently from usual, flying into a rage and abusing her; almost at once he became frightened at what would happen next. The teacher, however, controlled herself, understanding the importance of the event, and to her surprise the aggression checked itself spontaneously without her intervention; then he picked up paper and pencils with which to make several pictures. After his first drawing—a horrific face with enormous mouth and horns—he made others, but these were less dramatic; as he made them he became calm and by the time he arrived at the clinic he could put the aim of the first creative image into words: "For frighten people," he said and stumped off. Later he told me that the horns were devil's horns, that the eyes flashed fire, and that the name of the figure was "Witch-devil".

I interpreted his behaviour to myself as a statement that he knew he could be dangerous, and that I had been warned of it by him; this degree of consciousness, if true, was quite new. When I looked more carefully at the picture I noticed that, though he meant the picture to be horrific, the eyes expressed the pathetic look which I had seen in his own on numerous occasions, and when I turned the paper over, I was not altogether surprised to find kisses at the bottom, while above them were a number of mandala-like figures and letters of the alphabet, the latter filling the main part of the paper. As he learns at school it seemed likely that the letters were to help restore his broken relation to the teacher, and the kisses were to express love and gratitude to her for not hurting him and for remaining whole and not being damaged.

One emphasized feature of the drawing was the mouth, whose significance had come out clearly before. The ears, now very large, were united with the head for the first time, while the convention that he had used to depict them before had now been turned upside down and converted into a nose. The other feature which associated with his earlier behaviour was the horns on the figure's head. These aggressive objects represented the instruments of penetration which he wished to have on his own head when he tried to get inside my body through the hole that he believed to be there. It is further likely that he had fantasies of making such a hole, for in his play he regularly made "hills "or "castles" of sand into which he would burrow, scooping out the interior and looking inside for a dangerous object, usually an animal, until the sand superstructure eventually collapsed.

The picture marked a clear-cut stage in his development and numerous changes took place in his behaviour. He started to come into the playroom on his own; he listened to what was said and could be more readily deflected from any particular destructive purpose he had in mind. Further, he developed games which were recognized for the first time as "pretend"; he would *pretend* to frighten me and turn me out of the room, or alternatively he induced me to assert that I was too frightened to let him into the playroom and I was to shut the door against him so as to make the game more real; then he would burst into the room and take possession of it, asserting that I was the bad "Witch-devil" myself and must in turn be removed to the passage outside from which John had entered. He had discovered that I, and at the same time the fearful archetypal figure, could be influenced, or even controlled, by him.

Another sign of development was revealed by the following

incident. He brought a "bomb", a lead tube filled with pastry which his mother had given him, and threw it with an experimental air on to the stone floor, at the same time putting his hands over his ears "because of the explosion". Evidently he wanted to stop the noise causing him distress inside his head; this was the first direct indication that noises meant anything to him. Next he developed his experiment with other noises: he himself started shouting and screaming, sometimes holding his hands over his ears and sometimes keeping his ears open. Thus he showed me that he had discovered the difference between noises inside his head and those outside, for if ears are covered, shouts and screams become much more internal.

## DISCUSSION

There are two headings under which I want to discuss this turning-point in the child's analysis:

### 1. *The Symbolic Nature of the Episode*

The archetypal content of the picture was evident and the child's name for it, the "Witch-devil", indicated its hermaphroditic nature, of which there were other signs in the mouth and horns. Of great interest is the time of its emergence and the fact that it expressed the uniting process characteristic of a symbol; it clearly took part in holding together and partially transmuting instinctual impulses deriving from the earlier as well as from the present life of the child, apparently at the same time contributing to bring about greater control over them.

I have suggested elsewhere (Fordham, 1957*b*) that Jung's definition of a symbol implies that it is not in itself representable but is rather the entity whose manifestations can be witnessed in the uniting of psychic elements. The symbol, in this rather particular sense, I went on to maintain, is essentially related to the self. From this point of view the whole episode at school and the relevant content of John's analysis may be included in any account of the symbol's contents. In another contribution (Fordham, 1957*c*) I applied Jung's idea that the self lies behind ego development in infancy, and this has been applied to middle childhood by Lewis (1954) and to adolescence by Hawkey (1955). Since John's ego grew I would interpret its development as the consequence of the self's synthetic activity. Such an interpretation can have an air of finality about it which I want to avoid by pointing out that though the self is transcendent and so in a sense defies description, its effects in the ego are subject to analytic assessment.

John, it will be remembered, had often attacked me with violence before the occasion on which he started to launch his self-terminated attack upon his teacher. What interested me most was this: nothing that occurred with me had been as transforming as the events at school; the analysis had indeed been characterized by gradual changes alone. I therefore want to compare the two experiences.

(*a*) At school the rage was spontaneously inhibited by the child before any bodily contact had been established. This was not so with me, I had to use physical control.

(b) The object of his attack was a woman, whereas I am a man. I believe this must have been important even though some of his behaviour showed that he did not always distinguish between male and female very clearly.

(c) Drawing was part of the curriculum at his school. In his analysis it was allowed and drawing materials were available, but John was not making much use of them at this time.

These considerations show that the main similarity is in the child's aggression and the non-aggressive attitude of the adult. Since he was violent first with me and then with his teacher, it may be that my not retaliating violently, as his father did at home, was a necessary preliminary to his outburst with the teacher at school, and that he did not hit her partly because violence with his father is more familiar than with his mother. That his teacher, like me, had controlled his activities often, though unlike me she had not been attacked, would seem to be explained by these personal considerations. In support of this is the observation that in his analysis John's violence was consistently more difficult to control after his father had smacked him.

## 2. *The Role of the Image*

It will be remembered that in his rages during analysis the child became quasi- or, as I believe, actually hallucinated. Then as the consequence of my restraining intervention he related the hallucinations to parts of my body in such a way that I was compelled to frustrate him.

At first, it must be assumed, the hallucinatory image had been, from time to time, projected into his teacher's body and had frightened him too much for him to get into a rage with her. But gradually my analytical work had lessened his fear and a time came when he could test out the effectiveness of his aggressive defence against the fearful image.

I now want to suggest that a further factor contributed to the change. The passive attitude and sex of the teacher made it possible for him to detach the hallucinated and terrifying figure for the first time. This happened not only because of sexual differences but also because John was able to match the hallucinatory content of the image against reality, a process which he had begun in his analysis and which could be continued at school because of the uniting of sexual differences in the image.

As a next step he made the terrifying figure objective by drawing it, and in this his ego got brought into closer relation without needing to identify with it defensively. The nature of the figure, which he also used as a sympathetic magic, thus preventing the danger which my body had represented before, is interesting enough, but even more so is the fact that he had constructed it. This showed how much his ego had gained in strength and could now not only control his emotion but also allow the restitutive processes already described in his second picture, made on the back of the first, to express themselves.

It is the changed attitude of the ego, I conceive, that was most instrumental in changing hallucination and physical violence into imaginative activity, a sign that preconscious ego fragments, originating in the de-integrates of the self, had become more closely related to and partly built into his ego nucleus. A further confirmation of this view is the increased capacity to distinguish consciously between what is internal and external to himself and greater differentiation of his internal world. The latter is shown by the fact that before the picture he only knew that he had "bombs" inside him, afterwards he knew that there were not only the noises made by bombs, but also shouts and screams which he could keep inside or release into the outside world.

The greater range of play activity and the understanding of "pretend" is further evidence of ego growth if that be needed.

From this, it appears, there are four interpenetrating stages in consciousness which have been gone through, all related to the same image. First: hallucinations closely related to physical instinctual object relations, which must be classed as *pre-symbolic*. Second: only when this had been recognized, worked through and interpreted did imaginative activity result and induce the third stage: a uniting symbol which then operated so as to induce the fourth, in which ego fragments were integrated into the child's main ego nucleus.

## A LATER DEVELOPMENT

Though the symbolic miracle brought about a change, it did not by magic resolve the child's anxiety. Much consolidating of his gain was needed and further regressions might have been anticipated. Later, indeed, another crisis arose presaged by the child wandering from home; in the analysis his oral sadism came more to the fore and his attack became clearly directed to my chest on which he could imagine—not, I think, hallucinating this time—an evil breast. Again the concrete pre-symbolic instinctual imagery appeared; its object—the breast—was specific and needed to be understood as concrete. In this analytic interview John was taking up with me what he had partially experienced with his teacher, whose breast it was that he wanted to preserve and love. Thus the hermaphroditic image made it possible to work through pre-symbolic activities and I got treated as a mother even though I am male. It was interesting that this time there was no picture but, since once again his ego became stronger, symbolic activity may be inferred just the same.

## CONCLUSION

The material considered and discussed above went far to convince me of the need to distinguish between the archetypal image and the symbol, for to make an image symbolic John needed to find a special attitude of mind. At first he lacked it and so the capacity for symbol formation; then he developed it, lost it, and regained it once more.

It seems apparent that the adults in John's immediate environment had an important but limited part to play in this and that they could only create good conditions for the symbol to come into being. John himself had to develop far enough on his own before the conditions could be made use of and so become effective.

## REFERENCES

FORDHAM, M. (1957*a*). "A Child Guidance Approach to Marriage", *New Developments in Analytical Psychology*. London, Routledge & Kegan Paul.

FORDHAM, M. (1957*b*). "Reflections on Image and Symbol", *New Developments in Analytical Psychology*. London, Routledge & Kegan Paul.

FORDHAM, M. (1957*c*). "The Origins of the Ego in Childhood", *New Developments in Analytical Psychology*. London, Routledge & Kegan Paul.

HAWKEY, L. (1955). "The Function of the Self in Adolescence", *Brit. J. med. Psychol.*, **28**, 1.

LEWIS, E. (1954). "The Function of Group Play During Middle Childhood in Developing the Ego Complex", *Brit. J. med. Psychol.*, **27**, 1 and 2.

# 6

## *DIE MUTTERFIGUR IN DEN PHANTASIEN EINES FRÜHVERWAHRLOSTEN KNABEN*

W. ZÜBLIN, *Zürich*

ANALYTISCHE Untersuchungen an Kindern, die an einem Hospitalismus gelitten haben, sind nur selten möglich. Meistens werden solche Kinder pädagogisch betreut und nur selten tiefenpsychologisch behandelt. Daher scheint es sich zu rechtfertigen, wenn im Folgenden über eine Psychotherapie bei einem heute 15-jährigen Knaben berichtet wird, der seit seinem zehnten Jahr in Behandlung steht; dies um so eher, als das Problem des Hospitalismus, d.h. der frühkindlichen affektiven Verwahrlosung, eines der wichtigsten und aktuellsten der heutigen Kinderpsychiatrie ist.

Es handelt sich um einen Knaben, der—illegitim geboren—seine ersten zwei Lebensjahre in einem Kinderheim zubrachte, in dem er zwar gefüttert, gekleidet und gewaschen, aber affektiv nur sehr mangelhaft betreut und erzieherisch kaum gefördert wurde. Als er zwei Jahre alt war, konnte er noch nicht sprechen; er musste gefüttert werden, konnte sich weder ankleiden noch entkleiden und nässte und kotete ein. Auch körperlich war er nur sehr mangelhaft entwickelt. So wurde er als zwergwüchsiger Schwachsinniger, der überdies an einem Herzfehler litt, einer Pflegemutter anvertraut, die vor kurzem ihr einziges Kind auf tragische Weise verloren hatte und wünschte, ein besonders bedürftiges und bedauernswertes Kind in Pflege zu nehmen, um es später zu adoptieren. Ihr Mann hatte nichts dagegen einzuwenden, wenn er auch am Pflegekind nicht besonders interessiert war.

Obschon der Knabe wegen seiner körperlichen Unterentwicklung in den folgenden drei Jahren, also bis er fünfjährig war, immer wieder in Spitälern, Kur- und Erholungsheimen behandelt und gepflegt wurde, entwickelte er sich vorerst bei seinen Pflegeteltern erstaunlich gut. Der scheinbar Schwachsinnige begann sehr bald zu sprechen. Er wurde in seiner Motorik geschickter, konnte bald selbständig essen und nässte und schmierte nicht mehr; dies allerdings nur dank des intensiven Einsatzes der Pflegemutter, die ihn zeitweise nachts jede Stunde auf das Töpfchen setzte und tags weder mit guten Worten und noch weniger mit gutgemeinten Schlägen sparte, ihn sauber zu bringen und damit erst—wie sie es empfand—ihn für sich und seine Umgebung annehmbar zu machen. So schien seiner Entwicklung nichts mehr in Wege zu stehen, nachdem er sich auch körperlich erstaunlich erholt und seinen körperlichen Entwicklungsrückstand eingeholt hatte. Allerdings war der Knabe im Kindergarten ängstlich und scheu. Er blieb auch sonst am liebsten in der Nähe der Pflegemutter und suchte den Kontakt zu andern Kindern nicht, was man zu korrigieren suchte, indem man ihn immer wieder zu andern Kindern schickte, damit er mit ihnen spiele. Trotzdem blieb er der scheue, in der Kindergesellschaft unangepasste Aussenseiter, der aber seinen Pflegeeltern durch sein braves, folgsames und ruhiges Wesen und seine übergrosse Abhängigkeit von ihnen, die sie als Anhänglichkeit deuteten, Freude und innere Genugtuung verschaffte.

Die Zufriedenheit der Eltern hielt aber nicht sehr lange an. Schon in der ersten Schulklasse hatte der Kleine Mühe, mitzukommen, da er in seiner Verträumtheit, in seinem Konzentrationsmangel und bei seiner Neigung, sich durch geringste Kleinigkeiten von seinen Aufgaben ablenken zu lassen, dem Unterricht nur mangelhaft folgen konnte. Aehnlich intensiv wie seinerzeit bei der Reinlichkeitsgewöhnung widmete sich nun die Pflegemutter der intellektuellen Förderung ihres Adoptivsohnes. Dies ermöglichte ihm, die Klassen zwar mit Mühe aber ohne Rückversetzung zu durchlaufen, was eine um so grössere Leistung war, als schon in der ersten Klasse und später immer häufiger und stärker Bauchkoliken auftraten, die den Knaben zu Boden warfen und ihn immer mehr am Schulbesuch hinderten.

Während Jahren wurde versucht, die Ursachen der Schmerzen auf eine körperliche Störung zurück zu führen. Man konnte einzig ein spastisches Colon feststellen und keine medikamentöse

Behandlung hatte Erfolg. Dies gab dann Anlass, den Pat. im Alter von zehn Jahren dem Kinderpsychiater zuzuweisen.

Die psychiatrische Untersuchung ergab einen ausgesprochenen psychischen Infantilismus, eine deutliche Störung des affektiven Kontaktes und eine neurotische Herabsetzung des Appetits. Die Bauchkoliken wurden als psychogen gedeutet, wobei vermutet wurde, dass sie mit der forcierten Reinlichkeitserziehung und der Ueberforderung, der der Pat. später in der Schule und zuhause ausgesetzt war, zusammenhängen konnten.

In der Psychotherapie, die im Ganzen nicht geschildert werden soll, stand in den ersten ca. 150 Stunden das Problem der Mutterfigur im Vordergrund. Es wurde vor allem zeichnerisch und durch erfundene Geschichten dargestellt. Nachdem der Pat. zuerst seine Familie (Abb. 1) in einer fast rein intellektuellen Art gezeichnet hatte, entwickelte er mit viel Affekt die Geschichte "Vom Scheusslichsten was es gibt" (Abb. 2-5): Ein Krokodil und eine Schlange stritten sich miteinander (Abb. 2), wobei die Schlange vom Krokodil in Stücke gebissen wurde (Abb. 3). Aus Langeweile zauberte das Krokodil aus den Schlangentrümmern ein Pferd, das es aber erneut in Stücke zerbiss, um dann—da es allein zu langweilig war—sich selbst zutode zu beissen. Eine Blindschleiche bemächtigte sich nun des Zauberstabes des Krokodils, wurde dessen aber von einer Schnecke beraubt (Abb. 4) Die Schnecke zauberte nun zuerst die Blindschleiche, dann den Zauberstock zu nichts. Gleichzeitig verschwanden Blumen und Gras, dann sogar der Boden und schliesslich beleuchtete die Sonne die einzelnen Trümmer der auseinandergefallenen Schnecke (Abb. 5).

Ohne die Geschichte im einzelnen zu deuten, kann deren Sinn dahin zusammengefasst werden, das sie den vollständigen Zerfall darstellt, in dem die Welt zugrunde geht, da das aggressiv Weibliche das Männliche zerstört und damit sich selbst als dessen Gegenpol vernichtet.

Nach dieser Phantasie schien die schöpferische Fähigkeit des Pat. vorerst blockiert zu sein. Er wurde daher in eine Therapiegruppe aufgenommen, in der er sich zuerst passiv verhielt, bis er beim Spiel einer Familienszene der Mutter Gift ins Essen mischte.

Dieser Akt scheint die Phantasietätigkeit des Pat. erneut in

Gang gebracht zu haben: Er malte "Die Geschichte von der frechen Frau", wobei er beim Erzählen zwischen "Frau" und "Mutter" keinen Unterschied machte: Ein Mann hatte eine freche Frau. Als sie zusammen einmal im Auto fuhren, schwatzte sie so lange, bis er in ein Haus fuhr. Das Auto wurde zerstört, der Mann wurde schwer verletzt: Messer, die hinten im Auto deponiert waren, fuhren durch die Wucht des Aufpralles nach vorne. Sie stachen dem Mann die Augen aus, schnitten ihm Nase, Ohren und Hände ab. Die freche Frau blieb unverletzt. Sie trug den Mann nachhause, wo sie ihn im Dunkeln stehen liess, so dass er ganz bleich wurde. Sie überliess ihn sich selbst und darum versuchte er, sich selbst zu helfen. Er fand in der Küche Milch, die er trank. Die Milch war aber nicht gekocht und daher giftig und trieb dem Bedauernswerten den Bauch enorm auf, was ihm grosse Schmerzen verursachte. Da aber im gleichen Moment die Grossmutter der frechen Frau gestorben war, wuchsen die verlorenen oder verstümmelten Körperteile des Mannes wieder nach. Er konnte Hilfe herbeirufen. Der Arzt kam und liess ihm eine Brillenschlange durch den Anus in den Bauch kriechen, wo sie die giftige Milch aufsog, so dass der Mann gesund wurde. Er ging darauf zur Polizei und liess die freche Frau einsperren. Dann kaufte er sich eine Banane, die er mit Salzsäure vergiftete. Er gab sie der eingesperrten Frau, die sofort starb. Daraufhin nahm er eine liebe Mutter, die ihm nur noch gekochte Milch gab und kaufte ein neues Auto, in dem bei den gemeinsamen Ausfahrten die Frau nicht mehr ständig schwatzte.—Es scheint, dass der Pat. mit dieser Geschichte seine persönliche Vorgeschichte auf phantastische Art zu verarbeiten sucht, eüber welche er zwar nie mit Absicht aufgeklärt worden war, die er aber aus Gesprächen Erwachsener hin und wieder etwas erfahren hatte.

Mit Abschluss dieser Geschichte veränderte sich der Pat. sehr deutlich. Er arbeitete in der Schule besser, fand den Kontakt zu Kameraden und litt kaum mehr unter Bauchschmerzen. Dies bewog die Pflegemutter des Pat., die Behandlung gegen den ärztlichen Rat abzubrechen. Ein Rezidiv zwang sie aber nach ungefähr einem halben Jahr, ihren Pflegesohn erneut zur Therapie anzumelden. Es begann damit eine beinahe zwei Jahre lang dauernde Phase, in der fast ausschliesslich Hexengeschichten erfunden, im Sandkasten dargestellt oder nach Art eines

Psychodramas mit dem Therapeuten gespielt wurden. Die Hexengeschichten folgen anfangs ganz der Konvention: Eine Hexe raubte und frass Kinder, wurde gefangen und hingerichtet, worauf sie im Fegefeuer schrecklich gemartert und zerstückelt wurde (Abb. 6). Sie erstand nach erfolgter Busse jeweils wieder, um ihr altes Treiben vorerst weiter zu führen.

Schliesslich aber begann sie sich zu ändern. Sie wurde zur ambivalenten übermächtigen Mutterfigur, der "guten Hexe", die zwar wie ihre Freundinnen, die andern Hexen, Kinder fing, sie aber bei sich im Hexenhaus kräftig verwöhnte, sie nicht in die Schule schickte und ihnen jeden Wunsch erfüllte, und zwar, indem sie aus ihren Fäces die Gegenstände, selbst Häuser, Schlösser und—nachdem sie die alte Welt vernichtet hatte—eine ganz neue Welt hervorzauberte. Wegen dieser Zauberkraft hiess sie auch die Scheisshexe (Abb. 7). Nachdem sie so während einer Reihe von Therapiestunden ihr Wesen getrieben hatte, wurde sie vom Pat. plötzlich anders gewertet. Er kam nämlich zum Schluss, dass die Hexe zwar gut, aber auch böse war, da sie die Kinder nicht zur Schule schickte und es ihnen nach Art einer allzu behütenden und einengenden Mutter unmöglich machte, erwachsen zu werden. Ihre Feinde waren dementsprechend auch die Erwachsenen, die sie bekriegte, anfangs aber ganz erfolglos, da sie nicht bloss auf sie Feuer vom Himmel fallen liess, sondern sie auch in ihrem heissen Urin mitsamt der ganzen Welt der Erwachsenen ertränkte. So wurde eine allgemeine Versöhnung beschlossen: Man kam überein, dass die früheren Freundinnen der Hexe, die bösen Hexen, verbrannt werden sollten, während sich die Erwachsenen der guten Hexe unterwarfen und ihr Tribut zahlten, womit die Herrschaft der grossen Mutter angebrochen war. Die überall errichteten Festfeuer erschreckten aber eine Anzahl Erwachsener so, dass sie in Ohnmacht fielen, so dass das vielversprechend begonnene Versöhnungsfest mit der Kriegserklärung der unterdessen erstarkten Erwachsenen an die Hexe endete. Es gelang nun auch, die Hexe zu fangen. Sie musste aber vorerst immer wieder frei gelassen werden, da sie in ihrem Gefängnis derartige Mengen von Urin und Stuhl produzierte, dass selbst Bagger und Bulldozzers nicht imstande waren, allen Unrat weg zu räumen, Leute darin ertranken und der Weltuntergang nur verhindert werden konnte, indem man die Hexe frei liess. Endlich aber kam einer auf die Idee, die wiederum gefangene Hexe in ein tiefes Loch zu versenken, in dem sie sich in ihren eigenen Ausscheidungen ertränkte. Sie trocknete dort ein und wurde bei einer Ueberschwemmung zusammen mit ihrem Kot und getrockneten Urin ins Meer gespült, wo sie von einem Walfisch verschluckt wurde, um per vias naturales als lebendige Hexe aufzuerstehen, diesmal aber mit eindeutig guten und bösen Eigenschaften: Sie gab zwar den Kindern, die sie eingefangen hatte, was sie wollten, frass aber jeweils einige von ihnen auf. Unterdessen war die Macht der Erwachsenen so stark geworden, dass ihre Bekämpfung immer erfolgreicher wurde, wenn auch ihre bösen Eigenschaften zu-, die guten abnahmen. Ihre Zaubermacht konnte sie nur noch zeitweise ausüben und schliesslich wurde sie nur noch böse, aber schwach, von einer guten Fee vernichtet.

Die Hexengeschichten waren allerdings nicht abgeschlossen. Damit, dass an Stelle der ambivalenten übermächtigen Mutterfigur eine böse Hexe und eine gutte Fee getreten waren, trat auch der Hexenmann auf, der sich mit der Zeit immer erfolgreicher der Hexe gegenüber behaupten konnte. Anfangs ein gewöhnlicher Räuber, den sich die Hexe geraubt hatte, um Kinder zu bekommen, wurde er schliesslich zu ihrem erfolgreichen Gegenspieler, der sich seine Männlichkeit von der Hexe raubt, sie überwindet und damit erst zum Mann wird, wie die folgende Geschichte zeigt:

Es war einmal ein Hexenmann. Dieser baute sich ein grosses Haus für mehrere Familien, das aber von der Hexenkuh berannt wurde und daher aufs schwerste gefährdet war. Der Hexenmann beschloss, gegen die Kuh vorzugehen. Als sie schlief, schnitt er zwei Zitzen vom Euter. Aus ihnen trank er sich Mut und Stärke. Der Kuh aber zog er eine Ziegenmaske über den Kopf. Darauf legte er sich zum Schlafen nieder und wie er schlief, frass ihm die Kuh die Haare ab. Er aber träumte, die Kuh habe ihn verschlungen und dann wieder ausgeschieden. So beschloss er sich zu rächen, und am andern Tag, als die Kuh wieder schlief, schnitt er die beiden restlichen Zitzen auch noch weg. Darauf wurde er sehr stark und als ihn die Kuh in den Mist warf, schnitt er ihr ein Horn weg. Die Kuh aber zauberte sich nach China und verwandelte sich in die Kaiserin. Sie lud sich den Hexenmann zu Gast.

Kaum angekommen, sah er sich von ihren Kriegern umzingelt und bedroht. Er erkannte den Verrat, schob seinem Pferd eine Zitze in den Anus, worauf es mit ihm in die Luft stieg, so hoch, dass ihn die Pfeile seiner Feinde nicht erreichen konnten. Da stürzte die Kaiserin tot um und an ihrer Stelle stand eine wunderschöne Prinzessin, die dem Hexenmann kund tat, dass sie von der Hexe in die Kuh verzaubert worden war. Darauf hin heirateten beide und wurden glücklich.

Damit trat das Thema des andern Geschlechtes und der Sexualität auf. Es folgten zwei Zeichnungen, den Mond mit seiner Bahn und eine Mondrakete darstellend (Abb. 8 u. 9), wobei aber der Pat. andeutete, dass er eigentlich damit ein männliches und ein weibliches Genitale gezeichnet habe.

Das Auftreten des Themas "Mann und Frau" schloss auch die Frage des Vaters in sich ein und es entstand eine Geschichte, die die Frage seiner Nachfolge betrifft. Es ist "Die Geschichte vom Burggeist": Es war einmal ein König, der wohnte in einem Schloss, das aus Stahl und Gold gebaut war. Einmal kam der Nachtwächter voll Angst zum König und berichtete ihm, es sei ein Geist über die Burg geflogen (Abb. 10). Der König glaubte es aber nicht und befahl dem Nachtwächter, die nächste Nacht in seinem Bett zu schlafen. Er wolle den Nachtwächter spielen, um zu beweisen, dass kein Geist existiere. Als er aber auf dem Turm Wache hielt, erschien der Geist und stürzte ihn die Treppe hinunter, so dass er starb. Der König wurde begraben und an seine Stelle trat der Nachtwächter, der nun die Königin heiratete. Einmal aber flog der Geist wieder über die Burg und ein Jäger schoss ihn herunter. Da erstand der König zu neuem Leben und der Nachtwächter wollte zu seinen Gunsten zurück treten. Der auferstandene König aber sagte, er solle das nicht tun, er sei schon damit zufrieden, dass er Nachtwächter sein könne, und so blieb der frühere Nachtwächter König.

Das Hexenthema war damit aber noch nicht ganz abgeschlossen. Es erstand ein letztes Mal in einer Geschichte, in der der Hexenmann seiner Frau, der alten Hexe, weglief, nachdem er ihr einen Plan, in dem die Lage eines versteckten Schatzes angezeichnet war, entwendet hatte. Er kaufte sich zuerst schöne Frauen, denen er einen grossen Teil des Schatzes versprach. Ohne es zu bemerken, kaufte er aber mit diesen Frauen seine alte Hexe, die sich verschönt und verjüngt hatte und eine Fee, die die eigentliche Besitzerin des Schatzes war. Sie fanden zusammen auf der Spitze eines Berges den Schatz. Doch versuchten Hexenmann und Hexenfrau unterwegs, die andern Frauen und vor allem die Fee umzubringen, worauf diese die Beiden mitsamt dem Schatz in die Tiefe stürzte und selbst durch die Luft entschwebte. Vom Schatz aber, der ursprünglich zur Verteilung an Arme bestimmt gewesen war, fanden arme Leute am Fusse des Berges und in seinen Schluchten manchmal ein Goldstück.

Das Verschwinden der gewaltigen Märchenfiguren und das stückweise Finden des Schatzes durch gewöhnliche, bedürftige Menschen entsprach auch einer inneren Umstellung des Pat. Er hatte seine letzte Geschichte schon nicht mehr mit der für ihn früher typischen Intensität erzählt und wandte sich nun, ungefähr altersgemässen, realen Dingen zu. Neben der Technik begann ihn vor allen Dingen die Geographie zu interessieren. Er schuf sich gleichsam die Realität, indem er Reliefs bastelte, die aber anfangs—für ihn selbst halb bewusst und dem Therapeuten gegenüber verbal angedeutet—noch stark symbolischen Charakter hatten. Dies galt für ein sehr naturalistisch gebasteltes Eisenbahntunnel, dessen klaffende schwarze Oeffnungen Anlass zu koprophilen Witzen gaben, wie auch für das Modell des Matterhorns, das in seinem Kern ein Gerüst in der Form einer weiblichen Brust enthielt, wobei der Pat. immer wieder freudig betonte, dass nur er und sein Therapeut wüssten, was "eigentlich" im Matterhorn stecke, mit andern Worten, was die äussere Realität einschloss. Schliesslich aber wurden die Reliefs ausschliesslich zur Darstellung einer Landschaft korrekt und genau von einer Karte übertragen.

Im Laufe der Therapie war das Bauchweh verschwunden. Der einst scheinbar Schwachsinnige war zu einem mittleren Schüler der Realschule geworden, der seiner Umgebung nicht mehr auffiel. Sein Infantilismus war weitgehend überwunden.

Immerhin ist es nicht sinnlos, wenn der Therapeut bei einer derartigen Therapie für sich deutet. Allerdings sind sinnvolle Interpretationen oft erst nach Abschluss einer Psychotherapie möglich.—Bei unserem Patienten steht natürlich die Ich-Entwicklung im Vordergrund. Die erste Geschichte vom Pferd und dem Krokodil, der Blindschleiche und der Schnecke ist für die Ich–Schwäche des Patienten bezeichnend. Eine Figur, die als Vertreterin des Bewusstseins interpretiert werden könnte, kommt noch nicht vor. Der Konflikt spielt noch ganz im Unbewussten resp. im Vorbewussten. Die darauf folgende Geschichte vom Autounglück zeigt die Schwäche des männlichen Bewusstseins und dessen Abhängigkeit vom verderblichen Unbewussten, die zu Verstümmelung und Hilflosigkeit führt. Erst Intervention Erwachsener, nämlich des Arztes und der Polizei bessert die Situation. Der Patient hat sein schwaches Ich durch Identifikation mit hilfreichen männlichen Autoritätsfiguren gestärkt. Die Beziehung zur mütterlichen Frau wird adäquater. Allerdings verhindert dann der Unterbruch der Therapie das Weiterbestehen der zur Individuation nötigen Identifizierung mit der Vaterfigur (auf der Objektstufe mit dem Therapeuten), was zum Rezidiv führt.

Nach Wiederaufnahme der Behandlung ist daher die Mutterfigur in ihrem negativen Aspekt, nämlich die Hexe, übermächtig. Sie bleibt es selbst dann noch, nachdem sie sich in die "gute Hexe" verwandedt hat. Als solche kann sie zwar die kleinkindlichen Wünsche des Patienten befriedigen. Vor allen Dingen gibt sie ihm Geborgenheit. Sie verhindert aber gleichzeitig die Bewusstseinsentwicklung: Die Kinder, die die Hexe bei sich gefangen hält, werden zwar verwöhnt, bleiben aber unmündig. Sie gehen nicht zur Schule und wenn sie später selber einmal Kinder haben, so gehören diese der Hexe.—Im Laufe der Behandlung nimmt aber die Kraft der Hexe ab. Schliesslich tritt eine Differenzierung in eine böse Hexe und eine gute Fee auf, was natürlich die Auseinandersetzung des Patienten mit der Mutterwelt erleichtert und seine Individuation einleitet. Demzufolge tritt nun in den Geschichten die Figur des Hexenmannes auf. Anfangs ein schwächlicher Mann ohne eigene Rechte und ausschliesslich dazu bestimmt, mit der Hexe Kinder zu zeugen, wird er im Laufe der Behandlung immer stärker und aktiver. In dieser Figur bekämpft der Patient die alles beherrschende Mutterwelt. Er besiegt sie schliesslich; seine Beziehung zum Weiblichen ist nicht mehr die des abhängigen Kindes zur überwältigenden Mutter sondern die von Partner zu Partner. Diese Entwicklung ist in der Geschichte vom Kampf gegen die Kuh ausserordentlich eindrücklich dargestellt. Die Kuh wird schrittweise durch das Abschneiden der

Euterzitzen entmütterlicht aber auch gleichzeitig kastriert. Der Held der Geschichte raubt sich von der phallischen Mutter die Männlichkeit, wird im Kampf dabei einmal verschlungen und als viel stärker neu geboren. Schliesslich wird dem Helden auch das Geistige, dargestellt durch den Flug auf dem Pferd, zugänglich. Damit stirbt die alte Hexe. Die Prinzessin, also die erotische Beziehungsfähigkeit zur Frau, ist erlöst.

Diese entscheidende Veränderung in der Beziehung zum Weiblichen lässt nun vorerst die Problematik der Beziehung zwischen den Geschlechtern zurücktreten. An ihre Stelle tritt das Problem des Vaters. In der Geschichte vom König und vom Nachtwächter wird ein Thema behandelt, das normalerweise zur Problematik eines drei- bis fünfjährigen Knaben gerechnet werden muss. Der Nachtwächter stellt das neue Ich dar, das die kritiklose Identifikation mit dem Vater überwindet, von seiner Bedrohung durch Inhalte aus dem Unbewussten weiss und sich dementsprechend verhält.

Noch handeln diese Geschichten aber ganz im Magischen. Es sind reine Märchen. Ihre Personen sind archetypische Figuren und weisen kaum individuelle Züge auf. Der Uebergang zur Realität (im Sinne des Bewusstseins des Gegensatzes zwischen eigenem Ich und äusserer Dinglichkeit) erfolgt erst in der letzten grossen Geschichte vom Schatz der Fee, in der die Märchenfiguren teils einfach zugrunde gehen, zum andern Teil entschweben, währenddem der Schatz von Menschen gefunden wird, das Ich also bereichert d.h. gestärkt wird.

Damit leitet diese Geschichte in die Endphase der Therapie über. Die äussere Welt wird erobert. Anfangs allerdings ist sie nichts als das Projektionsfeld des Patienten, der nun im wahrsten Sinne des Wortes sich seine Welt schafft und gegenständlich (d.h. sie aussenstehend) macht, ahnend, dass damit auch gleichzeitig Dinge hergestellt werden, die seine persönliche Problematik beinhalten (so z.B. bei der Konstruktion des männlich aufragenden Matterhorns, das im innersten Kern eine weibliche Brust enthält.) Schliesslich entsteht daraus die Entwicklung eines altersgemässen Realitätsbezuges mit der üblichen Problematik des Pubertierenden, die die Eroberung der äusseren Welt zum Inhalt hat.

Damit durchlief der Patient in fünfjähriger Therapie eine Entwicklung, die beim Normalen fast die ganze Zeit bis zur

Pubertät beansprucht. Damit verlor er auch seine Fähigkeit, Märchen zu fabulieren, was der Erfahrung entspricht, dass solche in seinem Alter nur von sehr ich-schwachen Kindern erfunden werden können, währenddem normale Knaben seines Alters realistische Geschichten wünschen oder erfinden, wobei sie diese (z.B. als science-fiction oder Abenteuergeschichte) dazu benutzen, sich als Held zu fühlen, der die Welt erobert, ein Unterfangen, das unserem Patienten ohne die geschilderte Behandlung wohl kaum je möglich gewesen wäre.

## *THE MOTHER FIGURE IN THE FANTASIES OF A BOY SUFFERING FROM EARLY DEPRIVATION*

ANALYTICAL study of children suffering from institutionalism is seldom possible, since such children are usually handled by educational methods and are seldom treated by depth psychology. This alone might justify the following report on the psychological treatment of a boy, now aged 15, who has been under treatment since his tenth year. Generally speaking, the problem of institutionalism, that is, of affective deprivation in early childhood, is one of the most important of modern child psychiatry.

The boy in question, an illegitimate child, spent the first two years of his life in a home, in which he was, indeed, fed, clothed and washed, but emotionally most inadequately cared for and educationally practically neglected. At the age of two he still could not speak, had to be fed, could neither dress nor undress himself, and wetted and soiled himself. So, classified as mentally deficient and physically backward, and in addition suffering from cardiac weakness, he was entrusted to a foster-mother. She had recently lost her only child in tragic circumstances, and wished to take charge of a particularly needy and unfortunate child, with a view to later adoption. Her husband did not object, but he was not particularly interested in the foster-child.

Although for the next three years, until he was five, the boy, on account of his physical underdevelopment, was constantly being sent to hospitals and to nursing and convalescent homes, he developed surprisingly well under the care of his foster-parents. The so-called mentally deficient child soon began to speak. He became more adroit in his movements, was soon able to feed himself, and no longer wetted or soiled himself: the latter improvement was however only due to the intensive efforts of his foster-mother who, for a period, put him on the pot every hour at night, and during the day spared neither encouraging words nor well-intentioned slaps to train him and thus in her opinion make him acceptable to his surroundings. As he had made a remarkable physical recovery and had overcome his physical retardation, nothing further seemed to stand in the way of his development. However, at the kindergarten he was nervous and shy. He also preferred to stay close to his foster-mother, in spite of constant attempts to make him join in with other children. Nevertheless he remained the timid outsider, unadapted to the society of other children. But at home his good, obedient, quiet nature and his exaggerated dependence, which his foster-parents interpreted as affection, gave them great pleasure and inner satisfaction.

This satisfaction, however, did not last very long. The little boy had trouble in keeping up with even the first class at school, since his dreaminess, his lack of concentration, and his tendency to be very easily distracted from his work, made it difficult for him to follow any course of instruction. The foster-mother now applied herself to the educational development of her adoptive son with the same intensity as she had given to his bowel training. This helped him to get through his classes, with difficulty but without relegation, which was a considerable achievement, since the stomach colic that had affected him even in the first class became more frequent and serious, sometimes causing him to collapse with pain; this, naturally, prejudiced his school attendance.

For years the cause of these attacks was attributed to some physical disturbance. The only physical symptom was a spastic colon and no medical treatment brought relief. For this reason the patient was referred, at the age of 10, to the child psychiatrist.

Psychiatric investigation revealed a marked psychological infantilism, a considerable disturbance of affective contact and a neurotic loss of appetite. The colic was diagnosed as psychogenetic and it was suggested that it was related to high pressure bowel-training and the excessive demands subsequently placed on the patient both at school and at home.

We shall not describe the entire course of treatment: during the first 150 hours, however, the problem of the mother-figure was the central point, expressed mainly in drawings and in stories invented by the patient. At the very outset of treatment he drew his family in an almost purely intellectual manner (*Plate* 1); he developed, with considerable affect, the story of "the most horrible thing there is" (*Plates* 2–5): a crocodile and a snake are fighting (*Plate* 2) and the snake is bitten to pieces by the crocodile (*Plate* 3). The crocodile becomes bored and conjures up a horse out of the pieces of snake, but bites it to pieces again, only—because it is bored at being alone—to bite himself to death afterwards. A slow-worm then takes possession of the crocodile's magic wand, but is robbed of it by a snail (*Plate* 4). The snail now spirits away first the slow-worm and then the wand. At the same time the flowers and grass disappear, even the ground itself, and finally the sun's rays fall only on the remains of the disintegrated snail (*Plate* 5).

Without going into details it is clear that these pictures show a total collapse, in which the world falls to pieces, because the aggressive female destroys the male and thereby, being his opposite pole, destroys herself.

After this fantasy the creative activity of the patient appeared at first to be blocked. He was therefore included in a therapeutic group, in which he at first remained passive until in playing out a family scene, he put poison in the mother's food.

This action seemed to free the patient's fantasy. He then painted "The story of the Impertinent Woman". In relating the story he made no distinction between "woman" and "mother". A man had an impertinent wife. Once when they were out driving in a car she chattered so much that he drove into a house. The car was smashed, the man seriously injured; knives that had been put in the back of the car were thrown forward by the force of the impact. They gouged out the man's eyes and cut off his nose, ears and hands. The impertinent woman was unharmed. She carried the man home and left him lying in the dark so that he became quite pale. She left him to himself and so he tried to help himself. He found some milk in the kitchen and drank it. But the milk was not boiled, and therefore was poisonous. It made the unfortunate man's stomach swell and become very painful. But as the impertinent woman's grandmother died at that moment, the lost or mutilated parts of the man's body grew again. He was able to call for help. The doctor came and made an adder crawl through the anus into the man's stomach where it lapped up the poisonous milk so that the man got better. Then he went to the police and had the impertinent woman locked up. Then he bought a banana, which he poisoned with hydrochloric acid. He gave it to the imprisoned woman, who immediately died. Then he took to himself a dear mother, who gave him only boiled milk, and bought a new car, in which they both went for rides, and the woman did not chatter ceaselessly. It seems that the patient was trying, through fantasy, to assimilate his own early history, which had never been deliberately explained to him, though he had been able to learn something about it from the conversation of adults.

After this story the patient changed considerably. He worked better at school, made contact with his comrades, and suffered hardly at all from colic. This induced the foster-mother, against medical advice, to break off the treatment. After six months, however, a relapse compelled her to bring him back for a phase of treatment that lasted almost two years and consisted almost exclusively of witch stories, either modelled in the sand-box, or played out with the therapist like a psychodrama. At first the witch stories were conventional: a witch stole and devoured children, was caught and hung, after which she suffered the torments of hell-fire and was broken to pieces (*Plate* 6). But after due penance she always rose again to carry on her old tricks.

Finally, however, she began to change. She became the ambivalent overpowering mother-figure, the "good witch" who indeed captured children, like her friends, the other witches, but kept them and spoilt them in the witch-house, never sent them to school, fulfilled their every wish, and out of her faeces created a completely new world, including houses and castles, when she had destroyed the old one. Because of this magic power she was also called the shit-witch (*Plate* 7). After she had pursued this existence throughout a series of sessions, she was suddenly given a different valuation. The patient, namely, came to the conclusion that the witch was indeed good, but also bad because she did not send the children to school and, like an over-protective and restricting mother, made it impossible for them to grow up. Her enemies were therefore the adults also, who made war on her, at first entirely without success, for she not only brought down fire from heaven on their heads, but also drowned them, with the whole grown-up world, in her hot urine. So a general reconciliation was arranged: it was agreed that the witch's former friends, the other witches, should be burnt, while the adults should be subject to the good witch and pay her tribute, thus inaugurating the reign of the great mother. But the bonfires that were lit everywhere in celebration so alarmed some of the grown-ups that they fainted, so that the promising feast of reconciliation ended with a declaration of war on the witch by the adults, who had meanwhile grown much stronger. They were now able to catch the witch. But first she had to be set free again because she produced so much urine and stools in her prison that not even dredgers and bulldozers were able to clean up the mess: people were drowning in it, and the end of the world could be avoided only by her release. Finally someone hit on the idea of dropping the witch down a deep hole so that she would drown in her own excrement. There she dried up, and during a flood was swept, together with her excrement and dried-up urine, into the sea, where she was swallowed by a whale and then *per vias naturales* was born again as a living witch, this time with obviously good and bad qualities. She still gave the children she had kidnapped whatever they wanted, but from time to time ate some of them. Meanwhile the power of the grown-ups had increased so much that they were more and more successful in fighting her, even though her bad qualities increased and her good ones decreased. She could only exercise her magic power occasionally, and finally she became all bad, but weak, and was destroyed by a good fairy.

But this was not the end of the witch stories. After the ambivalent, overpowering mother-figure had been supplanted by a bad witch and a good fairy, there appeared a witch-man, who was in time able to stand up to the witch with increasing success. At first an ordinary robber, whom the witch had kidnapped in order to have children, he finally became her successful antagonist, who recovered his manhood from the witch, overcame her, and thereby became a man, as the following story[1] shows:

Once there was a witch-man. He built himself a great house for several families, but it was blockaded by the witch-cow and brought into great danger. The witch-man decided to attack the cow. As she slept he cut two teats from her udder, and from them he drank courage and strength. Then he lay down to sleep, and while he was asleep the cow ate his hair away. But he dreamt that the cow had swallowed him and then expelled him again. So he determined on revenge and on another day, when the cow was sleeping again, he cut off the two remaining teats. This made him very strong and when the cow tossed him on to the dung heap he cut off one of her horns. But the cow magically transported herself to China and turned into the empress. She invited the witch-man to visit her. Scarcely had he arrived than he found himself surrounded and menaced by her warriors. He realized he had been betrayed and thrust one teat into the horse's anus, whereupon it rose with him into the sky, so high that the enemy arrows could not reach him. Then the empress fell down dead and in her place there stood a very beautiful princess, who explained that she had been turned into a cow by the witch. Then they married and lived happily ever after.

Here the theme of the other sex and of sexuality appears. Shortly afterwards there followed two drawings showing the moon with its orbit and a moon-rocket (*Plates* 8 and 9), which the patient declared actually represented the male and female genitals.

The introduction of the "man and woman" theme also brought up the question of the father, and only a few interviews later there came a story dealing with the question of his successor. It is "The story of the Castle Ghost". There was a king who lived

[1]This story was developed about one year after treatment had been recommenced, and two years after treatment first began.

in a castle built of steel and gold. One day the night-watchman came to the king in great panic and told him a ghost had flown over the castle (*Plate* 10). The king did not believe it and ordered the night-watchman to stay in bed the next night. He would play the night-watchman himself, to prove that no ghost existed. But as he kept watch on the tower of the castle the ghost appeared and threw him down the steps so that he died. The king was buried and the night-watchman took his place and married the queen. But one day the ghost flew over the castle again and was shot down by a hunter. Then the king came to life once more and the night-watchman wanted to retire in his favour. But the risen king refused, saying that he would be quite happy to be the night-watchman, so the former night-watchman remained king.

But the witch theme was not yet quite exhausted. It appeared for the last time in a story in which the witch-man ran away from his wife, the old witch, after stealing from her a plan showing where a treasure was buried. At first he bought himself beautiful women, to whom he promised a large share of the treasure. But without noticing it he had, with these women, also bought his old witch, who had rejuvenated herself and become beautiful, and a fairy, who was the real owner of the treasure. Together they found the treasure on the summit of a mountain. Then the witch-man and the witch-woman tried to kill all the women, particularly the fairy, but they resisted and threw the pair, with the treasure, down into the valley, and then themselves floated away through the air. The treasure had originally been intended for distribution to the poor and many gold pieces were afterwards found by poor people at the foot of the mountain and in its ravines.

The disappearance of the powerful fairy figures and the piecemeal recovery of the treasure by ordinary, needy humans, corresponds to an inner transformation in the patient. In telling his last story he had no longer displayed his former typical intensity and was now turning towards real things, approximately corresponding to his age. Apart from technical subjects he was above all interested in geography. At this time he began to build up a reality for himself by modelling reliefs—half consciously, as indicated verbally to the therapist—of a highly symbolic character. This was true of a realistically modelled railway tunnel whose black, gaping orifice gave rise to coprophilic jokes: also a model of the Matterhorn that was built up on a frame the shape of a woman's breast, of which the patient frequently and happily remarked that only he and the therapist knew what was "actually" inside the Matterhorn, in other words what the outer reality enclosed. Finally however the reliefs were exclusively used to reproduce a landscape with complete exactness from a map.

In the course of treatment the stomach trouble disappeared. The formerly mentally deficient boy became an average scholar, no longer out of place in his environment. His infantilism had been largely overcome.

Nothing was interpreted during treatment either by the patient or by the therapist, but in such cases there is a certain value for the therapist in interpreting the material for himself. In any case, a meaningful interpretation is often only possible after the conclusion of the treatment. In this patient's case the most important aspect was his ego development. The first story of the horse and the crocodile, the slow-worm and the snail, illustrates his ego-weakness. There is as yet no figure that could be interpreted as representing consciousness. The conflict takes place in the unconscious or the pre-conscious. The next story about the car accident shows the weakness of the male consciousness and its dependence on the destructive forces of the unconscious, which leads to mutilation and helplessness. The first adult intervention, that is, by the doctor and the police, improves the situation. The patient has strengthened his weak ego by identification with the helpful figures of masculine authority. The relationship to the motherly woman becomes more adequate. But here the breaking off of the therapy hindered the identification with the father (on the objective level, with the therapist) that is necessary to individuation, and there was a relapse.

When the treatment was resumed the mother figure had therefore taken on a negative aspect, that of the overpowering witch. She remained thus even after she had turned into a "good witch". As such she could satisfy the patient's infantile wishes. Above all she gave him security, but she hindered the development of consciousness: the children the witch keeps imprisoned are indeed spoilt but remain minors. They do not go to school and when subsequently they themselves have children, these belong to the witch. Finally there is a differentiation between a bad witch and a good fairy, which naturally makes it easier for the patient to come to grips with the mother-world, and embark on the path to individuation. The stories continue with the appearance of the witch-man. At first a weakling with no rights of his own and solely designed to raise children by the witch, he later becomes stronger and more active. In this figure the patient struggles with the dominance of the mother-world. Finally he conquers it. His relationship to the feminine is no longer that of a dependent child to the all-powerful mother, but that between partners. This development is shown remarkably clearly in the story of the struggle with the cow. By the cutting off of her teats the cow is progressively dematernalized, but also at the same time castrated. The hero of the story steals his manhood from the phallic mother, is at one point swallowed up in his struggle with her, and is born again in greater strength. Finally the hero gains access to the spiritual, represented by the flight on horseback. Thereupon the old witch dies. The princess, that is, the capacity for erotic relationships with women, is set free.

This decisive transformation in the relationship to the feminine makes the problem of relationship between the sexes recede. It is replaced by the problem of the father. In the story of the king and the night-watchman we have a theme that normally appears amongst the problems of a three- to five-year-old boy. The night-watchman represents the newly found ego that has overcome an uncritical identification with the father, knows of the dangers arising out of the unconscious, and behaves accordingly.

Hitherto these stories have been purely magical, pure fairy tales. Their personages are archetypal figures and display hardly any individual features. The transition to reality (in the sense of the differentiation between the ego and outer reality) first appears in the long, final story about the fairy treasure, in which some of the fairy figures simply perish on the ground while the others float away: the treasure is found by men, and the ego thus enriched, that is, made stronger.

Here the story leads into the final phase of the treatment.

The outer world is conquered. At first it is the screen for the patient's own projections, since he has, in the truest sense of the word, to create his own world and objectivize it (that is, externalize it), realizing at the same time that he is producing things that also express his personal problems (for instance, the male, erect Matterhorn containing in its interior a female breast). From this point onwards there finally develops a sense of reality corresponding to this age, with the normal problems of puberty concerned with the conquest of the external world.

Thus the patient, in the course of treatment lasting five years passed through a period of development that in normal cases requires nearly the whole period up to puberty. In the course of this development he lost his capacity to invent fairy stories. This conforms to general experience that this capacity is found, at that age, only in children with weak egos, whereas normal boys of his age prefer or invent realistic stories (for instance, science-fiction or adventure stories) and use them to make themselves feel like heroes who can conquer the world, a task that our patient, without the treatment we have described, would have been hardly competent to undertake.

# 7

## A CONTRIBUTION TO THE PSYCHOLOGY OF THE MOTHER-CHILD RELATIONSHIP

ROBERT MOODY, *London*

I SHALL begin by describing an incident that occurred during the puerperium of a patient in analysis. This patient had come to me at the age of 36, suffering from anxiety attacks and a profound loss of confidence. She has a compulsive, obsessional personality; from early childhood her emotional and instinctual reactions had been severely inhibited and replaced by a strong drive to adapt to the demands of the environment.

She had two children and became pregnant for the third time after starting her analysis. When she told me of the pregnancy she also told me that she had had a dream that she had cancer of the uterus. This was a paradoxical state in which creation and destruction, life and death, were associated with the same organ and at the same time.

She was a mother to whom pregnancy was a particularly desirable state because it was the only time the felt she was really a woman. During pregnancy she felt contented and relaxed, she could have a loving contact with people around her and she was sexually more responsive than at other times. But after the birth of the first child she had become depressed and after the second she had actually had a breakdown, leading to a stay of several months in a psychiatric hospital. It was after her discharge from this hospital that she came to me for analysis.

During her third pregnancy, which occurred during the second year of analysis, she was very contented and relaxed most of the time. But she had attacks of anxiety which she came to associate with her cancer dream and with her fears of damage to the baby;

and these attacks became more frequent during the course of the pregnancy. Even so, at the time of her return home, after having had the baby in hospital, she was still very well and showed no symptoms of puerperal depression.

However, one evening several days later her husband telephoned me to ask if I could come to his home, as his wife was in a very agitated state and he could do nothing to calm her. On arrival I found her looking pale and distressed. She told me that during the day she had had several premonitions of something going seriously wrong. It was the same kind of feeling that had ushered in her previous breakdown. She continued in the following vein: "I can't do anything about it. You can't help me. I can hardly feel you are there. I cannot even cry. It's no good, I'm afraid it's all finished now. I feel empty and isolated and dead. I feel all broken to pieces inside. Thoughts rush through my head but they mean nothing. I am sure I am going mad again." I sat with her for half an hour, but could do nothing. It then occurred to me that the baby asleep in its cradle in the next room might succeed where I had obviously failed. I asked the nurse to bring her in and put her in her mother's arms. She gazed at the baby for a long time, as though she could hardly believe that it was real. Then, slowly, there was a change and she began to weep. She slept through the night with the baby in bed beside her. During the next few days one could see quite clearly that, so long as she maintained a close physical contact with the baby, she was free of anxiety: but, as soon as the baby was taken from her, the anxiety returned. Moreover, the anxiety was so acute and so like that experienced during her previous illness as to suggest that, unless this contact with the baby had been maintained during this critical period, she would again have broken down altogether.

This mother's reaction to separation from her baby made a deep impression on me and led me to formulate some of the ideas on which this paper is based.

There is a wide variety of psychic changes associated with pregnancy—changes that are dependent upon a complex interaction of physiological and psychological factors. Of the many different reactions that occur, a particularly interesting problem is presented by the woman who has had neurotic symptoms of many years duration and finds that during pregnancy they disappear, only to appear again after she has had the baby. Such a woman may experience an unusual sense of well-being and contentment.

In seeking to explain how pregnancy can produce such an effect in a neurotic case, I had first to clarify my ideas about the psychology of pregnancy in general. Jung's concept of the bipolar nature of the archetype is particularly applicable in interpreting the phenomena of pregnancy; for the psychology of pregnancy is intimately related to its physiology. We are dealing with a psychosomatic totality—in fact, with archetypes. And it seems to me that it is the archetype of the creative mother, that is, of the great mother in her creative aspect, and the archetype of wholeness, that is, of the self, which predominate at this time.

In the non-pregnant state the ordinary woman presents a mixture of feminine and masculine qualities and functions. But during pregnancy her biologically and psychologically maternal side is reinforced, with the result that she both feels and is more essentially and exclusively feminine than at any other time. Often this change may be observed even before she is aware that she is pregnant—a fact that emphasizes the physiological basis of the increased activity of the archetype.

In the non-pregnant state a woman may feel relatively "whole", either because she is a normally unconscious ordinary woman whose natural sense of wholeness has not been destroyed by neurotic conflict, or because she is a woman who has worked through her neurotic problems to achieve a state of relative wholeness that was previously alien to her. But, in either case, pregnancy has the effect of producing an enhanced sense of wholeness, and we may associate this with the archetype of the self.

During pregnancy the self may be experienced in two distinct though related ways: on the one hand, directly through the inseparable unity of the mother and the unborn child; on the other hand, through the mother's projection on to the unborn child, which may thus become a symbol of the self. But, in so far as pregnancy may be said to constellate the self, it does so through the body; the psychic experience of wholeness is dependent upon the physical fact of wholeness. When the child is born this comes to an end. Mother and child become separate entities, and there takes place in the mother a progressive de-identification from the archetypes.

In the case of a neurotic woman such as I have described, pregnancy may give her the only experience of femininity and wholeness that she has been able to achieve. Through identification with the archetypes she is temporarily released from her neurotic problem. Broadly speaking, this problem is connected with destructive impulses with which she has been unable to deal. In pregnancy she lives her creative side, and her destructiveness becomes unconscious. In this way an almost complete psychic split may occur. In consciousness she is identified with the archetypes activated by pregnancy; whereas in the unconscious the archetypal opposite—the essence of her own unresolved problem—is constellated and becomes progressively powerful.

A careful inquiry into the state of mothers after childbirth convinced me that mild degrees of puerperal depression—often unrecognized as such—are extremely common. The depression usually begins after the mother's return home from hospital. The reason for this delay in onset may be that the loss of wholeness sustained by the mother, through the birth of the baby, is not felt at first because she herself is still contained as a child in the maternal arms of the hospital. It is only when she returns home and has to be the mother that she is left unprotected against her inner destructiveness and its accompanying depression.

These depressions occur most frequently in women of the compulsive-obsessional type. It is these women who may be most aptly described as "possessed by the negative animus". During pregnancy they experience relief from its hold and from the neurotic symptoms to which it may give rise. But the value of this formulation is limited unless it is appreciated that, in spite of its superficial association with the father and the masculine world, the origin of the negative animus lies in the realm of the devouring mother. This is the archetypal opposite which becomes constellated in the unconscious during pregnancy.

In the case I have described, the initial constellation of the unconscious opposite is shown in the cancer dream that occurred at the beginning of the pregnancy; and its growing strength is suggested by the anxiety attacks and fears of damage to the unborn child, which became increasingly frequent. The emergence of the archetypal opposite into consciousness occurred in a dramatic way in the incident with which I began my paper.

From observation of the mother at this time it was clear that close physical (and emotional) contact with the child had the immediate effect of allaying her anxiety. One must therefore conclude that the child, or the mother-child relationship, was acting as a defence against a threatening danger. In considering the nature of this danger, I will remind you of my patient's description of her state of mind: "I feel empty, isolated and dead. I feel all broken in pieces inside. Thoughts rush through my head, but they mean nothing." This must refer to the dangerous state against which the mother-child relationship was acting as a defence. Moreover, the description suggests that the state is associated with some kind of destructive process that has taken place, as it were, within the organism. One is reminded here again of the dream about cancer of the uterus—another reference to a similar process.

This picture of internal destructive processes is by no means confined to puerperal depression. It is very common in many cases of the compulsive-obsessional group of patients in general. Its frequency and the sudden alarming onset of symptoms in puerperal cases are due to the very deep level of infantile experience that is activated by the actual process of childbirth and its sequelae.

Typical dream imagery referring to these processes is that of a dark enclosed place, the back room of a house, a cellar, an underground passage or cave, quite frequently a butcher's shop, slaughter house, or torture chamber. In this dark enclosed place, sometimes irretrievably cut off from the outer world, various forms of destruction have occurred or are occurring. The victims of this destruction may be animals or human beings, or parts of either. The destruction may take place by cutting, squashing, tearing apart, by fire or by other subtle means. One is reminded here of the popular theological conception of hell, to which it is undoubtedly related. A typical dream is the following: "I am investigating a torture chamber underground. A dictator has been running it. The place is full of male bodies that have been sliced up; and I am one of them." This happens to be the dream of a young man, and I mention it in order to emphasize that the psychology of these destructive processes is common to both sexes. In this case it was quite clear that the dictator referred, in the first instance, directly to the father (and to the analyst) but, at a deeper level, to the destructive aspect of the mother.

There is a basic form common to all dreams of this kind. There is an *aggressor* and there is a *victim*; and both are contained in an *enclosure*. There is also a basic meaning in that, in spite of derivatives from later sources, fundamentally they all refer to the mother problem at its deepest level. Out of a consideration of the form and meaning of these dreams I evolved a concept of what I shall call the *primal complex*. Such dreams and the psychic states associated with them may then be regarded as expressions of the activity of this complex.

I suggest that the conflict between aggressor and victim refers to the *original* conflict between mother and child; and that this conflict has become encapsulated or enclosed by an act—both real and fantasied—of swallowing; and that this gives rise to the image of the enclosure. It is possible to conceive this conflict in terms either of the child or of the mother, because both child and mother may be equally and reciprocally involved. Thus, the aggressor may be the child and the victim the mother; then the enclosure would be the child's belly. Alternatively, the aggressor may be the mother—or, more specifically, the mother's negative animus; then the victim would be the child and the enclosure would be the mother's belly. In fact, one can think of the enclosure as a function either of a devouring mother or of a devouring child. This act of swallowing is the somatic image that lies behind the abstract concept of repression and accounts for the universal way in which repressed feelings are located in the belly and become associated with urine, faeces, and babies. Although this act may be regarded primarily as a function of the child, it is also operative in the mother, who is probably dealing in a similar way with the feelings (especially the hostile feelings) that the child provokes in her. In fact, it might sometimes be more appropriate to say that a "swallowing-up" occurs in the mother-child relationship and it may not be possible to attribute this to the mother or the child individually. It could then be conceived of as an archetypal event in which both mother and child are involved and in which every mother and child is always at some time or another involved.

The primal complex manifests itself in many different ways and at many different psychic levels. Initially the victim may be the mother's breast and the aggressor the child's teeth. Later the victim may be the boy's penis and the aggressor the castrating mother. And, at a still later stage of development, the aggressor may be the father and the victim the child or some part of the child.

The primal complex, although derived from the child's negative relationship with the mother, may be projected on to an otherwise untraumatic act of parental intercourse. Then the mother is experienced by the child as the victim of the father's aggressive attack, in the so-called "primal scene" fantasy.

The basic pattern of the primal complex may be seen in the act of suicide or of homicide; and especially in the case of infanticide, where the infant appears so clearly as a projection of the victim.

The primal complex can be seen also as the operative factor in many, if not in all, forms of psychosomatic disorder—the attack of asthma, the attack of ulcerative colitis, the attack of migraine, the heart attack. The very expression "attack" implies both aggressor and victim. In this case the victim is a bodily organ and the aggressor is either the mother, i.e. the mother's destructive animus, or the child's hatred of the mother, which comes to the same thing. The father certainly may enter in; but, even though his role may be of predominant importance as the aggressor in a particular case, he is never first on the scene. The pattern of the primal complex has always been laid down in the mother-child relationship.

The primal complex becomes active in early infancy. In ontogenetic terms one can say that it originates at this time through the personal interaction between the mother and child. In phylogenetic terms one can speak of it first manifesting itself at this time. Archetype and actuality are here, as always, inextricably bound together. Thus, the primal complex, once formed, becomes modified in various ways as a result of the child's later experiences. Throughout life it can be seen to operate in many contexts and at many different psychic levels.

The three components of the complex may be derived from many sources, and may undergo many modifications in successive stages of development. I have already indicated how the aggressor, though first derived from and projected on to the mother, comes to be closely associated with the father at a later stage. And it is then that it becomes more easily recognizable in terms of our idea of negative animus. Then again, the enclosure, though originally derived from a real or fantasied act of swallowing associated with the mother, may be strengthened in later stages of development by inhibitory influences coming from other sources.

The three components of the complex may be regarded as invested with libido, which varies in quantity and distribution from case to case, and from time to time in the same case. In some cases the strength of the aggressor predominates; there is then a constant risk of breakdown, i.e. of the breaking through of destructive impulses in one form or another. Whereas sometimes the enclosure is so strong that relations with the external world are kept relatively stable, though without emotional content, while the inner world is broken up. Sometimes the victim is so well endowed with libido that there is, in effect, no victimization. This would imply a degree of emotional health that is rarely found.

Though it is beyond the scope of this paper to enter at all fully into the many manifestations of the complex, it can be said generally that it gives rise to various patterns of disturbance according to whether it is projected on to the outside world, on the body, or on to other psychic contacts. It may also be added that the complex itself may be affected by external events and situations in various ways according to which of its three components are most strongly activated or reinforced.

Finally, it may be said that the relation of the complex to ego-consciousness depends upon the "permeability" of the enclosure, which is variable and is never complete.

I would like to end my paper by giving you two short illustrations of the primal complex from two widely different types of patient.

The first patient was a young woman of 25. Her behaviour was impeccable but she was chronically depressed and isolated.

She was an obsessional, depressive, schizoid personality. At the time when I first saw her she wished only to be dead. She came to see me regularly for two years or more. I told her relatives in the end that I could do nothing for her and that she would almost certainly kill herself. With deliberation, and with characteristic care for the feelings of other people, she committed suicide. Shortly before her death some ten to twelve years ago, she brought me a picture (see *Plate* 11). It was only after I had thought out this paper and my idea of the primal complex that I looked up my old notes on this woman and I realized that this was a picture of the primal complex almost exactly as I had conceived it, and in its most malignant form. The aggressor, depicted by a black phallic object, was smashing up the victim, represented by red fragments, within a dense black enclosure that was almost totally impermeable. There was no way out; external expression of the complex was impossible and symbolical transformation of its contents was inconceivable.

The second case was of a woman of 33, the patient of a colleague. She was essentially hysterical and had had about two years of analysis. She had the following dream: "There is a garden. In it is a round flower-bed. It is my parent's home. In the middle of the flower-bed is a tree, but the ground is covered with huge volumes of the *Encyclopaedia Britannica*, like my father had in his study. I remove them and find the grass just beginning to grow underneath."

Here the complex presented itself in a benign form. The enclosure is the garden. It is a protection and not a prison. The aggressor is her father's intellect (his books) which is inhibiting, but not lethal. And the victim is the grass, which has suffered, but is essentially healthy and capable of growth.

In these two contrasting examples, the basic form is the same, but the content is different. In the first it is primitive, destructive, and incapable of integration. In the second it is developed, formulated, and on the point of integration.

In conclusion, may I remind you of the cancer dream to which I have already made several references. On the one hand, this dream presents a picture of the primal complex; the uterus is the enclosure, the cancer is the aggressor, and the victim is, by implication, the newly-conceived foetus. On the other hand, we know that cancer is a symbol of the devouring mother. Thus, once again, it is clear that the primal complex is a manifestation of the activity of this archetype.

My idea of what I have called the primal complex emerged inevitably, as it seemed to me, out of my clinical experience. Though I realize that this formulation has some affinities with the concepts of Klein, Winnicott, and others, it is, in fact, an expression of the only way in which I personally could approach an understanding of the various problems that presented themselves. But, as an analytical psychologist, I have been concerned all the time to understand how this formulation is related to Jung's psychology of archetypes. And I hope that my hypothesis of the primal concept may contribute to a clearer understanding of some of the ways in which the archetype of the devouring mother presents itself in clinical work.

# 8

## HEALING IN DEPTH
## THE CONCEPTION AND ITS APPLICATION

CULVER M. BARKER, *London*

### INTRODUCTION

A SERIES of revealing analytical experiences has led me to a specific conception of healing in depth, a special development of therapeutic method and approach. As a pupil and student of Jung, I would like to say that, though this work is based on his findings, his insights, and his teaching, it has arisen out of my experience and, as I hope to show you, adds a new therapeutic aid to the current procedures of psychotherapy.

Many of us may have had the experience of personalities of a high quality coming to seek our help who, despite outstanding work and achievement, are feeling empty, barren, frustrated, without a sense of meaning both in themselves and the world, and are often in despair: the solicitor famous for his care and sensitiveness in dealing with marriage problems and feeling hopelessly caught in a crippling marriage situation, or a most successful woman gynaecologist who had no relation to her instincts and, in her own words, had from childhood onwards hated the lower part of her body. Think of the many psychiatric and welfare workers, teachers, preachers, and, last but not least, psychotherapists who give to others what, basically and unconsciously, they vitally needed themselves.

Thus giving to others what he himself would need most, the present-day adult becomes more and more impoverished and empty. By tracing the causes of a present conflict and its pattern back through the various phases of a patient's life, I have time and again come to experiences and events that happened in what I call an area of critical hurt. I have found that in the cases of deep-seated disturbances this area of critical hurt is traceable and can be healed. Its treatment and healing, however, I find, require a special approach, insight, and method.

## AREAS OF CRITICAL HURT

My conception of healing in depth is based on a re-valuation of the significance of unconscious areas of critical hurt. Occurring usually within the formative period of growth, hurts are critical when the individual's instinctive nature, the feeling of himself, his image of himself, or essential values of his life have been damaged. I have found that such damage is to be looked for at a juncture where ego-consciousness buds off the instinctual matrix. Such a buried wound in the personality results in blocking the continuity of the flow of libido within the stem of the personality up through all subsequent turnings of the spiral of growth. Areas of critical hurt create a blockage because, in order to hold the shock, the area is numbed off. At this moment vital units go, so to speak, off into limbo, the safe place of the unrecognized, the unaccepted, the rejected. In severe cases a total amnesia may be the reaction because such a place of hurt is literally unbearable to consciousness, so unbearable that it is sometimes blacked out completely. To stand the strain of this unbearable situation, to protect this most sensitive area, a kind of iron curtain comes down as a desperate device of self-protection and self-preservation. This sort of iron curtain is often made of mentally developed coldness and objectivity towards oneself and frequently also towards others. Such impersonal coldness all too often indicates the guarding of an unbearable hurt, of insecurity, a sense of inferiority which if exposed would lead to overwhelming despair and panic.

Such *areas of critical hurt*, however, *contain not only traumatic experiences* that require attention *but also live energy that got blocked*. This is energy of a particular kind, *dawn energy* close to the budding of a new phase of growth *which, like nascent hydrogen, holds special power*. Here suspended moments of time, instead of dying, by one of the wonders of nature and life survive with all their potential energy and vitality, miraculously retaining, maybe for decades, their original charge of specific libido.

Unfortunately *this energy is not available* to the present-day personality who would need it badly. For, these units of live energy are shut off, remain *suspended in the shadow*, cocooned parts of the earlier healthy personality. This cut-off area is not under the control of the ego, of the individual's will-power, his consciousness, and has all the possibilities for *good and evil* which are a characteristic of the shadow area.

How then, since they are so deeply concealed in the unconscious, can we know of them at all, relate to them, hope to modify them and get them out of their darkness, constructively back into the stream of life? These concealed dynamic centres are, as one might put it, sending out radioactive interferences. They exert a determining and often *fateful influence, seemingly irrational* and without cause, *on every subsequent phase of development* right up to the present. For the analyst, however, it is *this trail* of seemingly irrational occurrences that *guides* him *in tracing the existence of such areas of* critical hurt, and in assessing their depth, severity, and prognosis. This is also of special significance in short-term diagnosis and treatment, which will be referred to later.

For instance, the *field of work* that the adult either chooses or finds himself in *is often patterned according to these invisible influences*, which, so it seems, tend to manifest themselves whenever there is a chance. I think of a very competent young woman doing excellent work who lost one job after another because, unknowingly, she created in the office setting a crisscross of tensions reflecting her unhappy family situation and expected her boss and colleagues to bring her the personal fulfilment she felt deprived of; it was as if the family pattern interposed distorting lenses between her and the actual situation so that, despite her friendliness and efficiency, people resented her projection.

At the same time you see here a clear example of how such *areas of critical hurt come out as projections* and thus can become recognizable with appropriate help. As a matter of fact I was able to help this patient and several others in similar circumstances by relating their present-day calamity, for such it was, with the interfering reactions of their deep-seated damage.

On the other hand, the feeling of distress caused by such recurrent, apparently "irrational" interferences can bring about a sense of urgency that will lead the sufferer to seek the help that we psychotherapists try to bring.

## THE PROCESS OF HEALING

How, then, can healing in depth be brought about? What we have to do is to contact the human being at that period of critical hurt and shock. For, at that period, the personality became divided within itself: the one that lived on in the outer world carries within him the shock, the fear, of the fateful experience, whereas the younger part detached itself and remained suspended in the shadow area. This *suspended unit has the healthy naïveté, zest, vitality*, sense of wonder, and much more that is *necessary for life*. When it does come out, it will often be with the voice, the vocabulary, and the imagery of that age. These inner figures may emerge from dreams, fantasies, etc., in human form as a child, a beloved figure, etc., or may present themselves in the shape of what at that time held the greatest value—the cat, the dog, the teddy bear, and so on.

*Basic conditions for their emergence*, however, are that the therapist, more even than we usually have to in deep analysis, has proved a trustworthy person and a safe place to relate to and also that he can hold the apprehension, the guilt, and the terror that still assail these patients whenever an experience in the here-and-now activates the old wound and situation. First supported by the analyst, then gradually transferred, "weaned back" to the care and attention of the adult patient, *a continuous, compassionate and highly responsible relationship to these human figures has to be achieved.* This is *a healing process, a synthesis which differs decisively from* the so-called *reductive analysis* although including it.

It is *to the living being* of such *long-past moments of hurt* that *healing awareness needs to be directed.* A most sensitive and painstaking awareness, a specially tuned consciousness are called for. It is like winning back a child whose trust has been broken. Only something comparable to the most loving, understanding, and firm parental care can restore its confidence. And this has to be done over and over again—often a concern of years, in all sorts of circumstances. The hurt one will test you time and again before it will dare to relate, to come out of its retreat, and to join once again with the mainstream of life.

You may have noticed that, in describing the shut-off, cocooned part of the personality, I took care *not* to use the term "*split-off*" —in order to avoid the suggestion of schizophrenia. Besides a deep yearning and a sense of urgent necessity for greater wholeness, besides being willing to do all they can to achieve a fuller life, these people I refer to need to be of strong fibre, with an ego of courage and integrity while working under their handicap, and healthy enough to relate with continuity both to the analyst and to their own inner figures as they emerge. For they *have to learn to hold their own adult consciousness* under the impelling fascination and the often disintegrating impact of these highly charged submerged units.

### TWO EXAMPLES OF HEALING IN DEPTH

To illustrate a significant part of the treatment I would like to take you with me now to living situations in which the recovery of a lost portion of personality took place.

The first of these was a professional woman between 50 and 60, efficient, conscientious and sensitive but complaining of a sense of hardening of her feelings, with some relevant psychosomatic symptoms. In the early part of her analysis one of the memories which came up was of herself at the age of 16 saying goodbye to her boy friend who was going away to the war. She had a vivid and most distressing picture of herself standing on the platform and watching the train disappear round the bend. This picture came up repeatedly during the analysis, sometimes several months apart, always with a tremendous sense of overwhelming despair and hopelessness. One Sunday afternoon I had a telephone call. She said that this "picture" had come back to her that afternoon; she had seen this girl waiting and watching the train disappear round the bend. This time she felt *she was* that girl, and at the same time *she was with* that girl, and she put her arm around her and held her closely and warmly, thus taking away the feeling of lostness and aloneness.

Now here something quite new had happened: the adult person had gone back herself within herself, had found this young girl within herself, and had given her the recognition, the sympathy, and understanding for which she herself had been waiting all along. Throughout these decades, she had unconsciously been trying to get from outside a corresponding satisfaction, yet no outer achievement could compensate for the lack of this basic inner relationship. So this young girl would have remained there for evermore, as a frozen part of herself, if the older part had not during her analytical work gained the experience to relate to this inner figure and found the compassion to go back and, finally, *herself* fetch her into the warm life of the here-and-now.

I myself was the parental, the significant mediating figure. To my astonishment this patient, always a most considerate woman, felt it urgently necessary to ring me up on a Sunday afternoon to tell me her news and share it. It was important to receive this message with an appropriateness that many errors, as well as successes, have helped me to develop.

The next example I want to present to you is taken from work with an engineer, a sensitive man of strong fibre and high intelligence, in his mid-thirties when he came, now an executive in a large international concern. He came in need of help for difficulties in settling down to his work and for dissatisfaction in his sexual relationships, which, though quite normal, lacked the sense of fulfilment. His parents were of incompatible temperament: the mother a passionate, chaotic, wildly intuitive Latin type; the father a steady, rational Scottish businessman who desperately tried to maintain a sense of order and sanity in the house. The boy felt shamed by his mother's eccentricity and the complete mess in the household where he could never ask a friend in. And so, by one of the almost unbelievable devices of young hurt life, he took it upon himself to become her knight, confessor, and protector, thus jumping his natural age and its needs of play and appropriate companionship. His mother wanted him to be there for her own sake—as he put it: "Mother never saw me as me."

Eventually the engineer was able to confide in me what was deeply troubling him: the fear that he might be homosexual. He felt fascinated and deeply stirred by healthy boys of about eight years old and had the greatest difficulty to hold his adultness and not to jump and hop with them down the street. After making sure that no more or less overt sexual activity had occurred we could concentrate on the boy within him, the very age he had missed living.

There is no time to show you how, one after another, unlived ages of life emerged down to four and up to fifteen and later. More astonishing still, once he had gained sufficient security in a particular age, its feminine counterpart appeared in dream figures or attached to memories of the past. Nor can I illustrate the fascinations exerted by actual people reflecting and activating his own unlived age groups, and the often dramatic experiences by which, gradually, he learnt to deal with them. I wish to give you, however, from his own notes, one example, out of many impressive ones, of the important stage of healing in depth that is experienced by the reunion of the ego with a suspended part of the personality.

For some days the engineer had felt contact with what he called "the younger one". This to him was a very big experience, a state of renewal, or newbornness, filling and warming the whole of him. This younger one in him seemed to get tired easily, in his words, "like a new-born calf, a bit dazed and uncertain and not quite safe on its legs"; it had "great wonder and intensity and then, rather like a child, wanted to go off to sleep".

He had been together with this younger part within himself now for several days, with a feeling of himself vitalized by that age, both in his personal life and in his work. But he became quite upset because he found his sleep was being disturbed. He too got easily tired.

Then one day he came to his session much brighter. He had found out how he could help this sleeplessness. Following up some suggestions of mine given in previous sessions, he had talked to this portion of himself—he has acquired a great facility of intelligently, maturely, but most naïvely talking to those suspended entities, to these particular aspects of himself that his life is forcing him, urging him to get into relationship with. He had discovered that his restlessness was really, as it were, the younger one trying to get near him. Thus when, instead of resisting this discomfort and taking a sleeping drug, he concentrated on and held the restlessness with great care, devotion, and adult consciousness, then it was as if the young one materialized. He felt his presence and began to feel him, actually, first his toes, his feet, his legs, his knees, and finally his whole body, until gradually the young one became incarnate. Then the embodied young man merged with him, the adult one, with great intensity and feeling; he finally could relax and go to sleep.

I would like to say here that I was greatly impressed when within the same week a woman patient told me of a similar occurrence and achievement.

To come back to the engineer: at another time he told me more about a further experience: "It was a tingling all over my body, and it was as if the tingling one were a different person that takes over my body, like a shadow person occupying the same body and shape, exactly as I do. This shadow-form takes over all my muscles and a tingling takes over, grips my muscles and becomes him. This new thing, him, is the same as me, only it is a third one."

There are evidently two that have come together, and a transcendent "third" that has come into being and been synthesized out of the older and the younger. He goes on: "It is as if the new thing is my young side, coming into its own, getting embodied in and united with me. That is, the shadow person or form has now become the young one. It is very important for me to feel this in my body and limbs. In the early stages, now some months or even years ago, this first presented itself in dreams. Then when the reunion took place there was a paroxysm in my limbs as this took over, something takes over and the something that takes over brings about this effect, this paroxysm in my limbs."

I have given you the description of this experience of regrowth, the beginning of healing, in his own words which in a man of uncommon ease and facility of expression still reflect a groping for words to convey an experience that all but defies verbal expression. It is a transforming moment of life, a moment of consummate fulfilment and highest significance.

And yet this is something which the patient has to experience, like any new phase of growth, over a period of time, again and again, in different circumstances, until it is well rooted, undoubted, complete, secure.

In order to counterbalance the consuming concentration on, and strain of bringing about, the opus, such patients need the discipline of daily work in the outer world, to some extent comparable to the demands of the psyche. It means attending to dreams at 3 a.m. and still getting up when the alarm clock goes by 7 a.m. to go to work.

For the analyst in this specially exacting and unpredictable work the constant check is whether and how the patient's inner and outer world respond to this endeavour.

*Culver M. Barker*

### THE CONCEPTION OF AREAS OF CRITICAL HURT VERSUS REDUCTIVE ANALYSIS

I would like to add the following general remarks about the tracing of such deep-seated injuries. The necessity for an anamnesis has always been accepted, but in my opinion the critical incidents and constellating environmental patterns in the childhood of the patient are often not recognized in their full significance and extent, let alone is the necessity seen to reconnect where possible the adult with the healthy younger part of the personality. Even if recognized, such units are allowed to recede into the background instead of being carried forward. Altogether they tend to be treated predominantly, almost exclusively, as aspects of the historical past, rather than as living energetic parts of the present adult personality on which, although unconscious, they are continually exerting their influence.

If this situation is handled by superficial analysis, inappropriate interpretation, will-power, or so-called rehabilitation, a certain amount of adaptation may be achieved. Two decisive factors, however, will be amiss: (i) the patient is working against the tension potential of his basic instinctual pattern, and so undue energy and will-power are required to operate such adaptation; and (ii) the original pattern in the depth, because never related to consciously with the mind and feelingly with the heart, remains essentially unmodified. Hence it is ever ready to overcome, to swamp the new adaptation with an uprush of revengeful, repressed instinctual energy.

### THE CONCEPTION AS AN AID IN ASSESSMENT, PROGNOSIS, AND TREATMENT

I now wish to indicate how the conception of the critical hurt areas can lead to a short-cut diagnostic tracing of the chief interferences with the life-stream.

In my approach, after getting the patient at ease and establishing the necessary rapport as we always try to do, you start to be alerted for signs of an interrelation between the difficulties of today with moments of comparable emotion and hurts in the past. In listening to the patient's story you take the present situation as potentially symptomatic, as a surface expression of something possibly much deeper. You look for the relationship between the patient's recurrent difficulties of today, with special attention to his pattern of work and its vocational significance, and an earlier unsolved difficulty or pattern. In other words, you allow for the difficulty of today being constellated by the unsolved, unhealed, recurrent problem of the past—an area of critical hurt. In this case the present-day situation happens to mirror more or less an earlier situation that critically challenged the individual. It induced a defence reaction (including repression), which at the time saved the situation. This became habitual, but at least now in adulthood no longer serves the individual's life.

It is most likely that the *deep hurts* that affect subsequent periods may have this *critical* quality *because the disturbing event coincided with the emergence of an archeptyal situation* or tension at a moment of growth.

In checking on the importance and severity of this hurtful event or experience, by keeping one's ear very close to the message of dreams, including early nightmares and fantasies, as well as of fears, apprehensions, and feelings of guilt, one discovers the same imprint or pattern in earlier or later events of the patient's life. Such recurrence points to the deep-seated, the original hurt (the first one spotted is not necessarily the original one). I am *often guided to areas of critical hurt by the fascination exerted by their reflection* in a present person or situation.

This scanning, checking, and assessing helps to trace the track the patient's injury has taken right through the years to the present as well as the complexes involved and constellated. By noting and feeling the type of reaction that he brings to stress situations—for instance of the withdrawing schizoid, the victim paranoid, the hysterical, or the obsessional type—we get a quickened sense of the diagnosis.

Out of this sensitive anamnesis we can judge some *factors essential for assessing the possibility and type of treatment and the prognostic outlook.* I would emphasize the health and quality of the substance; the stamina of the personality, its resilience or brittleness; the effort and persistence put in to reach the unconscious, and its response to it. Next I would mention the importance of environmental factors and their impact in particular on the hurt area and the shaping of the defence pattern. Of equal importance for the possibility of re-growth where possible is the integrity of the ego, however young and immature it may be in the adult of today, and his capacity to mature in due course and take over responsibility, not only for his outer but also for his inner life. In the external reality you check the degree of security in the environment, the range and daring of experience, the counterpoint in work, in the family, with friends, the rootedness in one's own sex and the healthy relationship to the opposite, and you try to estimate the degree of isolation.

The comparatively early or late occurrence of the critical hurt area, the degree of health below it, the more or less complicated reaction pattern built over the wound may help the establishment of an *early tentative prognosis* as to chances of "cure", to assess the type of therapy, the probable duration, and the frequency of treatment indicated.

Altogether *this conception ranges from the dilemma of today down to the original hurt and back again*—a span that is, as it were, radioactive in a complex psychological sense in its influence on the present day. It *provides an additional means*, a ray that may guide you more directly to such critical areas. Together with the many other aids of analytical psychology, it *gives an added wavelength* or special beam to the therapist engaged in such pioneering endeavours.

### WIDER APPLICATIONS

In encouraging and supporting a healing process by directing the adult's consciousness to those suspended personalities of an earlier age, I feel I got nearer to the process of growth and of re-growth of healing, than I had ever been able to do before. From the scientific point of view, I regard such experiences as most valuable opportunity for *research* and discovery of hitherto unrevealed aspects of the human psyche.

The labour put into this work and the attitude it leads to will, apart from being worthwhile in themselves, also help one with other patients who are not fated to travel the length and depth of the whole journey.

The insight I had to gain, the ways and sensitiveness I had to develop, have helped me to see in much *milder but more concealed cases* a similar process at work and to go more assuredly and quickly to such key places where real healing was possible and was achieved.

In what I should like to call *short-term treatment* I have found my conception helpful for the immediate relief of tension in acute anxiety states, in dealing with suicidal tendencies, and in tension leading to severe somatic pain. The therapist's insight into the basic pattern of recurrence will, if grasped by the patient, indeed often bring almost spontaneous alleviation to the sufferer beyond that of an ordinary abreaction.

In *long-term treatment* I have applied this conception to very disturbed and isolated patients, including one who needed mental-hospital care, with results that suggest that further application to such severe cases would be a promising line of research.

Beyond the clinical field there is a far *wider area* where this conception may be applied. I should have liked to show you some of these applications, first and foremost in vocational work, then in everyday life, in understanding people one meets, etc.

### THE ANALYST'S HYGIENE

As in all such deep work, special attention has to be paid to the analyst's own inner hygiene. When we who are workers in this field deal with other human beings without being sufficiently aware of our own place of need, we are actually using this most sensitive critical place of our own as a tool, an instrument, and often do not give it its own rightful recognition and care. We may think we are working securely behind a wall of objectivity, but sensitive "personalness" is passing through this permeable wall of our psyche. It is this which directs us and takes us to those aspects of our work which carry the glint of fascination—or the opposite, repulsion. If we are working with such a most personal part of ourselves without knowing it, without conscious awareness, this may ultimately damage us severely.

On the other hand, the patient must really feel both consciously and instinctively that we, the analysts, have been in and at least close to comparable experience and challenge. More than ever in this deep work we must realize that we are mediators or archetypal powers, ourselves under the divine auspices and in the service of healing mediators and not magicians.

# 9

## *HUNGRY PATIENTS*

### *Reflections on Ego Structure*

A. PLAUT, *London*

DURING the past five years I have come across a number of patients whose psychic structure differed considerably from that of the usual run of neurotic patients. In calling these patients hungry, I am deliberately choosing a common characteristic on which my observations have centred. Naturally, I cannot hope to introduce two of these patients to you as individuals within the limits of this paper. In fact, the most I can hope for is to describe how I got into theoretical difficulties and reached some tentative conclusions. I shall refer to the patients only to illustrate my points.

I am using hunger in a specific sense here, yet I want to make it clear that none of the patients considered themselves hungry when they were first seen. However, the subject of food and eating took a prominent place in their analyses. Both patients were under 30 years of age, and were immature personalities suffering from considerable ego weakness. The main burden of this paper will be to expound what I mean by ego weakness, a term which has been used increasingly by analysts writing about the psychodynamics of schizophrenia (e.g. Metman, 1956, 1957, 1958; Freeman *et al.*, 1957).

These patients had to be studied more through their behaviour in the analytical sessions than by other evidence of unconscious activity, e.g. dream analysis and active imagination. They *did* dream, but their interest could not be got by dream interpretation: other manifestations were more urgent. A modification of what might be regarded as classical analysis was therefore required.

In the abstract of this paper I referred—rather loosely—to the relations between hunger and sexual instincts. Much work has been done of recent years on the subject of instincts by ethologists, who now look upon instincts as whole sequences of behaviour. Regarding this topic Lorenz (1950, p. 261) says:

> "What formerly was very simply conceived of as 'an instinct' is shown by the advance of analysis to be a *very complex mechanism of very distinct and very different constituents* such as endogenous automatisms, releasing mechanisms, taxes, kineses and, maybe, quite a number of further as yet unrecognized particulate functions . . ." However: "The conceptual distinction of constituent parts and of their particular qualities does not in any way preclude the fullest cognizance of the general mutual interdependence and interaction and these parts."

It follows that if I wanted to satisfy an ethologist I would have to tell you whether, by speaking about *hunger* (or thirst) in my patients, I was referring purely to the *appetitive experience*, to *physiological phenomena*, e.g. contraction of stomach walls, parching of membranes, etc., to *appetitive behaviour*, e.g. search for food, specific sign stimuli, or *consummatory behaviour*, e.g. sucking, chewing, biting, swallowing. Fortunately, instinct is a biological concept with psychological implications, and I shall therefore regard it as good enough for my purposes to use the constituent parts of the instinct "hunger" as they turned up and without discrimination. It seems to be the fate of concepts that at the time of their invention they seem strikingly self-evident. Through frequent and often diverse usage the term gradually tends to become meaningless. Alternatively the formerly single concept becomes more detailed and complex. The more super-ordinate the concept the more certain is this to happen.

Therefore when we come to an important psychological term like "ego", the principle which Lorenz outlined in the passage I quoted may be applied—Jung has periodically reviewed and revised the terms which seemed most important to him. Thus he refers in *Aion* (1951, *Coll. Wks.*, **9**, 2, p. 3 f.) to the ego as a complex factor having both a somatic and a psychic basis, both of which consist in turn of conscious and unconscious factors.

According to his orientation my observations refer to those endosomatic stimuli which hover on the border of consciousness. These do, in my submission, make an important contribution to the structure of the ego and their importance in some cases seems to me considerable.

The first case is that of a young married woman who came in an agitated and depressed frame of mind after interviews with a priest and sedation by her general practioner had failed to give her relief. She suffered from feelings of unreality and depersonalization. Although a strong, sexually toned transference established itself fairly soon, this only shifted the symptoms to feelings of persecution, anxiety, and guilt, particularly after those sessions when she had dared to tell me about her feelings about me. Either she turned up depressed and neglected in her appearance, and would show me that nothing I could do or say was the slightest bit of good; or she would dress well and sit there gazing at me in a fashion which I could best describe as devouring me with her eyes.

In this state she would not speak, but chewed at her finger or pulled threads out of my cushion with her teeth or nails, or rubbed it against her mouth and nose. When I went away on holiday, she took this cushion home with her. Sometimes she would also take off parts of her clothing and gaze in the direction of my genital. After the attempts at seduction had failed, she acknowledged with genuine distress that she did not really want to have intercourse with me, but just wanted me in her mouth, and this desire was overwhelmingly strong; on several occasions it looked as if she was going to faint with the strength of the impulse.

The story was that her mother—a woman of extremely violent temper and most un-motherly disposition—had drunk herself to death at an early age. The patient, who was beautiful and intelligent, had attracted her husband, who compared her to the leading lady in the play *I am a Camera* by Christopher Isherwood. However, my patient's main interest centred on her brother, who shared his promiscuous sexual exploits with her in great detail. She herself had had premarital sexual relations with men, from which she dissociated herself to such a degree that she did not know in some cases whether or not she had had intercourse with her partners.

By analysing the transference it was not difficult to see that the content of her apparently sexual transference was only superficially a "brother-transference". More correctly it was a transference to the brother's penis, and this in turn was a substitute for her mother's breast. As she was capable of sincerity, the patient admitted later that the feelings for me which she had so fervently declared were just an overwhelming longing to practise fellatio and that real "heart-feelings", as she put it to distinguish them from her desires for sensation, were more than she could stand. In fact she had never had such feelings for any human being so far as she knew.

This patient illustrates how sexuality can be the cloak for an oral fixation. I prefer to call it oral fixation (with the breast as the central object) rather than a mother fixation, since it appeared that the patient had not yet developed the capacity to relate to whole persons or images of persons but only to parts. She often sat gazing at her fingers and wondering why they looked as they did, and was perplexed that people in the street had the shape they had, i.e. she did not see them as people but as noses.

I hope that this sketch will provide sufficient background against which to outline my notions of the ego's structure, the relations of its component parts, and the nature of a particular ego weakness, i.e. to mistake a "sign stimulus", the breast, for the penis, and to be helpless in the grip of the appetitive response to it.

My patient's situation may be summarized as follows:

(1) There was an inability to appreciate complete images and, consequently, to relate to people.

(2) A sense of wholeness was brought about with the help of very strong sensations referred to various parts of the body.

The fixated part-object remained essentially unchanged, although it could attach itself to various carriers (male or female). Looked at superficially, it may appear as if a development had taken place, e.g. from breast to penis, i.e. as if a genital ego element had been firmly established. This was, however, not the case.

(3) There was an absence of ego boundaries, i.e. a state of magical identity in which there was no distinction between "I" and "you". She was unable to believe that I ever felt or thought anything differently from herself.

(4) The patient was living in a continual state of anxiety caused by fear of losing her identity (such as it was) and by feelings of unreality.

The situation I have just described forms the basis of my concepts on ego structure, and I should therefore exemplify and illustrate it in the following manner: the sum total of an infant's awareness is in his mouth while feeding. In that condition he is unable to distinguish between mouth and nipple, let alone between himself and his mother, and neither space nor time are apprehended. I think it is possible to assume that this state of wholeness which depends on adequate oral localization is the forerunner of the later, more differentiated experiences of the self. However, while the infant is neither feeding nor sleeping, he develops responses which would indicate that he can also be aware of things happening around him and in him, and this capacity is independent of zonal excitation. I ascribe it to the formation of a central ego nucleus, able to anticipate situations and to experience fear and hope. As contrasted with the stimulus bound awareness characteristics of zonal ego elements, the nucleus is capable of developing a spatio-temporal continuity of experience. With the help of it there develops the possibility of appreciating images of whole objects. By this I mean the possibility to apperceive archetypal images other than those vested in numinous parts of the body. It is an important function of the nucleus to create an ego boundary, i.e. to integrate the component parts of the ego in such a way that under optimum conditions the ego is sufficiently unified to distinguish between itself and others, between an inner and an outer world.

However, this nucleus is extremely vulnerable to adverse influences, for example if the experience of wholeness remains exclusively linked with a zonal ego element and its corresponding objects, e.g. mouth and nipple. This threat goes a long way in accounting for my patient's fear of loss of identity and persecutory anxiety whenever she came near to having the sensations for which she most craved, especially in the presence of an observer.

But who is this observer in terms of the patient's psychology? I think that we may regard him as a representative of her own self-awareness, i.e. of the ego nucleus, which gives warning of danger. This identity between analyst and patient's ego nucleus may explain why the analyst at this stage is liable to appear as a forbidding or persecuting figure. If the relations between the zonal ego elements and the ego nucleus are disturbed in the manner described, hindering a properly organized and unified ego from functioning, undue emphasis will be placed on the development of a pseudo-ego or, to use Neumann's term, an emergency ego (*Not-Ich*). The emergency ego can *control* archetypal situations, thereby protecting a vulnerable nucleus against too powerful affects. The destructive potential of archetypes is checked for the time being but, on the other hand, no fruitful relationship between ego and archetype can be established in this way.

In the case of my second patient, a young single woman, this emergency ego was sufficiently well developed to enable her to get an academic degree and pursue a professional life. However, her hunger being much more severe than that of the other patient, it had forced her to resort to another form of defence, that of denial, i.e. of hunger. The result was that she was emaciated to a degree and lived in almost complete isolation. She spent most of her time under a blanket in her room, did not speak to anyone more than was necessary to keep herself alive, and never went to the lavatory if there was the slightest chance of anyone noticing her, nor would she eat when others were present. In analysis she hardly spoke at all for the first 18 months and sat stiffly in her chair, refusing to take her coat off or to put her handbag down. At this stage her hunger could be inferred from the loud and rumbling contractions of her intestines.

My point in mentioning this patient is that she was in a more obviously regressed condition and psychologically speaking much closer to an intrauterine existence. Until analysis started she had never allowed herself to become fully aware of her bodily needs. Although present, the zonal ego fragments had never become centres of pleasurable awareness. When she did talk she told me of dreams—I think her emergency ego had told her that was the proper thing to do in analysis. The dreams were mostly about the elements—wind, fire, water, and earth; rather violent events took place, frightening the dreamer, but otherwise there were no "dramatis personae". There were apparently no associations to these dreams.

Had it not been for her strongly developed emergency ego, I think the second patient would have been much closer to the type of patient whom Perry (1953) describes, i.e. living in a world of archetypal images, a kind of prenatal wholeness. In this condition hunger has not yet become a significant experience and it may apparently be left to the spontaneous activity of the unconscious to produce a psychic birth. Naturally the observer's orientation plays an important part in therapy, but I feel that the state of the patient's ego may also account for such differences in therapeutic approaches as we see in the case of Perry on the one hand and myself on the other.

It has been assumed that the prenatal wholeness as we imagine it, or even the post-natal states of integration observable in earliest infancy, are due to the presence of the self and prior to the appearance of an ego. Both Neumann (1955) and Fordham (1957) make this assumption. This has the obvious advantage of making comparison between the early integrated states and the phenomenology and experience of the self in later life possible. However, Neumann asks the very important question: Who is it that experiences anything if there is as yet no ego? He answers the question with the help of another concept, that of the ego-self axis. As I understand it, this means that the self can stand proxy for the ego while the latter is temporarily out of action or has not yet come into action. The concept of the ego-self axis is modelled on the Son-Father analogy which Jung used in "Transformation Symbolism in the Mass" (1942).

My difficulty is to conceive how the experience of strong affects, like anxiety about loss of identity, persecutory feelings, etc., can be ascribed to the presence of anything that is non-ego, e.g. the self. I should prefer to conceive of the self at this stage as an archaic ego component and postulate that other component parts, like the zonal fragments and the reflecting ego nucleus, are either added to or split off from this archaic ego. In favourable circumstances, the components are integrated into a unified if unstable system: the ego to which we commonly refer. On the other hand, the inclusion of something comparable to an ego from the earliest moment of life *in utero* would be in keeping with the principle of a continuity of development (*natura non facit saltus*) and does not do violence to observations concerning the probability of some awareness in the embryo, as Gesell (1945) reports at 32 weeks.

If we allow for the continued existence of an archaic ego as a constituent part of the whole ego system which can never become fully conscious and yet exerts an influence on the rest of the ego structure, then the relationship of this component to the self will have to be considered carefully. In "Transformation Symbolism in the Mass" Jung (1942) certainly states that the self is the father in that it forces us all the time to overcome unconsciousness. But he also says that the self is created by our making ourselves conscious and to that extent it is our son. This clearly implies a reciprocal relationship between ego and self. I doubt, furthermore, whether we are justified in assuming the existence of the self in the form of integrated states in infancy before at least an oral ego element has been established as a focal centre.

Rascovsky (1956), in a recent paper entitled "Beyond the Oral Stage", adduced some psychological and mythological evidence for the existence of a prenatal ego nucleus. I choose the word "archaic" in preference because I assume that it continues to exist throughout life, because its functioning may well be related to certain midbrain structures, and also because observations like Gesell's were made on foetal infants, i.e. prematurely born infants from the age of 28 weeks onwards. (I have refrained from calling it "primitive" because of the slightly derogatory flavour of this term.) Although one may argue that the fact of life being extra-uterine invalidates Gesell's observations, one also has to consider that an artificial environment had been created simulating the womb closely enough to support life. Such observations as we have on these infants make the notion of prenatal bliss and integration a myth rather than a physiological fact. Clear distinctions between activity and rest are impossible at this early stage: while the foetal infant is apparently drowsing peacefully facial muscle groups are active "as so many different workshops" to quote Gesell (1945, p. 114).

To return to my "hungry" patients, it was striking how definitely their expectation of wholeness was linked to body zones which had remained numinous. A fixation having occurred to an area which at one time stood for the whole world including themselves, this state of affairs had not changed materially, despite all sorts of other events. I assumed that if the bodily experiences of infancy were—for some reason or another—not satisfying, no separation between zonal ego element and its object occurred and that the ego nucleus could not become fully operative.

In this precarious situation, excitement as well as anxiety were aroused in the nucleus whenever it was threatened by overactivity of a zonal component. The latter was striving for ascendency over the nucleus and this may well be the reason why the true state of affairs could not come into the individual's consciousness. Hence patients wanted to still hunger or thirst but at the same time dared not agree to the fulfilment of such a dangerous wish.

The therapeutic implication is that feeding of the patient must keep in step with the development of the whole ego structure. Although my conceptual model is surely an over-simplification, in that innumerable anastomoses between the component parts occur, I hold that it is possible to observe which of the component parts of the ego is dominant at any given time.

In conclusion, it would seem as unwise to treat the origins of the ego which may be traced back to foetal life as if they were "the ego" as it would be to look upon moments of infantile repose as evidence of "the self". Undifferentiated states in which neither ego nor self are clearly discernible seem to come first. However, qualities of awareness, particularly very early evidence of anxiety, bear a closer relation to that ego component which I called archaic than to the self. Its relation to consciousness is remote compared with that of the ego nucleus. Yet, in states of stress and exhaustion, in sleep or in illness, and also at the very beginning and end of life, this archaic ego component seems to come into its own. It registers on behalf of the individual what is happening and reacts to events without being able to focus sharply enough to make one feel the space-time continuity expressed in "this is happening to me now". As I see it, none of the ego constituents vanishes or ceases to function altogether. The following may illustrate in a lighter vein what I mean:

An analyst—considering himself mature—may suddenly find

that during a session with his patient he has run out of tobacco. If I may be allowed to regard this as an oral gratification to which he is habituated, it may easily be imagined how this deprivation may disorganize the rest of his ego functions. Under the influence of this stress the vulnerable nucleus is weakened and his emergency ego may attempt to control the situation. This brings with it a lack of contact with the archaic ego and a loss of relationship with archetypal contents. If his ego nucleus should make him aware of this state of affairs and if he is still unable to get hold of his tobacco, he would be wise to let his archaic ego component have some say and stop talking as if he knew what was going on.

## REFERENCES


FORDHAM, M. (1957). "The Origins of the Ego in Childhood", *New Developments in Analytical Psychology*. London, Routledge & Kegan Paul.

FREEMAN, T., *et al.* (1957). "The State of the Ego in Chronic Schizophrenia" *Brit. J. med. Psychol.*, **30**, 1.

GESELL, A. (1945). *The Embryology of Behaviour*. New York and London, Harper.

JUNG, C. G. (1942). "Das Wandlungssymbol in der Messe", *Eranos-Jb.* **8.** Trans. "Transformation Symbolism in the Mass" in *Psychology and Religion: West and East, Coll. Wks.*, **11**.

JUNG, C. G. (1951). *Aion*. Zürich, Rascher. Trans. *Coll. Wks.*, **9**, 2.

LORENZ, K. (1950). *Physiological Mechanisms in Animal Behaviour*. London, Cambridge University Press.

METMAN, P. (1956). "The Ego in Schizophrenia", Part 1. *J. analyt. Psychol.*, **1**, 2.

METMAN, P. (1957). "The Ego in Schizophrenia", Part 2. *J. analyt. Psychol.*, **2**, 1.

METMAN, P. (1958). "The Trickster Figure in Schizophrenia", *J. analyt. Psychol.*, **3**, 1.

NEUMANN, E. (1955). "Narzissmus, Automorphismus und Urbeziehung" in *Studien zur analytischen Psychologie C. G. Jungs*, **1**. Zürich, Rascher.

PERRY, J. W. (1953). *The Self in Psychotic Process*. Berkeley and Los Angeles, University of California Press.

RASCOVSKY, A. (1956). "Beyond the Oral Stage", *Int. J. Psycho-anal.*, **37**, 4-5.

# 10

## EGO INTEGRATION AND PATTERNS OF CONIUNCTIO

GERHARD ADLER, *London*

In order to define the scope of my paper, I want to say at the beginning that I have tried to deal with my subject only from the feminine aspect. My material is, with one exception, taken from one particular case. With its help I shall try to illustrate the unfolding of the archetypal pattern of the coniunctio as starting from and based on the archetype of incest. I shall further try to show how the individual situation actualizes this archetypal pattern, in a negative way as frustrating it or in a positive way as constellating it. In all this it has to be kept in mind that the paper was originally given as a twenty-minutes lecture, and that I have kept it here to its original content. It should thus be regarded as a sketch of a problem capable of considerable enlargement.

The case is that of a woman in her early forties with agoraphobia. In her case, as in other cases of agoraphobia, I found that the symptom was due to a very early disturbance of the primal relationship to the mother, of what Neumann has called the *Urbeziehung* (Neumann, 1953, p. 4), plus an incestuous problem on the side of the father. First of all, the absence of the maternal temenos has produced the menace of the open space. The actual mother has proved insufficient, and has thus constellated the negative great mother. Then the infant finds it too difficult to identify with mother and suffers from lack of primal containment. In the end the infant has not succeeded in producing a secure enough ego, and the ego is, as it were, left without its proper skin, without its own protective temenos. Thus, on the one hand, it is constantly threatened by flowing away into the environment symbolized by the void of the open space; and, on the other hand, as a secondary phenomenon, space constantly threatens to intrude into the confines of an unprotected and too incoherent ego. This danger of intrusion gains even more reality in connection with the incest fantasy, and the latter assumes an overpowering character where the father's unconscious incestuous fantasies exert pressure from his side.

In itself the incest fantasy of the child is an archetypal pattern. It has its forerunner in a pre-incest situation in which the infant experiences a primal coniunctio in containment in and identification with the relationship of the parents. In my opinion this is, strictly speaking, a pre-ego state; and in this sense, as far as the ego's partner-role is concerned, the incest fantasy represents the basic pattern of the coniunctio. With its content of countersexual polarity, this positive incest, as I would like to call it, is full of integrative potentialities. For the girl it is the primal archetypal experience of the creative spirit, but naturally on an unconscious level. This experience turns, on account of the personal father's unconsciousness, into a negative incest fantasy. The latter is characterized by its menacing and hostile character to which the child stays fixated. The fear of—and repressed desire for—the masculine sex in general, and incest in particular, have been adduced as a basic element in the symptomatology of agoraphobia (Fenichel 1945, pp. 196, 208); to me it seems only a secondary although vital feature in the situation. The first condition is the faultiness of the maternal temenos which—in consequence—lays the child too wide open to the invasion of unassimilable contents, to the attack by the father's unconscious fantasies.

The case in question runs true to form in that the individual mother was an immature and self-centred woman, who could not relate to the child in a natural way. She was dominated by an exceptionally gifted husband. On the conscious level, the father had an excellent relationship to the child; it was, however, as analysis showed, vitiated on the unconscious level by a strong feeling problem of the father and an anima projection on to his daughter.

The first eighteen months of treatment had been dominated by infantile material relating to the image of the "bad mother".

Analysis brought to the surface how abandoned and isolated the infant had felt as a result of the faulty primal relationship. Very gradually analysis had produced a compensatory effect by creating a transference relationship in which I was experienced as the containing mother on whose undemanding love and patience she could rely. I cannot here go into the stages of the restoration of this maternal temenos, but a dream, about eighteen months after the start of analysis, will show where we had arrived at that stage, In the dream,

> she leads me, the analyst, through a flight of rooms into an inner, central hidden room where she has something very important to say. The room is very beautiful, warm and quiet, with soft light. I look very much as in reality. But suddenly I plunge my arms brutally down the opening of her dress and rape her. This "I had to do".

The two relevant facts of the dream are the "inner room" and the "rape". As to the latter, the dream was a real trauma. It terrified her; she could hardly tell me of it, and she was deeply disgusted with me for my action in the dream.

But equally important was the drama which takes place in the "inner room". In this central, beautiful, soft room we have the restored and secure maternal temenos. It is the archetypal womb, the krater, inside which the feminine ego can go through a critical experience. Thus the room symbolizes the positive great mother. She can now identify with her, and in this identification the feminine ego has been established. In this sense the restored maternal temenos and the patient's redeemed feminine ego coincide. Now the incestuous relationship can be faced. At this point the father image, the male element, is constellated.

The negative incest fantasy, which had been activated by the faulty father-daughter relationship, has to be redeemed in the transference. The projection of the incest fantasy on to the analyst thus does not just raise the negative incest fantasy with the father into consciousness, but, just as important, it is a stepping-stone beyond it: out of the negative into the positive incest, thus anticipating the coniunctio.

From the inner development of the dream it is evident that the very thing she has to communicate to me is just this experience of rape. The dream is important because it shows how inside the maternal temenos the attack of the male can be tolerated. In fact, it is an inevitable step on the way towards individuation. The "inner room" represents the position achieved; the rape the stage continuing it. But at this point the encounter with the male is still experienced as highly ambivalent: it is both the creative and desired act, and the unexpected, traumatic assault. The male "intruder" cannot yet be fully accepted since the feminine ego is still largely identified with and contained in the great mother: the patient still wants to remain the daughter. From a different angle the ambivalence expresses the constant ambivalence of the purposes of the ego and the self: the ego is still frightened of, and may be not yet fully prepared for, the purpose of the self.

Only in parenthesis I want to add that with this dream her sexual relationship with her husband began to improve. Whereas, previously, there had been a considerable problem of sexual adjustment in an otherwise happy marriage, now, after one and a half years, the physical relationship became a source of enjoyment and pleasure.

To return to the dream, it seems that before the male intruder can be more fully accepted, a further step in ego integration has to be achieved. This step appears to be de-identification from the great mother. It is indicated in a further dream, about six months after the rape dream. In the dream,

> she is a little girl watching other children play in a field. Suddenly a boar rushes into the field; she is terrified, but there is a house where she knows she can take refuge. In front of the house an old woman is standing quietly; without words the woman knows all about her, and she feels safe.

First of all, the dreamer experiences herself as a child. I should like to come back to this point later on. Then there is the threatening boar, the elemental, destructive, phallic power of the great mother. On the archetypal level this destructive power is symbolized in the killing of Attis or the Zeus of Crete; on the personal level it manifests itself as the negative animus. But at the point of crisis the other pole to this destructive aspect of the great mother is constellated; the guardian and goddess of the house, of the protective maternal temenos, appears. There is, however, a very different side to the ambivalent situation. John Layard, to whom I am much indebted in this respect, has drawn my attention to the positive significance of the boar, confrontation with whom is, as he put it in a written communication, "one of the great transforming situations of archetypal significance". To put it very briefly, the boar is also the archetypal male and the encounter with it represents the confrontation with positive incest.

On one level the old woman is the manifestation of the positive great mother who protects her, but on another level she would be the devouring mother who holds on to the child, and, by drawing her from the open field into the house, would prevent her encounter with the male. The dream then shows a great uncertainty and hesitation on the part of the feminine ego: at this point either she may still be unable to cope with the boar and therefore be in real need of the protection of the great mother; or she may simply cling to her protection in order to avoid the next step—that is, confrontation with the creative great father in the act of positive incest.

In spite of the manifest fear and hesitation, the dream takes the pattern of the coniunctio a stage beyond the rape-dream. For one thing, in the boar-dream the ambivalence, and with that the reality, of both female and male archetypal powers, are fully realized; for another, the female encounter with the male, though not yet consummated, is no longer bound up with the person of the analyst. True, it is still an incestuous situation in that the dreamer experiences herself as child; but, on the other hand, the male is, in the figure of the boar, experienced as elemental archetypal power.

The ambivalence of the dream indicates an unfinished situation, and points towards an encounter with the male as transpersonal power; an encounter yet to be accepted. The fact that the dream-ego appears as a child expresses a basic ambivalence: on the one hand, the ego is bound to feel inferior to the archetypal force of the non-ego; but, on the other hand, there is also the indication that the child can no longer depend on maternal protection in her encounter with the male. In this sense the sexual experience with the analyst in the rape-dream had been a rehearsal for the next stage of the coniunctio in which the frightened but established ego has to step out into the open. Now it has to maintain itself in its independence; identification with and containment in the great mother have to be sacrificed.

I want to point out only in parenthesis the significance of the enclosed space in the first dream and of the open field in the second with regard to the problem of agoraphobia: here again the encounter on the open field represents an important step beyond the protection of the inner room.

A remark which the patient made a short time after the last dream was characteristic of the inner development initiated with it. She expressed her feeling that a new stage in analysis had been reached. She described it by saying: "My interest in mother seems exhausted, and I know that now 'sex' is the important thing." With "sex" she meant to convey something much wider than the physical experience; as it were, "Sex" with a capital S, symbolizing the encounter with "Father"—again with a capital F—and with the male in general.

How real this new stage of realization and ego-integration was showed itself when, several months after the boar-dream, the patient was able to go out on her own for the first time since the start of the analysis. She had learnt to face and accept the male without running back into her mother's arms.

A new phase and a new pattern of the coniunctio manifest themselves in another dream about eight months after the boar-dream. In the dream she is lying in bed, nobody else is in the room, but then quite unexpectedly, something incredibly strong, like an electric current or a whirlwind, completely penetrates and seizes her whole being, rapes her, but without any negative connotation of the word: it is like an invasion by something superhuman, to which resistance would be both impossible and senseless. In the dream she said the words: "Now it can happen." The experience was so strong that she shook uncontrollably.

Here again we have an experience of rape, of invasion. The patient herself connected it with the first rape-dream. She felt the last dream to continue and complete the first one in two respects. First, whereas the earlier dream had been traumatic, there was no feeling of trauma or any idea of resistance in the latter; in spite of its overpowering character it seemed wholly acceptable. Secondly, whereas the rape-dream was still bound to the person of the analyst, the current was impersonal and numinous in quite a new way. She felt the whole experience to be deeply creative. Perhaps we can say that at this point the boar of the previous dream had penetrated her with his tusk-phallus, no longer killing but fertilizing; the ambivalence of the destructive-constructive great father has been synthesized in the fusing current of the transpersonal male.

Both the creative experience and the inherent limitation of this stage are self-evident. On the one hand, in the encounter with the numinous invader, the patient can completely submit to the masculine partner, and in her feminine surrender she becomes transformed. On the other hand, she is as yet only a passive recipient for the power of an impersonal and completely dominant male opposite. Further development of the pattern of the coniunctio will have to go in the direction of gradual equalization of the two partners and a growing individualization of the relationship. I should like to illustrate two further stages by two dreams.

The first one occurred about ten months after that of the invading current. In the dream a man who had always been to the patient the embodiment of positive spirit, but of whom for this very reason she had been rather frightened and full of inferiority feelings, talks to her in a tender understanding way of her "Beauty". Again, like "Sex" in the previous dream, "Beauty" meant much more than the word as such conveys: it was the essence of femininity, and she felt deeply appreciated and recognized.

This dream shows shows an individualized relationship. It is also one of relative equality, although the initiative and preponderance of the man are still clearly marked. He is a kind of liberator who helps the woman to realize and accept her feminine individuality. With that a mature relationship is ushered in; the two partners become more and more equals, and a meeting of two individuals can take place. This is meant to include both external and internal relatedness: on the actual plane of outer reality two integrated individuals can meet in creative exchange, and on the symbolical plane of inner reality woman can experience man as an inner creative partner. This represents the final stage of the coniunctio which leads to the birth of the divine child, the self. On account of the mutuality of relationship the experience of man is on this level, *mutatis mutandis*, identical with that of woman.

For both its clinical and theoretical importance I would like to mention here the close correspondence of the development sketched out by the dreams with that given by Neumann in his research on feminine psychology. He starts off with the primal relationship, the *Urbeziehung*, in which the infant is contained inside the "maternal uroboros" (Neumann, 1953, p. 4). He calls this phase that of "self-preservation" which is ended by the invasion of the "patriarchal uroboros" (Neumann, 1953, pp. 10–15). In my material we have first the containment in the inner room of the maternal uroboros; this phase of self-preservation is challenged in the ambivalence of the boar-dream. It is finally ended with the invasion by the impersonal numinous current. As next stage Neumann describes that of the patriarchate (Neumann, 1953, p. 26), which is expressed in my patient's material in the dream of the man making her aware of her feminine "Beauty". After this, according to Neumann, there follow two further stages; that of the "meeting", *Begegnung*, between two individuals, and that of "individuation", of inner realization (Neumann, 1953, p. 51). I prefer actually to see his two consecutive stages as the two aspects, outer and inner, of one and the same pattern of the coniunctio.

I would like to illustrate this final stage by a last dream, this time of another woman patient, aged fifty-three, who, in an analysis lasting over five years, had gone through an intense process of integration. This is the dream:

> I have just been married; my husband is a prince, wise, gentle, and loving. He puts a gold ring with an engraved flower on the third finger of my left hand. Then we are searching for ingots of gold which have been buried in a field. It is the royal treasure which has been hidden during times of trouble. We search a square patch of ground; at the edges we find nothing, but in the middle are the ingots of shining gold.

There is no longer invasion or inequality, but a loving relationship concluded under the sign of the "golden flower". It is consummated in the common search for the gold which had been hidden during the troubled times of neurosis. The treasure is found in the centre of the square temenos, varying the symbolism of the "jewel in the lotus" (cf. Jung, 1944, *Coll. Wks.*, **12**, p. 104).

To conclude, I want to sum up my material in terms of comparative patterns of the coniunctio, i.e. of the relationship between ego and non-ego. I began by describing the negative incest relationship which is in itself neurotic. In it a rudimentary ego is confronted with an overwhelming non-ego in projection on to a negative father. It is redeemed in the positive incest relationship in which a small but intact ego is confronted with a large non-ego in projection on to a positive father. In our case the negative incest situation had to be resolved through the transference on to the analyst. In the rape-dream the ego, which by now has become more stable and coherent, experiences the ambivalence of the non-ego in projection on the father-analyst. This dream marks the transition from the negative to the positive incest-fantasy. In the boar-dream the containment in the maternal temenos is realized in its relativity, and the ego faces the ambivalence of both female and male archetypal powers.

After that, in the experience of the current, an ego which is now intact can be confronted with the creative non-ego, at this point no longer in projection but as inner spiritual power. Here the incestuous claim on to the father-analyst is sacrificed and transformed, and we have reached the stage of what I would like to call the "internalized transference". At first, in the invasion by the "patriarchal uroboros", the ego is still only the passive, recipient vessel to the power of the anonymous non-ego; but with the next stage of the "patriarchate" a progressive approximation between ego and non-ego sets in. The coniunctio reaches its final pattern in the stage of individualized relationship and individuation. Here female and male, ego and non-ego, meet as equal partners of creative relationship.

## REFERENCES

FENICHEL, O. (1945). *The Psychoanalytic Theory of Neurosis.* London, Routledge & Kegan Paul; New York, Norton.

JUNG, C. G. (1944). *Psychologie und Alchemie.* Zürich, Rascher. Trans. *Coll. Wks.*, **12**.

NEUMANN, E. (1953). *Zur Psychologie des Weiblichen.* Zürich, Rascher.

# 11

## AN ANALYST'S DILEMMA

HILDE KIRSCH, *Los Angeles*

I WOULD like to share with you an experience which happened some years ago in my analytical practice. It occurred most unexpectedly in my work with a woman patient whose conscious personality was very undeveloped. Her dreams had the quality of inertness and repetitiveness. There was little movement toward ego consciousness.

The anamnesis of the patient is as follows: she is 48 years old, married, English by birth, and came to the United States as a child. She is one of seven children. Her parents are of English aristocratic background but without the financial means to live up to the desired standards. Her mother was experienced by the patient as duty-bound, cold, a sexually frigid woman, and a terrible nagger. She described her childhood as "awful", without any kindness or love from her mother. She felt unwanted in every way. The mother had the Victorian idea that all pleasure is sin. The patient herself was also sexually frigid and regarded sex as a mere duty.

Her father was, according to her experience, a kind and tender-hearted person, but completely dominated by his wife. The patient felt close to her father when her mother was not in the way. Mother's word was law.

An exploratory pelvic examination by her doctor revealed a double uterus and she was told she would never have any children, that childbirth would be fatal. When pregnancy did occur, she thought she would die. Actual delivery was difficult but uneventful. The child, a son, had a heart lesion and was mentally retarded. Therefore she felt herself to be a failure as a mother. A clinic report by a social worker, accidentally seen by the patient, stated that her son experienced her as "firm, cold, and rejecting". This was a terrific shock to her. Two days later she felt "electric shocks" in her head and lost consciousness for a brief time. Evidently a strong complex had been touched in her.

The family religion of her parents is Episcopal. The patient goes to church regularly and teaches Sunday School. She feels wicked, though, because often she has very negative feelings about religion, church, and the minister. Her husband is a devout Catholic, a fact which produced a tremendous amount of tension and argument between them, especially in regard to the religious upbringing of their son.

As a young girl, she loved to paint. When her mother suggested to her that she make some money with her paintings and show them in an art gallery, she stopped painting. She was 18 years old when this happened. She never touched a brush again until she had worked in her analysis for over a year. In my estimation the patient is a real artist, has imagination and a sense of beauty.

The patient suffers deeply from the fact that she has very little money. She lives with her family in very poor surroundings with cheap furniture and so on. Her husband is a night-watchman. He studied in a night-school, obtained a diploma but could not bring himself to apply for a job in his chosen field. He is truly living her negative counterpart, not realizing his potentials either.

In her first interview, she had terrific headaches which she described as if "something had exploded in my head". She did not always finish a sentence, though she was not aware of that fact. She could not see well, could not focus at all, which made it very difficult for her to get any kind of work. The money for her analysis was earned by menial work as a cleaning woman and baby-sitter. She charged only a very small amount for her services. The severity of her symptoms induced me to insist on a medical examination including an electroencephalogram, which turned out to be normal.

The patient was referred to me by the C. G. Jung Clinic in Los Angeles. At our monthly staff meetings it was my turn to present a case. The incident I am going to discuss occurred, which struck me as rather fateful. I hesitated about presenting the case of the patient I described above because she was rather boring. Very little had actually happened in her analysis, in her dreams and in her conscious life. Nothing touched her. She was like a record, repetitively telling me always the same stories. The animus of the mother was so overpowering that nothing changed in her. By now I had great doubt that anything basic would ever happen to her.

While I was weighing all these considerations, Mrs. X brought me the following dream:

> "Mrs. Kirsch had returned from Zürich. We were having our first interview again. She came to my house. All the blinds were up, the livingroom was bright with sunlight. We did not talk but sat and looked at each other, it was very comfortable. Mrs. Kirsch was at the door about to leave, when the clinic-secretary said that she could tell me how to get the cuticle off my fingernails and the bump at the base of the thumbnail. Mrs. Kirsch turned and said emphatically: 'I have tried hundreds of ways and they did not work on her.' I did not think she would tell people how hopeless I am."

She brought this dream at her first interview after I got back from a two-month stay in Zürich. The dream *coincided* with my decision to present her case in our Clinic. I felt I had failed to help her and I hoped that the group discussion would throw some light on the subject which I had been unable to see myself. Her dream shocked me very much. The whole problem of the authority of the unconscious was constellated. My natural tendency would have been not to present this case to the Clinic, especially as I also know the attitude of the Zürich analysts and Institute about not presenting any material of an analytic process which is not yet finished. But I found myself handling it differently. First I was wondering if her unconscious really caught my feelings about her analysis, and whether she experienced my attitude as a betrayal. As I confronted myself with this possibility I had to admit to myself that I *really* had given up hope that anything decisive could occur in her treatment. Then I wondered if I had made a mistake in not telling her that I was using her material for a case presentation. But something held me back and warned me against telling her. Next I compared this dream with her former dreams with regard to the transference situation. She had had many dreams before this one about her relationship to me. For instance she would dream that she could paint beautiful paintings but hoped I would not see them because then I would know that she could really paint. Or she would meet a man she loved very much, with whom she wanted to have a relationship, but she was afraid to let me know about it, because then I might expect her to do something about the relationship. I do not feel that her attitude derived from a negative mother projection on me but rather feel that I stood for a reality function for her. By trying to hide her positive capacities from me, she could go on being split. Secretly she felt herself to be very valuable. This she would not reveal to anyone, because it was her life source. It kept her young, infantile, and inflated, the puer æternus quality. To reveal this would have pricked her inflation and she was not willing or capable of sacrificing her secret in order to attain a fuller life. I was reminded of Jung's experience at Burghölzli, that some patients resented terrifically being taken out of their fantasy life. I felt, in the dream I just quoted, that the transference had changed into a positive one. It took place on a deep level since in the dream we could "sit in the same room, look at each other, did not talk, it was comfortable". It also occurred to me that it might even be of particular value to this patient that I bring her material to a collective body, the Clinic. It might help her to disidentify from the archetype and enable her to establish an ego relationship to the archetype.

As I reflected on all of this, a fantasy was developing in me. In it I was taking a steamroller and going with it through a brick wall, it was as if an ironlike barrier broke down and finally I could get to the other side. I was deeply stirred by this fantasy, because it happened autonomously, and I was grateful that it had occurred. I did not push it down again. When I confronted myself with it, though, I suddenly felt free to go ahead with the case presentation and prepare the material for the Clinic. I certainly did not expect the dramatic development that occurred to her as a direct consequence of my active intervention. In the very next interview the patient was completely changed. She looked happy and free. Her headache was gone; she could focus again. The hard brick wall that had always surrounded her had disappeared. Synchronistically things were happening in the outer reality as well. A very fine department store of the quality of Harrods in London had bought some of her trays, which she had painted in beautiful colours. She also brought the following dream to this interview:

> "I dreamt that I was in a dark house. There was a dining-room containing a table and chairs, a hall and a living-room, bare of furniture, all very dark rooms. There were other rooms in the house. I knew they were dark too, but the doors leading to them were closed. There was a very dark woman in one of the rooms. She did not like me. She had a youthful and beautiful son. She kept him with her. She did not allow me to see him or speak to him. It was my duty every morning to go out on the porch and look towards the ocean to see if the boat had arrived. It came every morning, a small skiff. It carried the Virgin Mary and the Holy Cross. She stood towards the back of the skiff, covered from head to feet by some heavenly blue diaphanous draperies. The Cross, about two feet high, stood in front of her covered with the same material. This morning I saw that the boat was in, it was a beautiful scene, everthing was a lovely heavenly blue. I went into the house and knocked at the door, opened it slightly and told the woman that the boat was in. Her son came out of the room wearing a grey hood like a clansman. He went to the boat and brought the Cross into the living-room. As I was placing the chair, I decided that this time I would turn the chair at an angle so that it would not face the doorway. The glory and radiance seeing the Cross all at once was too overwhelming for me and I thought it might be too much for other people too."

She was very touched by this dream, the first that ever reached her emotionally. The brick wall, which must have been the archetype common to both of us, was broken down with the help of my active imagination. I assumed from this dream that her brick wall must have been her English and Christian dogma, Victorian as well as Puritan, which did not allow her to know of the dark side of her instinctive nature. Therefore her whole darkness was projected out and she experienced nothing but darkness in her outer life.

Her animus was completely identified with these collective concepts, her own feelings were dominated by this animus. Now she saw in her dream that the dark woman has a beautiful son. It was not yet possible for the dark woman to contact her directly, but in this dream, the animus, the young son, appears in his positive form, he is the mediator between light and dark, he carries the Cross, the symbol of reconciliation of the opposites, into her house. The ritual of carrying the Cross into the house apparently happens every day and it is as if the unconscious is bringing the Cross to her a little at a time, so that she may get accustomed to the *tremendum* of having a genuine symbol of God and religion in her own inner house. She is aware of the numinosity and its danger which this Cross radiates. It is powerful and awe-inspiring, as every truly experienced archetype becomes. She places the Cross in an angle, upon which the sun does not shine. The Cross belongs here to the dark side in her house and brings enlightenment in this darkness. The Cross is needed by her for comprehension of the opposites in her, of the dark and the light, or the Mary figure and the dark woman. The duality is also especially expressed in this dream through the fact that the Cross is two feet high.

Synchronistically life brought the Cross into her house that same week concretely. Her husband asked for an interview with me. In it he told me that he had an illegitimate son older than their own son. He had carried this burden through his marriage, but he was not able to carry it any longer. He went home and told her about it. Her husband's revelation would have been shattering to her prior to the previously described experience, but in a most miraculous and mature way she was able to suffer the shock and to become more human herself through it. The far-reaching effect of such a synchronistic event is manifested as well in the break-through her husband experienced. He was moved to expose himself to his wife at a time when she was prepared for it.

The end of the first dream: "I did not think she would tell people how hopeless I am," had posed a dilemma. Would my decision to present her material hurt or help her? By means of the active imagination the unconscious wanted to impress on me a course of action, namely to force the exposure by presenting the case. It not only reassured me in deciding to proceed, but it also provided me with the energy, the steamroller, to go ahead in the face of this conflict. If I had acquiesced to her fears by not revealing her present state to the light of conscious scrutiny, she would have remained in darkness.

Many dreams followed which had to do with the problem of the opposites, light and dark, black and white. In one dream she was scrubbing the floor of my office which consisted of black and white squares. White marble became visible after she cleaned it; she was glad to do so and to share it with me.

I would like to add that she stopped analysis after the following dream: "She was walking on a wide and broad road leading on and on. The road was bright and left and right was darkness. But she knew that this road was her way, she was warned not to go off this road."

I am aware that I am exposing a personal experience in this paper. Never before have I used active imagination on any patient's material or problems, nor ever afterwards has this occurred to me. Therefore this was a unique experience to me. I reacted with an active imagination because the patient's dream caught my own unconscious thoughts regarding the obstacle in the analysis. It had the effect of breaking through the brick-wall barrier. I do not therefore think it is accidental that I have been presenting this experience again to an even wider audience.

# 12

## THE MAGICAL DIMENSION IN TRANSFERENCE AND COUNTER-TRANSFERENCE

EDWARD C. WHITMONT, *New York*

THE principle that the libido of the transference should be made accessible to the patient's understanding through interpretation has been practically axiomatic in analytical psychology. Confrontation with and interpretation of the unconscious material are considered the basic means to this end, even when immediate acceptance of the material is still impossible for the patient. Usually, indeed, such interpretation, either reductively or prospectively in archetypal terms, leads to a transformation of the projected complexes and thus to a severance of the transference in its essential aspects.

There are, however, instances in which a certain affective dynamism of the unconscious is encountered, most usually, but by no means only, limited to work with psychotics or near psychotics, in which the interpretative approach seems inadequate to the purpose.

The obligation upon the therapist to meet such situations by expressing in his response the patient's individual mode of experiencing, rather than his own normal and rational mode, has been described by Sechehaye (1955, p. 13) in her method as "symbolic wish-fulfilment, a substitution for blindly psychotic satisfaction of a fully conscious satisfaction of those fundamental affective needs whose lack of satisfaction keeps those needs ever aroused . . ."

But, actually, because "for the schizophrenic, the method of presymbolic magic participation becomes the sole means of expressing his needs and basic desires" (Sechehaye, 1956, p. 8),[1] what Sechehaye's cases demonstrate is more than mere satisfaction or wish fulfilment; it is symbolic experiencing, symbolic realization, a direct experiencing rather than rational understanding of symbolic images and events.

Some specific implications of this therapeutic approach, as they affect the analytical dynamism of transference and counter-transference, are the subject of examination in this paper.

The material that serves as our starting point derives from a patient with marked compulsive and paranoid traits. These appeared in the transference as ambivalent feelings of intense hate and fear and violent sexual demands. All were impervious to analytic interpretation.

1. *Fantasy:* "I am three years old and my father places me on the kitchen table and has intercourse with me, all the while teasing and being playful with me. I am enjoying it immensely. When we are through he straightens out my dress and warns me never to let anyone but him do that to me, or he will kill them, and I promise. And he says to my brothers and to the family that is gathered around, very sternly, never to do that to me or he will kill them and they resentfully have to promise because he is the boss and they are only his vassal-sons. He is the tyrant whom everybody fears but me he loves and tells me I will always have everything I want as long as I am a good girl (in the above way).

2. *Dream:* I am in the bathtub, soaking. My father starts to come in. "Not now, not now," I call out, as I do not want him to find me there in the nude. But he is coming anyway, he begins to hammer the door knob in order to break it. His action tells me that I cannot lock him out. He has a stubborn expression as if to say I will not get rid of him.

I am running the streets, hatred in my heart for not being able to get my independence from my father. I have a scythe-like instrument in my hand or a giant barber-razor with blade

[1]Since for analytical psychology a symbol is an image through which archetypal meaning can become accessible to understanding rather than a product of understanding or thinking, like a sign or allegory, we could call symbolic what Sechehaye calls pre-symbolic.

extended which I keep waving like a scythe. The feeling within me is murderous hate and the sweetness of revenge.

3. *Dream:* I was lying on my bed reading and pressing my clitoris as I read aloud each word. It was as if I were typing or marking the words somehow . . . rather than sexual play. However, by the time I finished the article, I had aroused myself sexually and felt I would need to gratify myself.

Dr. Whitmont lay down beside me. Perhaps he was persuading me to masturbate while he looked on and I did not wish to. He asked me why I resisted, when we both knew very well that I had desired for a long time to masturbate in his presence. I believe he had just about convinced me when I woke up.

4. *Fantasy:* I was nailed to a tree like to a cross. Growing out of my head was my father; out of my feet my mother, out of either hand each of my brothers; growing out of my arms, attached by his penis was my husband. I was nude and cried to you to save me. I was rooted to the tree and unable to move because of the above attachments.

You stripped and approached me with lascivious movements and both of us saying "the word" over and over again, had a lecherous intercourse; during the course of which the growths just seemed to disintegrate and vanish into nothingness like a fire smothered by chemicals. And I stepped forward, free, my inertia seemed to vanish and I found myself wide-awake, alert and in good humour.

The first fantasy and dream express the nature of the dreamer's psychological disturbance. An elementary force comparable to a brutish tribal chief, an uroboric father figure (in Neumann's terminology, a patriarchal uroboros) holds the dreamer's ego in incestuous submission. There is both lustful adherence to the regressive dependence as well as a fearsome inability to break free of the incest. Consequently, the animus (the brothers) cannot be contacted and interpersonal relationship is impossible. The resulting feeling of impotence and rage is projected as hatred upon the environment and along with incestuous sexuality, upon the analyst.

The second dream points the direction of possible development. The dreamer associates reading with learning, with striving for understanding, in short, with awareness. This awareness is to be realized by what is symbolically expressed as typing upon her clitoris, or masturbating in the presence of the analyst. This is an imprinting upon the instinct experience, an instinctual self-realization (masturbation) in the actual analytical relationship (in the presence of the analyst). Needless to say, the analyst was not inclined at any time to encourage or even permit such activity in the literal sense. He hoped for a solution by the traditional interpretative method, but in vain.

The last fantasy goes a step further and depicts what seems to be a sexual wish fulfilment; however, it takes the form of a symbolic sexual ceremonial. This ceremonial is carried out in terms of the analytic relationship—by the figure of the analyst. A liberation of the patient's attachment to the tree, the enslaving magical power of the collective unconscious, is thereby achieved. (It should be noted that the cross is also a symbol of Hecate) (Jung, 1952, *Coll. Wks*, **5**, p. 370).

In literal terms, or in terms of wish fulfilment, the assumed need for such a procedure would confront us with a highly doubtful proposition. In wider, symbolic terms—of symbolic magical participation—we may, perhaps, be able to find practical therapeutic implications.

Psychologically, the incest symbolism expresses the overpowering attraction of the unconscious, the regressive tendency towards the total involvement of the nascent ego in the ecstasy of the uroboros.

The figure of the uroboric father is a composite one. In addition to the patriarchal trend toward logos-discrimination, it encompasses the chthonic man, a uroboric, magical, primitive, phallic, nature-instinct being, an ogre or dragon, who holds the maiden in his thrall. He is the archetype of the primitive magician and corresponds to an early state of consciousness, characterized by adualism, compulsive domination through instinctual drives, affect, primitive power impulses, and infantile instinct gratification. The ego consciousness in this state is relatively undeveloped and still overshadowed by *participation mystique*, magical group and world identity. In the development of individual consciousness the height of this phase is reached at about the age of three or four. (In the incest dream, the patient is three years old.) This magical state is probably also characteristic of the primitive. When it emerges and overwhelms the more fully developed ego, we have a psychotic regression.

The term, magic layer of the unconscious, used to describe this psychological phase in a former essay (Whitmont, 1957), has met with some objection. The word "magic" is usually understood in terms of Webster's definition: "The art which claims or is believed to produce effects by the assistance of supernatural beings or by a mastery of secret forces of nature." In this sense the term implies a manipulation of force rather than a specific energy phenomenon, as such. "Magic" as used in this paper, however, refers to certain *phenomena*, physical and psychological, which have been recognized in one form or another in every past culture. It postulates them, hypothetically, as *expressions* of a *specific energy field*—another dimension of experience—underlying our tangible familiar reality.

Thus it refers to a particular and typical dimension of psychological functioning. Its expression takes the form of magical participation, synchronicity, magico-religious rites, and transformation phenomena. In short, we are investigating the objective field effect of *archetypal dynamis.* This is not merely primitive and regressively inferior; it can also, creatively, extend and widen consciousness.

In Jung's words (1954, *Coll. Wks.*, **8**, p. 211): "The archetype . . . as well as being an image in its own right, is at the same time a dynamism which makes itself felt in the numinosity and fascinating power of the archetypal image. The realization and assimilation of instinct never take place . . . by absorption into the instinctual sphere, but only through integration of the image which signifies and at the same time evokes the instinct." Realization of the archetypal image means to experience it as an "image of meaning" (*Sinnbild*), rather than to become immersed in and overwhelmed by its *dynamis*. It means splitting the total experience into a subject confronting an object, which thus replaces the phylogenetically earlier adualistic identity participation. Such a dualistic confrontation presupposes a certain minimum of ego strength and separatedness, of which neither the infant, the primitive, not the schizoid patient is capable. When the archetypal dynamism cannot be experienced as *comprehension* of image-*meaning*, it is experienced as image-*drive*, which directly and compulsively activates and brings into expression the dynamism of the meaning. The energy of the archetypal "field of force" (Heyer, 1949) which is not, or cannot be, assimilated by understanding, operates directly as effectual numinous affect happening. As *mysterium tremendum*, it moves, compels, awes, overpowers, and constellates urgency (Otto, 1952, p. 12). The phenomena of synchronicity would seem to show that it affects the behaviour not only of living objects but even of lifeless things.

It is of practical importance for the psychologist that, in form and substance, the workings of whatever fragmentary consciousness are encountered in this magical sphere, differ greatly from our accustomed mental processes. They have a reasoning of their own not devoid of logic but of a different logical frame of reference.

If a relationship between therapist and patient is to become possible at all, it is absolutely essential for the therapist to be familiar with the formalistic nature of this magical "thinking". Let us now attempt to trace out its essential characteristics.

## FORMAL CHARACTERIZATION OF THE MAGICAL LAYER

1. *Lack of Ability to Abstract.* Inability to abstract is a basic characteristic of the minds of the primitive, the infant, and the schizophrenic. All three share an incapacity to think in terms of general classes of things, that is, to formulate concepts. All three are unable to grasp a common denominator, a separate entity to be pulled away from individual things (Latin *abstrahere:* to pull away from). For instance, when asked to define "house", a schizophrenic answered, "There are all kinds of houses—nice houses, nice private houses . . . ." (Arieti, 1955, p. 211).

Since non-abstractive experiencing is *per*ception rather than *con*ception it is determined by qualities and activities or predicates (Arieti, 1955, p. 194), rather than by the subjects or objects that we postulate as the carriers of these qualities or activities. The experience is established not by "house", but by "nice" or "private". To our accustomed way of thinking, this is an experience of a partial aspect (quality or activity) instead of the whole; it is *pars pro toto*. While, from the intellectual point of view, this type of experience is merely fragmentary, actually it is more immediate, more emotionally stirring and—in a different dimension—much more whole than our own conceptualized experience. Since non-abstractive experience is concerned with qualities rather than objects, the interrelationships between objects (identities and differences) are based on their partial qualities, for example, of likeness and unlikeness, that is to say, on correspondence rather than on comparison of their abstract concepts. What matters is not the "it is" of identity, but the "behaves like" or "does like" of association.

Thus for a schizophrenic patient, Jesus, cigar boxes and sex were identical. The common denominator or quality which led to the identification was encirclement. The head of Jesus is encircled by a halo, the cigar by the tax band, and woman by the sex glance of the man (Arieti, 1955, p. 196). A young child also fails to differentiate between image representations and things. It will feed milk to a doll or to a picture. It will clamour for food by calling "Hot, hot," the quality not the concept. The most extreme expression of this associative thinking is, of course, the schizophrenic "word salad".

This identification by quality we are familiar with as a fundamental principle of magic (Frazer, 1948, p. 12). In the magical *pars pro toto*, the partial aspect of activity carries and conveys the mana, the effective power of the whole.

Of the greatest practical importance is the fact that owing to the lack of differentiation between image experience and what it represents, the symbol also "is" that to which, in our concept, it merely alludes. There is, therefore, no difference between a symbol and its meaning. The symbol activates, carries, and conveys the whole affective dynamism of that which it represents. The symbol is immediate, effective presence and happening.

"To 'participate' (magically) means to confuse, to fuse the symbol with the signified, the word with the thing it expresses, and the thought with the object" (Sechehaye, 1956, p. 146). Thus, in the magical world, to know, to be able to pronounce the right or real name, gives power over the object or thing which that name denotes. The word, the name, is imbued with mana, in fact the word "is" mana. It is the effective expression of numinous power.

Since abstracting is a distilling of a mental meaning from an emotionally and intuitively charged total sensory experience, it brings about a losing, a repressing of affect libido through conversion into thought. An "objective" mental, relatively harmless, affect-free concept is substituted for the subjective, affect-charged experience. Conversely, where the abstractive ability is absent, no such objectivization is possible. Every experience mobilizes the maximum of affect charge. The schizophrenic, the infant, the primitive, each lives in a world of highly charged affectivity, of intense emotional involvement in subjective happenings. There is no discrimination between what we would call essential or unessential details. Any occurrence, image, symbol, verbal aside, or word may mobilize the total libido.

Let us consider now the practical importance for the transference of these characteristics, remembering that the differences that exist in our own thinking between symbolic and actual experiences are invalid for a patient who functions magically. To such a patient the therapeutic situation becomes effective through the symbolic events and occurrences *themselves*, rather than through their understanding. What occurs in feelings, thoughts, actions, and images has a direct effect. In this sense the therapeutic situation is dominated and determined by the magical direct dynamism of archetypal meaning rather than by comprehension of this meaning. Interpretation may puzzle and confuse, or inject an (in practical terms) irrelevant factor, and therefore be even positively harmful.

On the other hand, verbalization has not only a cathartic but a magical effect. Not only has translation of the unconscious into a communicable language a redeeming effect (Jung, 1948, *Coll. Wks.*, **8**, p. 315), but saying the right word, as such, can have direct therapeutic efficacy. Furthermore, as we all know, saying the "wrong" word, even inadvertently, may have devastating results. What matters is the magic of the words themselves, and not our attempt to interpret their meaning.

The libido is activated by association and correspondence;

whatever is resolved or complicated in affectively charged symbolic activities is therefore dealt with, *ipso facto*, also in the corresponding psychological dynamism in a like corresponding fashion. This refers as much to artistic or fantasy activities as to any acted-out or abreacted symbolic experiences. The therapeutic situation becomes a magical oneness, a telepathic identity, in which a symbolic drama of transforming effectiveness is enacted. This is borne out by the fact that also the form elements typical for telepathic functioning can be demonstrated.

2. *Telepathic Identity*. The mana field level is closely associated with telepathic or synchronicity phenomena. Jung has drawn attention to the fact that the occurrence of synchronicity phenomena is associated with intense affectivity as well as with the involvement of archetypal dynamism. In its symptomatic formalism, the magical dynamism is analogous to telepathic phenomena in the "scatter" phenomenon (Ehrenwald, 1948, p. 60). Both the percipient in spontaneous cases of telepathy as well as the schizophrenic tend to miss what we would call the central idea of a concept. They score "near misses" scattered around the fringe of the central idea. They fail to differentiate the essential from the accidental, the real thing from the symbolic representation (Arieti, 1955, p. 261; Ehrenwald, 1948, p. 69).

In drawing attention to the sensitivity of heteropsychic material of the schizophrenic to telepathic invasion, Ehrenwald mentions that these telepathic phenomena usually fail to occur when one's attention is focused upon them. They tend rather to manifest themselves when the observer is off guard and unprepared to pay attention; they are found scattered to the fringes of consciousness.

Moreover in telepathy also *pars pro toto* holds true, as an experiment mentioned by Ehrenwald serves to illustrate. An attempt was made to convey telepathically a picture of an airship moored in an aerodrome. The percipient drew merely a number of ladders leaning against the wall. His telepathic copy was a reproduction of the lateral supports of the aerodrome, and omitted the more essential parts (Ehrenwald, 1948, p. 62). The part was substituted for the whole.

These facts serve to draw our attention to the operation of

telepathic identity between analyst and patient whenever the field of energy of the archetypal numen is contacted. This telepathic identity is constellated in direct proportion to the absence of conscious attention and awareness. The analyst's unconscious fears, thoughts, hesitations, anxieties, and repressions become his patient's; in turn, the analyst is subject to psychic infection by the patient's complexes, fears, repressions, and anxieties.

Where the analyst is blocked in himself the patient will remain so too, the best professional knowledge notwithstanding. Whatever the analyst resolves in himself when the psychic infection makes him confront those problems of his own that had hitherto not been constellated, may thereby and simultaneously be resolved in the patient. In fact, in situations of this sort, sometimes the only way to elicit a therapeutic effect may be through confronting one's own corresponding difficulties, without having to explain or interpret anything about them to the patient.

3. *Subjectivity of Motivation*. The magical, primitive, infantile and schizophrenic mentality does not differentiate between causation, willing, responsibility and guilt. In this realm of non-objectivity, of lack of abstraction and division between subject and object everything is still "as though" subjectively determined. Underlying everything there are not objective causes but subjective motivations that have to be dealt with by taboo and ritual. To the primitive, "natural causation is a mere semblance and not worthy of mention" (Jung, 1949, p. 151). Whatever happens is said, felt, done, or experienced, has been willed by "them", "the others", or by a "power" and, when introjected, by the patient himself or, in therapy, by the analyst. In everything and anything there is seen a sign, an omen or intent, pregnant with some unknown meaning. Symbol and concrete reality are not differentiated; thus everything, even the most trifling objects and occurrences are like symbols, charged with mana and secret "meaning".

Consequently, any attitude, gesture, or remark of the therapist may appear deliberately aimed at the patient with some unknown or ominous intent. If the analyst does not participate in the patient's impulses, in his attempts to react, in order to try to establish contact between them; or if the analyst interprets instead of reacting to such attempts, or reacts "wrongly", it may produce the same effect on the patient as deliberate, wilful rejection. To be rejected, in turn, means that either the patient or the therapist—or probably both because they are magically identical—is "bad". This promptly results in self-condemnation and violent hostility to the analyst.

4. *Taboo and Ritual.* The instinctual response to the overwhelming anxiety-evoking power of mana and numen are taboo and ritual. Taboo is a sense of interdiction that becomes a compelling rule and compulsive automatism. "Either that which is taboo is holy and to be feared as the seat of mystic supernatural power . . . or the object is unclean and therefore taboo lest it infect man with its own evil nature" (*Encyclopaedia Britannica*, 1955, 21:732). Thus in the taboo, the opposites are still treated adualistically as equivalents. Taboo is passive interdiction to avoid guilt and danger; ritual however is activity, an established, efficacious formula which propitiates, affects, worships and reconciles mana and numen. Thus ritual has a transformative effect. Both, taboo and ritual, are of compelling necessity. They are determined by an autonomous, impersonal formalism which cannot be altered arbitrarily without loss of effectiveness. But whereas in taboo man is merely passively *exposed* to the compelling mana anxiety, hardly aware of himself as a self, in ritual he begins an active confrontation. Thus he opens the way to an awareness of "I" versus "thou", to transformation and relationship. Ritual thus constitutes a forward step. Historically-collectively as well as personally in the individual development it is the form through which the libido strives toward consciousness. A ritual happening arises from the unconscious spontaneously when the magical compulsiveness is to be overcome.

Every habit and obsession of the schizoid patient who is under compulsive taboo anxiety is like an inevitable law or a moral interdiction that he dare not, indeed feels forbidden to, transgress (Sechehaye, 1956, p. 40). For the therapist to question or overlook the taboo is useless, dangerous, and conducive to anxiety reactions. The road to freedom is over the ritual drama, and one may anticipate its emergence, even though often only in fragmentary or perfunctory form, at this phase of the analytic development. Ritual elements occur spontaneously as expressions of inner archetypal necessity; they are not willed or planned for by either patient or doctor. Their contents are archetypally not arbitrarily determined.

A therapist who is aware of these tendencies may further the transformation through an understanding participation. Whenever such conscious readiness is lacking, the inner necessity nevertheless prevails. But then the ritual "happens" in a relatively primitive and compulsive fashion. Dramatic incidents taking the form of irrational eruptions may not be recognized in their archetypal meaning by the patient, of whom one cannot expect it anyway, nor by the doctor. As rather awkward incidents they lead to confusions and recriminations, in transference and counter-transference, particularly in view of the primitive sexual character of what is likely to emerge on this level.

5. *Infantile Sexuality*. As outlined in more detailed form in an earlier essay (Whitmont, 1957), the developmental phase akin to the magical state is passed through during the first few years of life in the relatively space-time-less telepathic instinctual identity with mother and surroundings. During this period occurs the preoccupation with what Freud called infantile or pre-genital sexuality. The first measure of self-control and self-consciousness is gained as a first step towards that mysterious experience called "I" by establishing awareness and control of those automatic functions which, in the form of nutrition and excretion, mediate the relationship between the adualistic subjective state and the objective world of "being" and confrontation. The primary awareness of the instinctual drives is centred upon the body orifices, mouth, anus, and urethra.

The transition from magical taboo to ritual confrontation thus also occurs through primitive body symbolism. This fact explains the abundance of oral and excretory symbolism in psychotic fantasies as well as in primitive magical rites and customs.

Orality expresses dependence, clinging to support and protection, by grasping, taking hold, absorbing, contacting, and experiencing in identity (the mouth is the first organ of perception).

Anality, the first function brought under conscious control, represents the first victory over instinct automatism; it is the first primitive experience of choice and relative freedom. Thus it expresses self control, self-assertion, defiance, and aggressiveness. As primitive power egotism it represents power magic *par excellence*.

Freud did not define the urinary preoccupation clearly. I believe that it coincides with what he termed "phallic" as distinct from "genital" sexuality (Freud, 1949, pp. 29, 30). In both sexes it represents the experience of an outpouring active energy stream.

In primitive magic urination represents creative fertilizing mana conveying health, love, blessing, strength, and salvation. Rain is the urination of the divinity; salt and yellow colouring are added to holy water. As a drive outward of near-eros quality it marks the turning point from the subject-centred, basically egotistical, adualistic attitude of orality and anality to the thou-directed outgoing development which leads eventually to dualism and relationship in "genital" sexuality.

However, the actual point of transition is the masturbatory phase. Although masturbation is still a self-centred narcissistic activity, it marks the experiencing of one's own body as a "thou"; the body, in fact, substitutes for a "thou". At this point "I" and the world are still one but their dichotomy has begun. "Atum who indulged himself in Heliopolis, took his phallus in his hand in order to arouse pleasure. A brother and sister were produced, Shu and Tefnut" (Neumann, 1954, p. 19). Out of the encompassing one there arises the two in the masturbatory symbolism. When that dualistic experience of I and Thou, myself and world, subject and object is reached, the magical all-identity is overcome. Thus sexual symbolism is relationship symbolism. And masturbation expresses that final point of transition from "incestuous" adualistic participation to the relative freedom of dualistic consciousness. Masturbation "imprints" into the genital sexual sphere what was originally the evolving consciousness of oral and excretory symbolism.

Only now may we be able to interpret our patient's dreams and fantasies. They show that she cannot free herself alone from the "incestuous" involvement in the magical field, her defence by means of "taboo" and her compulsive rigidity are inadequate safeguards against the threat of psychosis (the father breaks her door in). Liberation may be accomplished through the symbolic typing on the clitoris, masturbating in the presence of the analyst and through the tree ritual—primitive instinctuality imprinted into genital sexuality. Thus autistic adualism may give way to dualistic confrontation and relatedness; taboo confinement may be transformed through a ritual-like experience arising from the analytic relationship (symbolized in the person of the analyst).

The implication of the ritual is, however, still puzzling. Referring, as it does, to the analytic process itself we ought to have a better comprehension of the elements which compose such a non-interpretative liberation through the transference relationship.

A dream from a later stage of this development helped the analyst's orientation:

"I was seeking rest and tried to find it in a cemetery among wire structures like crutches for amputated limbs. But that took my breath away. Then I saw a red pencil-like thing on the ground. There, with that I could find rest."

To the wire structures the patient associated clothes hangers, to that "red pencil-like thing" a phallus or a sort of small live creature. The obvious implication of the dream is that freedom from the compulsion is to be found not in the spirit-deadening suffocating atmosphere of persona crutches but in the red phallic dwarf, who, as a pencil may help to "inscribe" (this is analogous to the earlier "imprinting").

In my paper previously referred to, the importance of the phallic dwarf as the archetype of the magician was discussed. He is the personification of the first masculine consciousness principle, the son of the chthonic great mother, both opposed to her as well as mediating between her and the patriarchal world of heaven and spirit. Positively constellated, he leads out of the dangerous magical world, negatively constellated as trickster power demon and devilish goblin, he confounds, confuses, and leads to regression.

A specific form of the phallic dwarf in folklore as the little "red" man is the "alraun". And in the alraun ritual as described by H. Rahner (1945) we find specific "instructions" for transforming the magical demon from a dangerous fiend into a helpful guardian and protector against the dangers of the magical field.

"The little red man that sticks in the ground cryeth out: *Juva me et juvabo te*. That is a right alraun's cry and calling; make sure that thou tiest the root onto the dog's tail and then at once get thee away' " (Rahner, 1945, p. 201).

While still in the ground, the alraun or man's root, the mandrake, is under the power of Hecate and her evil demons. It is the source of sleep confusion and love madness. Extracted from the ground by means of the proper ritual (otherwise it kills), it becomes a source of deliverance, a protective talisman against the evil Hecate and thus a pharmacon of peace. Resembling a man without a head, it waits to be crowned with the head of Christ. Finding peace with the alraun "pencil" thus may be equivalent to gaining deliverance from the magical tree to which the patient is "rooted".

But one must know the proper ritual way to extract the root.

In the extraction ceremony all initiative and activity seem to come exclusively from the rhizotomist who in practical therapeutics probably is represented by the analyst. This is a one-sided situation compared to our usual conception of the therapeutic relationship as a partnership undertaking in which both sides have to exert their utmost efforts. Of such an active effort, however, the mana imprisoned person, particularly the psychotic or near-psychotic, is incapable. He is affixed, rooted, to the maternal tree, the magical mana field. His ability to communicate and to enter into a relationship with others and with external reality is impared, even though this has to be looked at not merely in the purely negative sense of loss, but rather as "an impossibility on his part and on our own to meet: the modes of existence of one and the other no longer coincide" (Sechehaye, 1956, pp. 25, 26).

The initiative must, obviously, shift to the therapist, at least temporarily, with the purpose of establishing a more equal partnership situation as the goal of the "rhizotomy".

However, a minimal involvement, a minimal participation of at least an unconscious, partial instinct aspect of the patient is indispensable if anything is to happen at all. And this limited participation of the patient seems to be expressed in the requirement of the extraction ritual that a "helper" has to dance around the plant and should murmur as much as comes to his mind of aphrodisiac things; the analysand has to help by verbalizing associatively whatever irrational elements the instinct pressure brings up.

In a dream coinciding with a particularly violent obsessive phase, the patient found relative peace and freedom through dancing a minuet, a stylized ceremonial dance. In dream No. 3, this irrational minimal instinct participation seems expresssed through the acts of typing on the clitoris and masturbating before the analyst. All these symbolic expressions further the development of consciousness. The primitive instinctual (excretory magical) nature of what these verbalization or abreaction phases may bring out is furthermore emphasized by the injunction to pour urine or menstrual blood upon the plant.

The helpful and protective character of these primitive expressions, when allowed into the therapeutic relationship, is also emphasized by the fact that the "helper", through his aphrodisiac dance, actually creates a fourth circle around the three which the rhizotomist, prior to the extraction, has to draw around the plant according to the ritual with an iron sword. The therapist's discrimination (the sword) forms a protective circle of understanding and discretion around the patient's expressions. As in a *vas alchymicum*, the libido is concentrated within the trustworthy insulation from the outside, which protects, by means of absolute discretion, whatever happens or is expressed in the privileged situation of the therapeutic meeting. The therapeutic meeting thus becomes almost a laboratory of existential transformation. But the dance of the involvement and of the participation of the patient's, albeit primitive, instinct reaction makes for an existentially real quaternio-wholeness of not merely the four circles but also of the four active elements of the process, namely, plant, dog, rhizotomist, and helper. Thus, the symbolism makes it apparent that it is the transforming power of the self that is invoked within this sheltering temenos of the magical circle.

The extraction has to take place at night; then the plant shines like a lamp and is easily found. This nocturnal light is obviously analogous to the *lumen naturae*, the instinct vision of the unconscious. The bright daylight of rationality does not help sufficiently to find the way to effective disentanglement from the enchanting power of Hecate. Good and sensible rules for dealing with the transference are of as little help, when rigidly adhered to, as any good advice. In this phase of darkness we have to rely upon the knowledge of our own instinct, which "knows" even though we are ignorant.

Nevertheless certain rules and precautions must be observed.

One has to face west to the seat of Hecate. In undertaking an active therapeutic involvement with the magical force field one has to face up to the risks one incurs. Only through full awareness of the dangers, both to the patient and to oneself, of being overwhelmed by the affective contents evoked, can the "consent" of the "mistress of those below" be gained. West is also the direction of the setting sun, of the *descensus ad inferos* of death and sacrifice. The "consent" of Hecate who, as the nether psychopompos represents the regenerating power of death (Graves, 1955, pp. 31-2) depends upon the readiness to forego, to sacrifice one's personal wishes, prejudices, and desires to the demands of the opus. This again is emphasized in the dog sacrifice.

The wind has to be guarded against. There is danger of psychic infection. The complexes that have not yet been consciously extracted may activate the analyst's own corresponding predispositions, predispositions which otherwise may have remained dormant. Also, this is a warning against identifying with "hunches" or intuitive convictions (of "smelling" this or that). Such premature diagnostic convictions are likely to be contaminated by the unextracted and, therefore, projected complexes and power drives, of analyst as well as of patient, merged now on the unconscious magical participation level. Especially when one is particularly sure that one "understands" the situation, it becomes most important to watch one's own dreams and fantasies for warning signals.

At the moment of actual extraction, one must hold one's ears tightly shut to protect oneself from the ghastly cry of the alraun. This is a warning against "forbidden compassion". The actual confrontation with the psychotic layer may impose sufferings upon the patient which can shatter the analyst's firmness. The counter-transference may take the form of compassionate and erotic feelings. As such, they may be unavoidable and even indispensable, as we shall see. But they may unconsciously involve the analyst and make him lose his ability to give a direction based upon his objective view of situation and goal. Then the alraun's cry kills. The analysis collapses.

First, the root has to be exposed by digging out the earth around it. The covering inhibitions and repressions have to be removed from the root-problem and from the affectively charged complexes. As far as the patient is concerned this demand is self-evident, provided it is at all possible. Since the symbolism stresses it, however, we have to consider this demand as it applies to the analyst himself. He ought to realize now what in himself has been called forth, as anxieties, resistances, aversions, or attractions and instinct drives, through the leavening effect of the concentration and interchange of affect libido within the magic circle. The essential nature of his share of the root, his counter-transference and its meaning, has to be consciously exposed to his consciousness before his libido may be used to "pull out" the root. What the analyst can accept only hesitatingly in himself may well point towards the corresponding or complementary problem in the patient. Dealing with his own resistance, he may help free the patient of his!

And now the plant may be extracted by tying it to a black dog's tail. It is the dog who, obeying the call of the rhizotomist, who has to step back, pulls out the plant. The dog is the animal of Persephone and Hecate, the dark side of the moon, complementary to the light aspect of the lapis, the shepherded aspect of the logos and the man's familiaris (Jung, 1955, pp. 27, 31, 143, 160, 162, 163, 291.) It separates the living from the dead and carries those aspects of the personality which are felt to be essential (ibid. p. 167).

The dog represents the *potentiae sensuales* (ibid, p. 161). As Cerberos, who guards the door of Hades, and Actaeon's dog, who tears his master to pieces, and also as the dog whose bite robs man of consciousness, it represents the dangers of the unconscious when it is neglected or improperly approached (ibid, pp. 170-1). "The Great Goddess . . . is a dog because of her promiscuity in love and because she is an eater of corpses; in her honour, as lovely Iris and Astarte, her initiates wear dog masks and in her honour, as deathly Hecate or Brimo, dogs are sacrificed where three roads meet" (Graves, 1946, p. 240).

Thus, the dog represents the paradoxical contradiction of our instinct world: sensuousness, desirousness, promiscuity, the potential ability of discernment, of realization, the destructiveness of anger, rage and aggressiveness. In transference and counter-transference it is this irrationality of the ambivalent level of drives, with all its dangers and potentialities, that becomes activated. In our special situation, in which the initiative rests with the analyst-rhizotomist, the "dog-forces" are to be sought primarily in the counter-transference.

Thus, it is the therapist's libido involvement, whatever in him becomes activated as *potentiae sensuales*—his drives, desires and impulses—which pulls out the root. Not professional skill but the risk of instinctual involvement effects the extraction. This is possible only, however, when the dog obeys the call of the rhizotomist, that is, when it is not identified with, but harnessed to, the analyst's conscious "call". As the guardian of the underworld of Hecate, the driving force of the counter-transference is not to be trifled with. It is helpful when faced and related to properly, but destructive when, through lack of awareness of its implications and its "magical" power, it holds us in compulsive sway. This is indeed a *cave*, a "beware of the dog", for anyone; it is particularly so for the beginner whose relationship to the demons of his own unconscious has not yet been sufficiently tested.

Finally, the dog has to be sacrificed in the man's place. It is the Great Goddess's, not ours. Although the involvement is personal, it is not meant for personal satisfaction. The therapist has to differentiate between himself and the dog, between his affect nature, which has to be sacrificed to the transpersonal value and to the objective needs of the patient, and the transformation mystery that encompasses both therapist and patient. The fact that the dog is a substitute offering for the rhizotomist emphasizes the fact that, psychologically, this differentiation between oneself and the affective content of the counter-transference and its dedication to the opus are the ultimate protection against falling victim oneself to the dangers of the unconscious.

The same motif is also expressed in the injunction to carry the root pointing downwards, to the earth, the great mother, to whom it is dedicated. Even when we have accomplished a difficult therapeutic step, we may not pride ourselves by considering it our own accomplishment. The therapist's inflation would soon result in a serious analytic setback.

The mandrake ritual mirrors one aspect of the individuation symbolism. As an inner happening, the individuation process is a confrontation and coming to terms of ego and self. But the self, as the wholeness of everything that does and will belong to one's life, encompasses also the meeting and contact with world and "Thou". Thus, also in the therapeutic meeting, the individuation problem may be constellated for patient and analyst with like meaning, albeit on different levels of awareness and maturity. The analyst especially may find his individuation problem constellated when he has to deal with transference and counter-transference. "The doctor knows—or at least he should know—that he did not choose his career by chance; and the psychotherapist in particular should clearly understand that psychic infections, however superfluous they seem to him, are in fact the predestined concomitants of his work, and thus fully in accord with the instinctive disposition of his own life" (Jung, 1946, *Coll. Wks.*, **16,** p. 177).

Thus, the individuation symbolism of the mandrake extraction applies not only to the individuation process in general but also to that special aspect constellated in transference and particularly in counter-transference.

## SUMMARY AND CONCLUSION

When the magical dimension is constellated, the therapeutic happening is determined by the direct effects of words, gestures, actions, and emotional attitude, particularly of the therapist and especially through the therapist's sufficient or insufficient conscious understanding and accepting insight into his own affect responses. The analyst's awareness and acceptance have to fill in what the patient still lacks of those qualities on this level. The patient's improvement is brought about not so much by his understanding, for which he may lack ability, as by synchronistic magical telepathic correspondence. Liberation from the magical entanglement evolves from taboo to ceremonial rite; from infantile primitive, via masturbatory, to genital sexual symbolism; from adualistic *participation mystique* to dualistic confrontation and relationship.

In this phase the transference cannot be effective therapeutically by appeals to reason or understanding or merely by symbolic wish fulfilment. What has been characterized as symbolic "rhizotomy" takes place. When the therapist is able to understand, accept, and consciously participate symbolically in the "extraction ceremony", the archetypally determined primitive ritual elements arising spontaneously may become factors that promote consciousness through "symbolic realization". The therapeutic relationship is thereby akin to an experimental alchemist's laboratory, in which compulsive dynamism is converted into stepping stones toward consciousness.

From the therapist this process requires a high degree of consciousness, emotional integrity, and strength, where his own instincts and affects are concerned, for unavoidably they are bound to be aroused as counter-transference. He must be capable of using the counter-transference as a therapeutic sense organ and tool without himself becoming bewitched by, or identical with it. The counter-transference imposes on him the enactment of a role similar to one in an initiation drama.

The "root of madness" is at the same time the "pharmacon of peace" and "symbol of divine love", according to the myth. It represents the archetypal field of the "divine healer", in whom illness, suffering of the physician, and healing are one. In this sense, transference and counter-transference may be likened to a therapeutic illness, the "imprisonment by the god" in the therapeutic ritual (Meier, 1949, p. 100).

Through awareness that the therapeutic meeting as well as therapeutic effort and result, transference, and counter-transference are subsumed in this archetypal field, the healing tranformation is channelled, *Deo concedente*.

## REFERENCES

Arieti, S. (1955). *Interpretation of Schizophrenia*. New York, Robert Brunner.

Ehrenwald, J. (1948). *Telepathy and Medical Psychology*. London, Allen & Unwin; New York, Norton.

Frazer, J. G. (1948). *The Golden Bough* (abridged ed.) New York and London, Macmillan.

FREUD, S. (1949). *An Outline of Psychoanalysis*. London, Hogarth; New York, Norton.

GRAVES, ROBERT (1946). *King Jesus*. London, Cassell; New York, Farrar, Strauss, Cudahy.

GRAVES, ROBERT (1955). *The Greek Myths*. Vol. 1. Harmondsworth, Baltimore, Penguin Books.

HEYER, G. R. (1949). *Vom Kraftfeld der Seele*. Zürich, Origo.

JUNG, C. G. (1946). *Die Psychologie der Übertragung*, Zürich, Rascher. Trans. "Psychology of the Transference", *Coll. Wks.*, **16**.

JUNG, C. G. (1948). *Über psychische Energetik und das Wesen der Träume*. (2nd ed.). Zürich, Rascher. Trans. "The Psychological Foundations of Belief in Spirits". *Coll. Wks.*, **8**.

JUNG, C. G. (1949). "Archaic Man". In: *Modern Man in Search of a Soul*. London, Routledge & Kegan Paul. To be published in *Coll. Wks.*, **10**.

JUNG, C. G. (1952). *Symbole der Wandlung*. Zürich, Rascher. Trans. *Symbols of Transformation*. *Coll. Wks.*, **5**.

JUNG, C. G. (1954). "Theoretische Überlegungen zum Wesen des Psychischen". In: *Von den Wurzeln des Bewusstseins*. Zürich, Rascher. Trans. "On the Nature of the Psyche." *Coll. Wks.*, **8**.

JUNG, C. G. (1955). *Mysterium Coniunctionis*. Vol. I. Zürich, Rascher. To be published in *Coll. Wks.*, **14**.

MEIER, C. A. (1949). *Antike Inkubation und moderne Psychotherapie*. Zürich, Rascher.

NEUMANN, E. (1954). *The Origins and History of Consciousness*. Bollingen Series 42. New York, Pantheon; London, Routledge & Kegan Paul.

OTTO, R. (1952). *The Idea of the Holy*. London, New York, Toronto, Oxford University Press.

RAHNER, H. (1945). "Mandragore, die ewige Menschenwurzel". In: "*Die* seelenheilende Blume". *Eranos-Jb.* **12**. Zürich, Rhein-Verlag.

SECHEHAYE, M. (1955). *Die symbolische Wunscherfüllung*. Bern, Stuttgart, Hans Huber.

SECHEHAYE, M. (1956). *A new Psychotherapy in Schizophrenia*. New York, Grune & Stratton.

WHITMONT, E. (1957), "Magic and the Psychology of Compulsive States". *J. analyt. Psychol.*, **2**, 1.

# 13

## THE RESISTANCE TO CHRISTIAN SYMBOLISM IN THE PROCESS OF PSYCHOLOGICAL DEVELOPMENT

RENÉE BRAND, *San Francisco*

This paper is an attempt to show the particular kind of resistance which Christian symbolism produces when a certain point in analysis is reached. I have observed this in both Christian and Jewish patients, so I assume that the problem is independent of the traditional Christian and Jewish views. I have to limit myself to one case illustrating this resistance.

The analysand is a Jewish woman in her thirties. She is married and has a two-year-old child. She has been in analysis approximately six years, with frequent necessary interruptions. As usual, the earlier phase of the work, which cannot be discussed here, dealt with problems of ego, sex, parental fixation, interpersonal relations, and with the relevant factors in the personal unconscious. The present material points to the necessity of a transition to a new psychological level.

The patient has a quick, sharp intelligence and grasp of her material, a good sense of humour, and works with intensity and dedication. She is an engaging and colourful person who easily overdramatizes her affective reactions. She has a powerful, often destructively self-critical animus.

She had been a performer with a promising but unstable career, showing the usual picture of intermittent success and failure, and lacking in security. Nevertheless, this career had given her a channel for her creative animus and her ego drive, and had supplied her with a well-defined and satisfying social-professional status. Her identity had been in this status.

While she was committed to pursuing her career, she also

wished for a full feminine experience of marriage and children, and had hoped to combine both. This seemed impossible after her first child was born, as her work had always been so engrossing, its importance so inflated, that she had no libido left for anything else. She felt she had to make a choice and decided to give up the career rather than allow it to threaten her family life. This decision left her with a deep conflict.

She soon found that her former professionally established identity became unreal, and she felt more and more like a mere appendage to her husband and child. Her demands on her marriage grew, as it now seemed to be the only source of fulfilment and meaning. But her husband was busy establishing himself in his profession, which demanded much of his libido. Over a period of four years, she found her marriage increasingly unrewarding, since it failed to compensate for what her career had offered. She criticized her husband for his lack of relationship, she felt left out in his circle of friends, and had lost touch with hers. There was no outlet for her animus, which demanded expression. Her husband is an introverted thinking type, while she is an extraverted feeling-intuitive, which posed additional problems between them.

She has always found it difficult, even before her marriage, to keep connected with the inner process and with her introverted feeling. Neurotic depressions have occurred regularly, characterized by loss of feeling and resultant emptiness and anxiety. Now these depressions are blamed on the marriage.

At the time of the dream series presented here, she was again in a period of depression, more severe than usual, as she was three months in her second pregnancy and found that her marriage was deteriorating. The pregnancy had not been planned; it was an accident. The expected baby was unwanted, as she had been thinking of a divorce.

I have selected several from a series of dreams occurring within a six-week period, and am focusing on a recurrent motif connected with the problems outlined and their potential solution.

> Dream: "I am standing in line waiting for two passports. Only one is available. My husband advises me to take the one, as the second is being worked on. I am carrying my child

while waiting and find that my husband is given three quarts of skim milk; the fourth quart of whole milk has to be waited for."

The dream implies the journey. The passport identifies the ego as she ventures into unfamiliar country. The second passport would presumably be for the other, new aspect of the ego. She carries the child; therefore the ego may be conscious of her responsibility for the new development. The husband as animus has three quarts of the nourishment for the child. The fourth is natural whole milk, untampered-with by the ego; it is still in the unconscious. The ego and the animus are co-operating towards the new development. The symbolism of the three and the one making four will occur again later.

Dream: " I and my husband buy separate cars."

This disidentification from her actual husband indicates that in her personal life she can now move under her own power on the external collective level, instead of being carried along as an appendage to her family.

Dream: "I am putting on a larger-size brassière, such as I buy when I am pregnant. It is still too large."

On the objective level, this dream gives an answer to the initial rejection of her pregnancy and marriage; on the subjective level, she is beginning to acknowledge her maternal feeling.

Dream: "I am inside a protected area. It is rectangular in shape; on three sides is a low stone wall. The fourth side is made up of a rectangular low stone house. There is a collective group of women and children in the area with me. There were men and women and children on the outside. A fight is going on. The people on the outside are throwing rocks at us, and we are throwing them back. A couple of them hit me with some impact. I don't like the fact that children on either side might be hurt. I sympathize with the mothers."

Her association: "He that is without sin among you, let him first cast a stone." (John viii, 7.)

The dream and associations suggest that she is recognizing her own animus aggression when criticizing her husband and his friends. Her feeling of guilt is expressed in a Christian context. This is the first emergence of Christian symbolism. But the basic conflict about Christianity comes up at the same time: she also sees the rock-throwing as anti-Semitic attacks, and Christians are blamed for not heeding Christ's teaching. The place where she begins to deal with the conflict is four-sided and implies the self. Her sympathy with the mothers against the animus is a protection for her newly developing feminine ego.

Dream: "I am in a New York hospital. I give birth to a hermaphrodite infant. I am heart-broken. I call the analyst and ask that she help me cope with the problem, for I feel helpless. The doctor asks what I want to have done with the child. At first I tell him to kill it or give it away or put it in an institution. I can't handle the responsibility.

Then I look at my husband, and I know I can't do any of those things. That I would lose something of the best part of me if I did. That this is what life has given me, and I cannot run from it."

This dream shows a first intimation of the organic duality of her feminine and masculine sides, which she cannot accept. She needs the analyst to help her cope with this problem, since the first reaction of the ego and of the extraverted collective mind is to try to annihilate the new insight. The introverted animus makes her accept the responsibility for this new life. This dream is a correction of the idea that she can turn herself into a one hundred per cent feminine mother-woman. She has to remember her duty to both sides, the masculine and the feminine. What her ego cannot achieve or accept, the self may accept. The image of the hermaphrodite again suggests the symbol of wholeness which we refer to as the self.

Dream: "My face breaks out. Then I walk out of prison."

She interprets the skin trouble as caused by an over-balance of female hormones in pregnancy. The new feminine development opens the door of her imprisonment by her neurosis.

> Dream: "I am in a car and being smashed in the face and body. There were two physical jolts, which I felt and which awakened me."

A sudden traumatic realization of her whole system of collective adaptation and power breaks in on her. This occurs after her husband states that her animus demands and criticisms are the major cause of their estrangement. The dream also gives a warning about a possible somatic involvement when it speaks of the two physical jolts. The patient actually had an ante-partum haemorrhage at this point, perhaps caused by too much activity in the unconscious and too much emotional turmoil, plus the intensity of the whole experience. This actual threat to her pregnancy was a turning-point. It changed her attitude. She now wanted the baby and also the marriage. Finding herself powerless and confronted by fate she had a deep emotional reaction, almost like a religious conversion.

These are her statements about it:

> "This made all discussions about the marriage working or not working academic. It had to work. It was as if the unconscious had said, 'Let's cut out the nonsense; you have no choice; you go this way.'
>
> "If the child is saved and born, it will always seem to me to be golden. Isn't that what the alchemists created out of dross? It would be a symbol of what happened here to me. If I lose the baby, it will make me very sad, but at least it won't have been created in vain.
>
> "So here is the self, and it says to me: 'You were so frightened of me that you wouldn't let me come to you. Perhaps this was the only way you would let me come, and that is why I had to do this to you.' The self appeared in the image of Christ. Now I will bear whatever happens."

Next dream: "The analyst and I are working. There is a shadowy girl in the room with us. Suddenly a blue glass rectangular tray appears in my hand. I say: 'Is it? Is it really a mandala?' I hold it up to the light. It is like a blue stained-glass church window. There is an image of Christ, and also one of the analyst. It is very beautiful. Then lots of children appear. Somehow the glass mandala breaks apart. It disintegrates quietly like a kaleidoscope."

The analysand had a somewhat euphoric expectation in this dream. It could be the hope that the analyst or the transference would solve her problem. To have the purely human, the analyst, in the same framework with the archetypal image points to a confusion. It may be helpful here to elucidate the state of her transference: she had earlier projected the parental complex and the self on the analyst. About three years prior to the phase of her analysis presented here, the transference had been analysed to the extent that the personal parents became differentiated from the analyst, so that I, as the analyst, became a more real and human figure to whom she could relate in a personal way, and my function became that of a helpful guide on her journey. Seeing the Christ image and the analyst together would imply the phase of her transference which needed to be analysed at this time.

The glass mandala is first something to be handled, a tray, which is utilitarian, and then looked at, something to be contemplated, like a stained-glass window. In this case, it is an ego-made aesthetic concept of the mandala and the Christ. The shattering of her expectations was necessary to make room for a more real experience, including the suffering and sacrifice implicit in the Christ image and left out in this smooth and brittle representation.

In an enantiodromia, the analysand then brought up her resistance to Christianity and the Christ symbol, probably contained in the shadowy girl in the mandala dream just quoted.

She stated with much affect: "I am Russian Jewish. I cannot change that any more than I can change the colour of my skin.

> I carry fear and dread of Christianity in my bones. It is the product of centuries of persecution and suffering. My father and father's father, etc. I cannot dissociate Christ from the later development of Christianity. Christ seems to stand for the individual conscience, yet in a Christian world the emphasis is on Christian law and conformity."

This incapacity to distinguish Christ from organized Christianity describes the obstacle to an acceptance of the original Christian teaching[1] which I mentioned in the beginning. The formulation of her commitment to Judaism resulted in a clarification of what she called her "Jewish roots". It emerged that she had a rather collective attitude, based on the need to defend herself against anti-Semitic attacks. In our discussion she realized with some surprise that she, too, was chauvinistic (was throwing rocks) and that her Jewish shadow contained intolerance of Christians and Christianity, together with an inflation of belonging to the "Chosen People", even though she had no knowledge of her cultural Jewish heritage.

In analysing the resistance of Jewish patients to Christianity, I find that in the individuation process, the essence of Christian experience and values has to be integrated, as a step toward wholeness. I am not making this demand but merely observing that in many cases their unconscious or self makes it in bringing up Christian symbolism recurrently and with insistence, as we see exemplified here. In trying to understand this curious insistence, I have thought that their resistance suggests the exclusion or repression of a fundamental spiritual experience of Western man in general.

The patient agreed that she needed to establish a relation to the Christ image as it was coming up from her own unconscious. But her resistance remained. In my experience, resistance to the figure of Christ in both Christians and Jews brings into focus a

[1]By "original Christian teaching" I refer to the psychological aspect of the essence of Jesus' teachings, as well as to the essence of the original psychological experience underlying the formulations of the Christian dogma, as interpreted by C. G. Jung (cf. Bibliography). This is to be distinguished from present-day "organized Christianity", referring to the various religious systems structured by the official Christian churches—collective institutions which for many individuals no longer provide direction or answer for their religious need.

more general spiritual problem, and the unconscious then produces compensatory material, often containing the rejected Christian symbolism.

All of the following is one long dream about this problem. I shall interpret it step by step, including the patient's associations.

> Dream: "It is a quarter to seven and not yet daylight. I am walking alone. I see my ex-husband, a rabbi, coming towards me. I just keep going on my way."
> Her associations: "The number seven indicates that this is a religious dream. I married my first husband, a rabbi, to find some sort of Jewish roots. But he wasn't rooted himself and was a limited, rigid, patriarchal figure."

A vicarious connection with Judaism through an animus whose patriarchal power attitude was unacceptable cannot help her to deal with her problem. She leaves such a possibility behind and goes on her way.

> Next episode: "I am prevented from crossing the street by a political parade. A beribboned car passes. In it are two politicians. They are lobbing the conversational ball back and forth between them, trying to impress the populace. It is all too silly and on an infantile level."
> Her associations interpret this episode clearly enough. She says:
> "Political parade would have to do with my collective Jewish intolerance of Christians and Christianity and my inability to dissociate the figure of Christ from the subsequent political and religious development of Christian churches. The lobbing of the ball back and forth is like the discussion we had about this, and my superficial attitude."

> Next episode: "I dart across the street; I go to Central Park. It is still barely dawn and ordinarily one wouldn't go into the park at such an hour. It would be dangerous."
> Her associations: "Central Park at dawn is a place of threat and danger, like a jungle. One would not go there at that hour; one risks one's life."

This is the place in the unconscious where her central problem is to be met. She risks herself by going there, although her ego might be attacked.

> Next: "I go two levels below the street, and there is a landing, rectangular in shape."

She proceeds down from the collective street to the cultural level of her unconscious, and lands at her destination. The four-sided place and Central Park both indicate the centre, the place of possible integration.

> Next: "A drab, poor woman dressed in brown is sitting on a bench at the left, as I approach. She is very respectable and dreary. She has come from the parade. She says, referring to the two politicians: 'They ought to do something about the places for the poor.'"
> Her associations: "This woman probably has to do with the poor that Jesus talked about, who are always with us." (Matthew xxvi, 11: "For ye have the poor always with you, but me ye have not always.")

*Interpretation.* She confronts her shadow. The drabness, dreariness, and brownness of the shadow represent the lack of a vital connection with instinct and indicate the negative earth principle, perhaps materialism. The shadow makes a humanitarian request: that the politicians should do something for the poor, thus falsely limiting the problem to a sociological, rational solution, and, because of the materialistic attitude, failing to see the real problem, the "inner" poor.

> Next episode: "The drab woman indicates a filthy old man who is sitting on the bench opposite her. He is ragged and encrusted with filth. He, too, wears a brown coat. He is like the dregs of humanity. While she is the respectable poor, he is the disreputable poor, beyond the pale of society, the outsider, 'the least among you'."
>
> "The man says, 'They ought to do something about the small animals.' I then really look at him. He is sitting on the

right-hand bench. Strewn on his lap are three dead rats, and one dead grey rabbit.

"I then see that his head is veiled by a cloud of gnats. They are all over his head, and in it, and in his nose and his eyes. At first, it looks to me like a halo. Rather than being horrified and running, which is what I would ordinarily do, I feel great compassion for him. The analyst says: 'This is Christ.' We decide to call someone to help him."

Patient's association: "The ragged man is unquestionably a Christ figure, probably having to do with my own inability to accept either a Christian kind of redemption or any redemption at all."

Perhaps I should mention that the patient interprets my attitude towards her shadow, her suffering, and guilt feelings as specifically Christian. Her positive image of Christianity is connected with tolerance and acceptance, and it was an important experience in her analysis to find her shadow accepted before she was asked to take responsibility for it. This may, in part, explain why it is the analyst who states that this man is Christ.

*Interpretation.* The man sits on the right side, opposite the shadow, indicating the corresponding masculine aspect of the problem. The brown coat of the man has the same depreciatory implication as that of the shadow. The image represents the neglected spiritual principle, the negative, materialistic animus of the patient. She admits that there is a deeper problem even than her conflict about Christianity, when she speaks of her incapacity to accept any kind of redemption, Christian or otherwise. However, her thought that this is "unquestionably Christ" paradoxically expresses the necessity for a specifically Christian redemption.

Through the analyst, the unconscious has stated that this man *is* Christ, but this statement seems to be contradicted by the description of a filthy old man. As I see it, the patient's negative concept of him must be transformed in order for him truly to *become* Christ. In this context, Christ may be interpreted as a process of sacrifice and suffering which produces spiritual transformation in man. For the patient this process started with a filthy, suffering old man, sitting on a park bench. The association to "the least of men" refers to Matthew xxv, 40—"Inasmuch as ye have done it unto one of the least of these, my brethren, ye have done it unto me." It is possible to see behind this "least of men" the process of transformation the patient needs to go through so that the archetype of the self as Christ will appear.

> Her associations to the animals on the man's lap: "Rats: the lowest, most vicious and most dangerous of the rodents, everywhere, disgusting, frightening.
>
> "Rabbits: fruitful, harmless, loved by children, Easter and resurrection symbol, also make good food. This section of my dream would indicate my problem with Christianity."

*Interpretation.* The four dead chthonic animals indicate that the matriarchal unconscious is cut off and needs to be reanimated.

According to Neumann (1955) and Layard (1942), the rat is a chthonic animal connected with the terrible great mother. It carries the ruthless, but necessary, instinct for survival and also has an aggressive phallic implication.

The rabbit is a "domesticated" form of the hare, an archetypal moon symbol, containing both the fecundating force and the sacrifice, and carrying the idea of redemption on the chthonic level (Neumann, 1955; Layard, 1944). It represents the fruitful powers of nature belonging to the chthonic world, in contrast to the harmful chthonic powers, the rats. These negative and positive symbols are found together on the man's lap in correspondence with the order of nature. The matriarchal unconscious does not make the distinctions that man makes. It accepts all living creatures, and only through patriarchal consciousness do we project positive or negative qualities.

*Three* rats indicate a kind of chthonic trinity, the negative great mother in her threefold aspect. *One* rabbit represents the uniting principle, associated with the positive lunar cycle, the idea of wholeness represented as one. This is a recurrent motif; there were three quarts of skim and one quart of whole milk, as here are three rats and one rabbit. The idea of the three and one is universal symbolism, pointing to the concept of redemption and wholeness.

The ragged old man says, "They should do something for the

small animals." "They" would refer to the politicians in the same way the shadow referred to them just previously. The men who run things should develop compassion. Patriarchal consciousness is projected onto this figure, showing that the analysand is still thinking in over-rational terms. But obviously "they" do not help. Only an individual act of sacrifice and suffering can bring redemption.

If the miracle of reviving the animals comes to pass, this would be distinctly different from the traditional Christian attitude, which excludes and depreciates animal nature. Through the man's request, the analysand's unconscious compensates and corrects the earlier Christian attitude in favour of a contemporary one which we owe to Dr. Jung and which becomes available through analytical psychology.

The cloud of gnats represents a disturbance in the autonomic nervous system, attacking consciousness and obscuring the true nature of this image. When there is a major crisis in the individual's life, a dual possibility presents itself, either of a uniting religious symbol giving new meaning to one's life—in this case the halo around the head of the man—or of being overwhelmed by the collective unconscious. The possibility of healing and unification had been glimpsed by the analysand when she first saw the halo, anticipating a possible transformation of this negative image. But the immediate dissolution of the halo into a swarm of gnats seems to make the transformation impossible.

In contrast to the earlier dream of the smooth, idealized glass mandala, the analysand now participates genuinely in the suffering and feels compassion. There are two moments in which the ego acts in a responsible and authentic way: first, when she really looks at the ragged man with the dead animals on his lap, and next when, instead of being horrified and running away from the swarm of gnats in and around his head, she feels compassion. Compassion leads to her recognizing the need for help and change. These are two individual acts: looking at the problem in order to become conscious, and feeling compassion. This is her charity and help, given to the least of men, and therefore to her own transformation.

The following dream episode, occurring the same night, shows a different picture:

> Dream: "I am in a beautiful field. There is brilliant sunlight. There are many beautiful children around. Then I meet the parents of the children. They are themselves beautiful. I ask the mother how come she has had so many children, so quickly. She says that they are Catholic. She had become converted when she was ten years old. She had had dreadful parents, and a brother whom she adored. At a certain point he had been converted to Catholicism, and in order to be with him she had become converted, also. She is extremely happy."

The associations brought up several significant experiences at age ten: a Christian servant secretly took her to church and she was so moved that she wanted to become a Christian. Fear of her mother's scorn prevented her. Paradoxically, she also had a traumatic anti-Semitic experience at that age which indirectly involved her brother, who is several years younger and for whom she had maternal feelings. A much older and threatening girl had challenged her to a fist fight which she took on, rather than risk the possibility that her small brother would become the victim. Her terror was so great that she has never stood her ground since then. This attack and a series of similar experiences cut her off from her deep feeling and its spontaneous expression, and her self-preservative instincts became paralysed. These experiences were at least partly responsible for the four dead animals and the threat of dissolution by gnats of the figure referred to as Christ.

It is understandable that the complex of anti-Semitism became activated when Christian symbolism appeared in her dreams and associations. The catharsis of relating these conscious but never verbalized experiences worked toward a resolution of this complex. She felt "as if a boil was breaking".

The patient's potential for a rich development with a catholic, that is, an all-embracing, universal attitude and a spiritual centredness is portrayed in the Catholic family with the many children on the beautiful, sunlit field.

> Next episode: "My girl friend, a singer, appears. The Catholic family wants her to make a recording for them. Soon I hear a most glorious voice coming from upstairs. She tells me that

she was taught to sing by a Russian man. It is beautiful Russian church music."

Her association: "This girl friend is a singer. But she likes most to sing for herself; for her, it is true self-expression. Russian music is part of my heritage, connected with my father. I respond very emotionally."

*Interpretation.* In this episode her introverted feeling which had been cut off, expresses itself (glorious voice singing) in relation to the Christian spirit (church music), and including her Russian Jewish heritage. It seems that she is on her way toward resolving her anti-Christian and anti-religious conflicts so that she will eventually develop her own spiritual values. This solution is indicated in a subsequent dream where she has a four-year-old blond brother, whom she is washing in the sink. This little brother she is taking care of represents wholeness and spiritual value, and may be a symbol of rebirth.

As pointed out by Neumann in his interpretation of the Psyche myth (Neumann, 1952) and in his article on "The Moon and Matriarchal Consciousness" (Neumann, 1953), it is necessary for the modern woman to reach below the patriarchal layer of the unconscious and the corresponding superimposed patriarchal animus in order to find a connection with the matriarchal unconscious. In the case of this analysand, the matriarchal unconscious was paralysed. The block was caused in part by these traumatic experiences and by painful contents inherited in the cultural unconscious. But the negativity of her personal mother, this mother's lack of earth connection, and her resulting anxiety were important contributing factors. The cut-off instincts in the lap and the damage to the head of the man in need of redemption, i.e. healing, are two aspects of the same problem. A transformation through feeling seems to promise a solution on both levels, the instinctual and the spiritual. While the resolution of her resistance was not yet achieved at the time of this dream, and while the dream has to be seen as compensatory to her conscious attitude concerning the problem with Christianity, her feeling did become available.

The point was made earlier that the difficulty for Jewish analysands in accepting Christian symbolism is part of a more general picture. In Christian analysands, the personal and cultural layers of the unconscious may contain an equally negative resistance to organized Christianity. The puritan preacher of childhood memory, the Sunday School teaching, the dogmatic and inhibitive parent all block the path. Similarly, we find the inaccessibility of the matriarchal unconscious, the cut-off, inactive instincts, and the refusal to relate to the spiritual principle as Christ. The historical and cultural reasons for this phenomenon may be different in Jews and Christians, but the results are the same. Many Christian analysands also reject Christ, and in most cases Christian symbolism becomes acceptable only when it is possible to integrate the repressed pagan contents.

The analysand of the dream series presented here had the same resistance any semi-conscious person has to becoming integrated and to accepting the life of the spirit. Everybody has the problem of sacrificing the supremacy of the ego to the self, and compliance with this request is only possible after all other ways out of a painful and threatening dilemma are barred. That suffering and pain and sacrifice are necessary aspects of human existence is not acceptable in this phase of resistance, and perhaps not even recognized as a premise. The erroneous modern equation of life with happiness, and of suffering with undeserved punishment may explain this attitude. The quest for happiness or pleasure, as a modern ego demand, makes it difficult to understand that the self may not be interested in happiness or unhappiness in human terms. The extreme picture of this Christ image in Central Park with the dead animals and the dissolving head is conditioned by individual neurotic factors. But beyond that it may accurately describe the suffering of Christ in our time, that is: the general collective neglect of the spirit.

## REFERENCES

Jung, C. G. (1948). "Versuch zu einer psychologischen Deutung des Trinitätsdogmas" (Chapter IV), in: *Symbolik des Geistes*. Zürich, Rascher. Trans. "A Psychological Approach to the Dogma of the Trinity". *Coll. Wks.*, **11**.

Jung, C. G. (1951). *Aion*. (Chapter V). Zürich, Rascher. Trans. *Coll. Wks.*, **9**, 2.

LAYARD, JOHN (1942). *Stone Men of Malekula*. London, Chatto & Windus.

LAYARD, JOHN (1944). *The Lady of the Hare*. London, Faber and Faber.

NEUMANN, ERICH, (1952). *Amor und Psyche*. Zürich, Rascher. Trans. Bollingen Series 54, New York, Pantheon; London, Routledge & Kegan Paul.

NEUMANN, ERICH (1953). Über den Mond und das matriarchale Bewusstsein", in: *Zur Psychologie des Weiblichen*. Zürich, Rascher. Trans. "The Moon and Matriarchal Consciousness", in *Spring* 1954. New York, The Analytical Psychology Club.

NEUMANN, ERICH (1955). *The Great Mother*. Bollingen Series 47. New York, Pantheon; London, Routledge & Kegan Paul.

# 14

## *FROM SCHIZOPHRENIA TO ART*
## *EXCERPTS FROM A CASE-HISTORY*[1]

HEINZ WESTMAN, *New York*

### THE CASE OF JOAN

"THE patient is on the borderline of a psychotic break which, should it occur, would probably be manic and severe in nature. There is evidence of marked paranoia and of being a split personality from early childhood."

Joan, the patient referred to in this summation by the testing psychologist, was nineteen years old at the time, the second of three daughters of parents of the middle class. Her father is a store-keeper, her mother a good housewife. Honest, well-meaning people, they were hopeful that Joan, like her sisters, would grow up healthy and happy, have a good job as a stenographer and marry quickly. After high-school, because she had a talent for drawing, she was registered in a commercial art school, but she did not go to classes. She ran away and roamed the countryside, came back to the city and lived like a derelict for nearly two years. When she appeared at the psychiatric outpatient department of a New York hospital she was, as the psychologist's report indicates, in very grave distress. She looked strong, she was well and solidly built, but she was shabby and dirty and she was wholly withdrawn; she had unusual facial mannerisms, a one-

[1]It has not been feasible to present in this publication the whole of this case-history, with the patient's sixty-two drawings. The complete case is presented as a portion of Mr. Westman's book, *The Springs of Creativity* (Atheneum Publishers, New York 1961).

sided smile, for example, which scarcely moved her lips, and her eyes were blank.

Joan was given a battery of tests. She rated 109 on the verbal scale, 113 on performance; her arithmetic score was very low. No evidence emerged of hereditary factors in relation to mental illness. Speaking of her parents during an early interview, Joan said she did not believe they loved her "beyond the sort of love one gives to something one owns". Later, her mother admitted having had difficulties nursing her from the beginning. Joan described her father as cold but intelligent. When he was told that his daughter had a remarkable artistic talent, he answered, "All what I got in her is a crazy artist, eh?"

She was asked during the testing period to draw a picture and she replied that she was an art student and so whatever she drew would be "just art". Coming from someone in deep depression, this was a highly significant reply and the decision to attempt to treat her by psychotherapy hinged upon it. It meant she thought she had to justify her interest in art by always drawing pictures the world would call "artistic", but it meant also that she somehow knew better, that her real need was to use her gifts in her own way, as she must, according to her own nature, never minding whether the picture turned out to be "art" or not.

One of the pictures she drew while undergoing the test was that of a woman in the rain (*Plate* 12); in referring to it, she said, "It's obvious as hell. She is obviously lost .... you could tell that."[1]

The difference between Joan's second drawing (*Plate* 13) and her first is immediately obvious. The first could not have been drawn by a psychotic patient; neither, in fact, could this, but it shows that she is perilously close. It is as though she had held onto herself just long enough to draw the woman in the rain in that disciplined, terse, economical way, and then, having found in the psychotherapeutic situation a mite of hope, simply let go. The line is shattered. The atmosphere is stark and menacing;

[1]Joan was seen during the first six months of her analysis for one session per week at the hospital. After that period she was treated weekly in addition to her visits to the hospital for one analytic hour at my private office. The portion of her analysis presented here covers a period of just over one year. In order to show the time elapsed between each stage of her development, the exact dates on which the drawings were made are printed next to the number of the plate.

the imagination is in chains. The drawing shows the direction her vital energies have taken and what she is going to suffer: it is a rendering of the first hesitant step into psychosis. The diagnosis of the testing psychologist is justified. There is not only great danger of a lapse into a severe catatonic state, but in a subtle sense that lapse has already taken place. Her hope is in the blades of grass and the flower. As biological symbols they are the only signs of life and they serve as a kind of point-of-view for the whole drawing, making it a rendering of an experience rather than simply the gifted scribblings of a girl *mentally ill*. They are symbolic of what remains of her shattered personality, that frail means by which up to now she has been, however wretchedly, related with existence. That she could draw them gave some hope for the re-establishment and growth of her personality.

To think of schizophrenia in terms of its etymology ("split-mind") is not very helpful. The psyche is, to some degree, always *split*, in the sense that it is a complex of energies and inertias variously conditioned and directed, released and dammed up, unused, unsuspected, repressed. Precisely as our cellular energies are directed toward the orderly and harmonious realization and functioning of the physical organism; precisely as cosmic energies work toward the harmony of the universe, the energies of the psyche in its ontogenesis work toward order, harmony, and wholeness. Neither in the physical organism nor in the universe nor in the psyche is there a discoverable *centre:* in all three the integration is ineffably mysterious. We can really only talk about the *means toward* that integration. As far as the psyche is concerned that *means* is personality by which man is related with the world and with the dynamics of his being. In mental illness this is what breaks down. In schizophrenia the various aspects of the personality split away from each other in radical dissociation that may exhibit many shades and gradations and may be quite systematic or wholly unsystematic. Joan's third drawing (*Plate* 14) pictures critical dissociation of the unsystematic kind. She draws herself in depression and utter bewilderment, holding her head in her hands in a posture exactly descriptive of the catatonic state threatened in *Plate* 13. Everything around her is out of joint. Outside, separate from her vision of herself as consciously depressed, weird figures grow one from the other, and strange shapes crowd into the scene with no hint of system or design. But on the head of one of the figures the blades of grass reappear.

Often during the schizophrenic process, depending upon the degree of severity, it happens that energy is channelled into a part or parts of the psyche and a kind of autonomy is established; a part rules the rest and the patient lives an aspect of his humanity as if it were the whole. In Joan's case, the figure throwing stones in *Plate* 15 is symbolic of a part of the psyche which intends to rule the rest. It first appeared in her childhood; here, at a very early stage, it re-emerges to become a kind of companion, accompanying her in many disguises throughout her treatment. Destructive, obstructive, negative, resistant, the figure as drawn is a realization of the archetypal shadow. Powerful as it appears to be and literally is, it is, by curious paradox, the product of the inertia inherent in the psyche which thwarts the personality in its growth. In the most subtle way, it is that inertia itself which is active here, presenting itself to the imagination in a symbol of power which is the very obverse of its nature. It is true that our most energetic and powerful actions are often no more than the products of our primal inertia and as such they are invariably destructive to the personality.

Joan wrote on the back of *Plate* 15, "the Descent". She was right. Her energies have turned downward or backward to the beginnings of the psyche (*Plate* 16), to that original state which is neither "dreaming innocence" nor "Paradise" but *chaos in simultaneity*. Everything is potential here, nothing is actual, nothing human, except in that it is *all* human, a picture of the primal ground (*Urgrund*) before, so to speak, the Word was uttered. She places herself within this chaos as the central figure at the bottom of the picture, and deepens the sense of what she said about the "woman in the rain": "It's obvious as hell. She's obviously lost."

Joan was not, when she drew this, *remembering;* it is not a matter of recapturing the past. As far as the psyche is concerned, time is the least of things. The original state is eternally present, it is the ultimate foundation of the instant, the locale within which we experience the timeless.

"When above the heaven had not (yet) been named
(And) below the earth had not (yet) been called by name;
(When) Apsu primeval, their begetter,
Mummu (and) Tiamat, she who gave birth to them all,
Still mingled their waters together,
And no pasture land had been formed (and) not (even)
a reed marsh was to be seen;
When none of the (other) gods had been brought into being,
(When) they had not (yet) been called by (their) name(s),
(and their) destinies had not yet been fixed,
(At that time) were the gods created within them."

*Enuma Elish*, Tablet I, 1–9

The *Enuma Elish* (Heidel, 1951) contains a great deal that is important in the understanding of Joan's case. It is apparently the earliest Babylonian creation myth, a kind of *Ur*-myth, and it is as directly concerned as is the *Book of Genesis* with the origins and growth of the psyche. Its dramatic motifs are prototypical of much that is familiar to us in other myths of other peoples.[1]

The primal ground, as Joan draws it, is analogous to that described by the Babylonian poets. The waters are still mingled together; the primal force is undifferentiated; there is no sexuality. The experience in the Garden ("And they saw that they were naked") has not taken place. There has in fact been no "seeing", no action on the basis of that *presupposition of our humanness* by which we enter the primal realm on our own terms in order to understand ourselves through ourselves. This is the true *original* human situation. It has nothing to do with conflicts between matriarchal and patriarchal culture patterns; such rationalizations may be useful to anthropologists and to some social psychologists but they remain "analytical" approaches to the deepest human experience and have next to nothing to do with it.[2]

Inherent in the original human situation is the original conflict, the conflict between the force which strives toward wholeness and, thus, toward creativity, and the inertia which strives to maintain chaos and thwart creativity.

[1]Not that the *Enuma Elish* is being considered here as the one, original source of these motifs; rather, what it deals with is a universal experience which it renders in symbols that seem to be inherent in us as archetypal patterns of individual development.

[2]Readers familiar with Erich Fromm's *The Forgotten Language* will see quickly that the following reading of the *Enuma Elish* is in diametric opposition to Fromm's.

"Apsu opened his mouth
And said to Tiamat in a loud voice,
By day I cannot rest, by night I cannot sleep;
I will destroy (them) and put an end to their way,
That silence be established, and then let us sleep!" Tablet I, 35-40

Apsu is crying out against the gods, his first-born, who have been disturbing "the inner parts of Tiamat, moving and running about in divine abode (?)" (*Enuma Elish*, Tablet I, 23–24). What the poet is really talking about here is his own experience of the primal conflict; the cry is the cry of his own inertia and it is very important that the father, Apsu, is made to utter it. Again and again the poets have chosen the negative parent as a symbol for inertia and they have symbolized the conflict between that inertia and their own creativity not as a situation of "love" between son and mother, but as the act of parricide. What is true of the other great pagan mythological dramas is true of the *Enuma Elish:* love as *motive* is non-existent.

When Tiamat heard Apsu's cry,

"She was wroth and cried out to her husband;
She cried out and raged furiously, she alone.
She pondered the evil in her heart (and said):
Why should we destroy that which we ourselves have
brought forth?
Their way is indeed very painful, but let us take it goodnaturedly." Tablet I, 42-46

But Apsu, like Cronos, went on plotting the murder of his children, only to be murdered instead by his son, Ea, as Laius was murdered by Oedipus. Then, like Jocasta, Tiamat took her son Kingu as her husband.

"She gave him the tablet of destinies, she fastened (it)
upon his breast, (saying):
As for thee, thy command shall not be changed, (the
word of thy mouth) shall be dependable." Tablet I, 156-157

The tablet she gave her "unique spouse" gave him the power to create reality by the spoken word. Then, to avenge Apsu, she got ready for war against his children. Marduk, her son, came forth as their champion. He had already proved to have, out of himself, out of his own individuality, the power the tablet of destinies was supposed to confer on Kingu.

"Thy power and authority, O lord, shall be supreme among the Gods.
Command to destroy and to create, (and) they shall be!
By the word of thy mouth, let the garment be destroyed;
Command again, and let the garment be whole!
He commanded with his mouth, and the garment was destroyed.
He commanded again and the garment was restored." Tablet IV, 21-27

Before the battle Marduk spoke to Tiamat, his mother, in a way very familiar to psychotherapists:

"Why dost thou act (so) friendly on the surface,
While thine heart is plotting to stir up strife?
The sons have rebelled (and) maltreat their fathers;
And thou, their bearer, hatest mercy." Tablet IV, 77-80

Tiamat lost the battle, Marduk killed her, and then:

"He took from him (Kingu) the tablet of destinies,
*which was not his rightful possession.*" (my italics). Tablet IV, 121

He assembled the great gods and asked:

"Who was it that created the strife,
And caused Tiamat to revolt and prepare for battle?
Let him who created the strife be delivered up;
The great gods answered him:
Kingu it was who created the strife,
And caused Tiamat to revolt and prepare for battle.
They bound him and held him before Ea;
Punishment they inflicted upon him by cutting
(the arteries of) his blood.
With this blood they created mankind." Tablet VI, 23-35, 29-33

The Babylonian poets probed to an astonishing depth into the human situation. They differ from the poets of the *Book of Genesis* in that they could not conceive of a time when there was *nothing but God* and had, therefore, to set down their experience in terms of cosmic events; nevertheless, from the psychological point of view, their work is not only one of humanity's earliest but one of its most valid efforts to reveal the way of the psyche in its ontogenesis. Apsu and Tiamat symbolize the primal state, the chaos of the potential. Kingu symbolizes that mode of action of the psyche through which it identifies itself with and depends wholly upon parental images. In him the Babylonian poets anticipate by some four thousand years Freud's hypothesis (i.e., identification with parental images as evidenced in the Oedipus complex), which is now taken to be "scientifically" proven. Kingu is, however, more than this: he is an extension of the Apsu-inertia motif and the poets rightly condemn him to death but, most significant of all, they knew mankind was created from his blood, knew, in other words, that what he represents is an inherent part of our nature. Marduk is a symbol of personality: in him as an ideal the poets anticipate that means by which the psyche becomes creative of its own accord. His destruction and re-creation of the garment by the power of the Word alone is symbolic of his individuality and of his independence. His battle with Tiamat is a dramatization of this independence and a testing of the power he demonstrated in the incident of the garment; his victory was certain before the battle started, but it was necessary that the psychic "fact" be experienced in the world of action. The signal difference between Marduk and Kingu is that the latter is guilty of hybris, that "overweening pride" which is truly an idolatry of the ego, and it leads him to accept from his mother what is not hers to give nor his rightfully to take. Behind his hybris there is the more "original" sin of inertia by which he depends upon a parental image for an identity whose power is symbolized in the tablet of destinies. Inertia often shows itself and its influence in modern life in such a symbol as this. It is original "sin" in that it thwarts the ontogenetic purpose of the psyche, hampers the development of personality and thus thwarts creativity and leads us to fail the Creation of which we are a part.

Marduk conquered himself and won the power of creativity and proceeded to impose order in the primal chaos. This divine act of creation is the poet's image for his own experience, for what he himself went through when order first came into the chaos of his beginnings, when, out of the inevitable conflict between the creative forces within him and the inertia that is their natural counterpart, he glimpsed in the order of the cosmos the possibility of order within himself and the hope of wholeness.

The conflict between creativity and inertia, this fundamental problem of our existence, is resolved in a markedly different way in the *Book of Genesis.* The key to the later, more radical and human resolution is in the idea of the One God and man's most intimate relation with him. There is no parricide in the Jacob-

Esau legend and there is no "identification" with the mother; there is rather the opposite. It is through the blind father's blessing and the mother's willingness to take a curse upon herself that the personality of the son is urged forward into action and, thus, the psyche urged toward wholeness.

The meaning of the *Enuma Elish* is directly apropos to Joan's case. She wrote a message on the back of *Plate* 15: "Don't feel a thing, am in an ugly mood now. Something has got to change. . . and soon . . . very, very soon. I will die this way. I am too lonely."

There is nothing lonelier than the primal realm of Apsu and Tiamat, and few descents are more dangerous to undertake. But there is another way to look at this picture: hesitant, tentative, even dim, it is, nevertheless a view from a different angle of the sacred precinct. This is not by any means an image of an experience suffered solely by the schizophrenic. In a very real sense, every artist "descends" in his own way, to varying depths depending upon his inner strength, into the primal realm where he experiences the "self-realizing and self-manifesting agency" of his origins. In doing so, he risks himself, and this is a very difficult and dangerous thing. To give up one's hard-won "objectivity" is very hard and fearsome; once it is gone what comes is a terrible anxiety about existence itself and the terror that we may lose that sense we have of *being*, of an individuality somehow related with the world inside and out. All of this is reflected in the temperament of the artist.[1]

In Joan's case it is a matter of extremity. Her anxiety was enormous and it was in every way healthy that she felt it. There was great danger that, having descended into the primal realm, she would never come out of it. The moment she entered it, she encountered a destructive "spirit" (*Plate* 14), a stone-thrower who threatened to become autonomous and prevent any possibility of cure. The stone-thrower corresponds to Apsu and he meant literally to kill her as a personality, to keep her, in other words, in his realm, inert at the centre of violent energies. This picture (*Plate* 15) is full of energy pouring out and spending itself in unnamed, mindless creation; the crowds of figures are simply events, things happening in the primal situation in which there is as yet no means by which the intrinsic individuality can relate itself

[1]See Andrew Lytle's fine and moving essay, "The Working Novelist" (1959.)

with the powers that sustain it. But the descent and the encounter with the stone-thrower were necessary experiences for Joan, as they are, to a degree, necessary for all of us. The stone-thrower is symbolic of a vital aspect of the "self-creating and self-manifesting agency". He appears demonic, but that is a part of life. It seems tragic to us that we must experience this "Behemoth" as a natural and necessary part of our being, but this is our task and when we accept it the sense of tragedy fades. The power of what the stone-thrower represents is not absolute but relative and to the degree that we experience this relativity we know our finiteness and our dignity. Our acceptance of the task is the decisive criterion; it is the way to the psyche's wholeness, to the realization of the ontogenetic purpose not only in ourselves as individuals but in humanity itself in all its potential grandeur.

Joan said about the next drawing (*Plate* 17): "These people are all dead." Pierre Janet referred to the experience she has pictured here and to what she has suffered as an *abaissement du niveau mental*. The level upon which the psyche is active with its surroundings has fallen toward a state of seeming nothingness, mere biological existence with little or no awareness of the intrinsically human or of possible access to creative energies. This is the true existential "Nothingness"; the nothingness of anonymity.

During the time these drawings were done, Joan wrote in her diary:

"I remember being me and being with Joyce (her sister) . . . and our friends were young, and maybe even Joyce was young . . . but I don't know, and I felt as if I had to be strong, and felt like I should never tell Joyce or even me what I felt because it was too soft and like the sky . . . and I was a clown and she laughed . . . and I *was* funny. I was the hardest, most cynical child in the world. I took pleasure from the fact that dogs and children disliked me. I felt three million years old. As I grew older I felt younger.

"I'm made, I'm made of solid stone . . .
hard . . . too brittle to break
I'm made, I'm made of solid stone . . .
of solid, solid stone.

I'm heavy like a rock lying bloodless and cold
I cannot speak or be understood
for people don't understand rocks.
My heart is made of solid stone
And no one knows the difference,
the difference
And no one knows the difference,
the difference . . . or cares."

In reply to a comment about the artistic quality of her drawings, she said:

"Artist, what a laugh, I only ease myself. All prostitutes should be able to draw, all idiots too, all weak disgusting people should be able to draw. I wish I could be eaten alive by vultures. I wish dark monsters could claw at me and pick the dirt from my bones. I want to be picked apart and eaten by the ugliest things alive. I wish I were a prostitute begging for love. I wish I were naked and disgraced. I wish I were in the cool earth. I am not disgusted now, I am disgusting."

Two months passed:

"Mind, you are incorrigible. I was afraid to draw. I don't trust my hand or my mind. They both doubted each other and it was a terrible feeling. I was so conscious of *doing* a drawing . . . It ruins the only thing that really means anything to me . . . my only way of living."

She withdrew. She could not, at this stage, go on with her remarkable explorations through the medium of her art. She wrote:

"Don't turn around
Don't let these eyes see
Don't look
Don't see.
Twist the mass of yourself inward . . . inward
There you are pure and safe.
Ah, sweet safety,
sweet safety.
Your body does not exist.
What importance is it?
Your self exists only for yourself

and there it sees only the light of fear.
This fear exists only for yourself
Therefore, it does not exist, you make it so.
How fine,
How very fine
Your fear does not exist even inwardly.
Outwardly you are quite untouchable,
Untouchable,
Ha, Ha,
Nothing can touch me
For I have negated the world
It is only a dream now
Tomorrow I can laugh at it
And although it touches me in a million different ways
and every moment of my most unimportant life
It shall never really touch me
It shall never really touch me."

"When I was young and my friends were gay and youthful, I condemned them with my hatred and my silence. I hated their joviality, their stupid gaiety . . . I only joined them when I could mock, when I could openly hate . . . not only them but myself. What a fool I am for writing on this paper now . . . if only the realization of what I say would not frighten me . . . and make me feel so hopelessly lost to everyone."

But something very vital took place during this period of withdrawal and her next drawing (*Plate* 18) reveals it.

*Choice*, the human presupposition and prerogative, becomes for Joan, with this crucial picture, a possibility.

"If only the realization of what I say would not frighten me. . . ."

Her fear is of choice itself, the unknown. She cannot imagine a state of existence in which she is *not* gripped by the brutal forces of her psyche; she cannot imagine beginning to feel and to act independently, as herself. She clings, and this is typical of most of us, to what she *knows*, no matter how destructive it may be to her growth.

"It shall never really touch me."

But in spite of herself, of her fear and her determination never to be touched, it happened that she was, and in this picture the event is rendered. She did not rationally grasp it or even really know of it: it happened in the primal realm, like revelation, and she treats it in terms of a cosmic event. The sky seems to have split; lightning strikes down. The three figures, full of negativity still, are yet caught up in attitudes of bewilderment and awe. The child, with an animal's head, clings to the mother: it is Joan herself in the very act of clinging to the Known. But the whole seems to be a picture of the birth of feeling, for, soon after, in referring to her next drawing, she was able to make a direct, emphatic statement of feeling:

"I *hate* the face looking up, but I *love* the girl that sees nothing."

Revelation is never anything but promise until it is manifested in action, and the same is true of choice. This drawing (*Plate* 18) is symbolic, therefore, of something decisive which has happened in the primal realm. If it had not happened, she would have been lost to the brutal forces of her psyche. As a symbol, the drawing states the possibility that the same event may now take place in consciousness. It becomes possible now for her to begin to feel in her own way, to react out of her own individuality, to breathe a different air. She *may* choose, and it is exactly this, the possibility of choice, which is necessary if any relationship is to be achieved with the autonomous, deterministic forces of the unconscious, and the way opened for the experience of individuality and the self.

Joan wrote at the back of the drawing reproduced as *Plate* 19: "The stones have blended together to become the stalks of growing things."

The quickening of the stones takes place in the presence of a most significant figure: the hermaphrodite, who appears in the drawing isolated from all the other chaotic events. The hermaphrodite is a collective symbol found in all cultures. What it stands for is a *natural activity* of the psyche, an insistent urge toward structure and form through which opposing energies and inertias are reconciled. Jung has written: "The symbol of the hermaphrodite in its functional significance does not point backwards but forward toward a goal which is not yet reached." It is, therefore, an archetypal symbol for *what is* within the psyche and for what *may be* since its aim is creativity.

This, one of the deepest of human insights, finds its purest expression in the symbol of Christ as hermaphrodite. In this image of Him who was God-man, the primal waters once mingled, then by the Word divided, are reunited in a higher awareness; male and female, yin and yang are joined in a *unio oppositorum* which is a vision not only of human experience of the divine but also of the psyche at the height of its creativity.[1]

For Joan, on the deeply personal level, the symbol of the woman with penis had another significance. It was a fact that, in her pathological state, she experienced her mother and father not as individual human beings but as one, locked together in a single unity. This "unity", the diametric opposite of the hermaphrodite, so loomed in the foreground of her existence that she could see and feel little else. But here, still face to face with this pathological reality, she draws what co-exists with it. With the appearance of the hermaphrodite, the psyche reveals the resources it has for its own cure. The hermaphrodite takes a central position and a new phase of her art begins. The imagination drops its chains, there is a hint of rhythm and form, and gradually she speaks in a different way about her work.

She wrote in her diary at this time:

"When I left your office on Friday, there was something I remembered after it was too late, and it is very important to me. Remember I told you once that I was impressed by a Van Gogh painting. It seemed to me that there was a force at the back of the painting which pulled everything into an intense order giving it form. I said that was what I was beginning to experience myself. On Friday in drawing class I painted a figure. I had to fight with the shapes, they all wanted to go back because this force was pulling so hard. I did not want them to. I felt that I would be left with a lot of over-simplified boulders. I also felt that perhaps this force was my unconscious itself, or my

[1]"The Church symbolism of *sponsus* and *sponsa* leads to the mystic union of the two, i.e., to the *anima Christi* which lives in the *corpus mysticum* of the Church. This unity underlies the idea of Christ's androgyny, which medieval alchemy exploited for its own ends. The much older figure of the Hermaphroditus, whose outward aspect probably derives from a Cyprian *Venus barbata*, encountered in the Eastern Church the already extant idea of an androgynous Christ, which is no doubt connected with the Platonic conception of the bisexual First Man ,for Christ is ultimately the Anthropos" (Jung, 1946, *Coll. Wks.*, 16, p. 306).

mother. I must add that the part of me that fights this force is very strong too. In this drawing many forms seem to rest on a plane, the space behind this plane goes into the distance. The lines always form a triangular shape. This drawing itself seems to be a sort of dead-end valley, surrounded by mountains, or a vagina. This is considering the whole drawing."

In writing this, she knew very well what she was saying on one level, but not at all what she was saying on another, deeper level. She knew nothing about the symbols and mythological motifs, she had no inkling of the significance of the archetypes they represent. Yet in her remark that "the lines always form a triangular shape," she expressed unconsciously her direct experience of the activity of an archetype. And she has felt the "force" at the back of the picture which gives it form!

She kept working at her drawing, but her inertia was great and dead-set against the new hopeful change that come with the appearance of the hermaphrodite.

"I think I am afraid that if I am real things will mean more to me and I will be ruined. How easy it is to say that nothing exists in the world . . . I am an animal with no understanding except a vague confusion . . . I see nothing . . . I do not want to be seen. I am strong. I can drop a flood bomb and singe your speaking shapes. If you want to die, keep knowing me. I don't want to have any more contacts with human beings . . . Never, never, never, I don't want them to kill me.

"I hate to draw now. I am too stuck. I have no feeling in me now but death, and I am sick and tired of it. I don't want to draw it anymore. Oh, shut your mouth, you cold dead fish, and I know what I am saying now: that, sir, is to say sometimes I just felt things, and when I spoke them I felt guilty, but now I understand and know I am a cold dead fish. Thank you, dearie, for the pretty justification."

The primal inertia—the true adversary—is now out in the open. She experiences it in "hating" to draw and in being afraid. "I am afraid that if I am real . . ." Speaking here out of the depths of her suffering, doesn't she also speak for her century?

Her very potentialities for growth seem to her a threat of annihilation. She is afraid that, if she is real, all she knew of herself before, no matter how pale and partial a summation it was, will be destroyed. She cannot see that what is really threatened is her identification with the parental psyche and her own inertia; that what is *not* threatened, what is in fact promised, is that existence which is individual and, ultimately, invulnerable. Her fear of cutting off her arms, or head, or fingers is a direct manifestation of the inertia which determinedly thwarts the development of her personality and, simultaneously, creates her anxieties.

During this phase, quite understandably, she offered great resistance to the psychotherapeutic situation.

On the back of the drawing reproduced as *Plate* 20, she wrote: "I feel there is something keeping me from drawing." Thus she begins, by being clearly conscious of her inertia, to differentiate herself from it.

The process by which the inner world becomes an objective reality continues, pressing toward a dramatic event. From the standpoint of the psychotherapist, the next drawing (*Plate* 21) makes secure all she had accomplished up to now and marks, therefore, the turning point from schizophrenia to neurosis. As a drawing, it is open; the sense of imprisonment, of containment within the dark realms of the psyche, is gone. Until this happened, nothing was secure. She wrote on the back a single word, "Foo!" an onomatopoetic expression of her great sense of relief. It is the sigh which comes with significant achievement.

Joan takes much better care of herself now (written May 1958). She dresses neatly. She lives with her parents under pleasanter circumstances than ever before, and she is capable of relationships with young men of her own age. She has a part-time job and earns enough to buy her art supplies. She draws and paints regularly. As is obvious from this study, her experience of psychotherapy did not stop or thwart or even threaten the creative process; rather, the very opposite. She has made great progress toward the establishment of that *means* I have called personality, by which she is related with the world and with the dynamics of her own being. She will always, no doubt, have her ups and downs, crises of hope and belief, and, to some degree, of inertia and despair, but it is her task to come to terms with them since they are natural to her human condition, her prerogative as an artist, one might say, and her privilege.

The whole course of her treatment was and continues to be governed by the fact that she is an artist, and that it is primarily through her art that the psyche reveals itself. This explains why there has been no mention of her dreams: they were of very little help. She so lacked, from the beginning, any relationship with the forces at work within her that, in effect, she lived her dreams in "reality". The highly complex problem of her father was never touched on by any dream; it had to be dealt with in dealing with the problem of the transference. The equally complex problem of her mother was projected in her dreams and everyday life into a relationship with a girl friend and so had to be met indirectly. It was in her drawings day by day that the truth of her situation came to light and it was through them that the psyche brought about its own cure.

## REFERENCES

FROMM, ERICH (1951). *The Forgotten Language*. New York, Rinehart.

HEIDEL, A. (1951). *The Babylonian Genesis*. Chicago University Press.

JUNG, C. G. (1946). *Die Psychologie der Übertragung*. Zürich, Rascher. Trans. "Psychology of the Transference", *Coll. Wks.* **16**.

LYTLE, ANDREW. "The Working Novelist", *Daedalus*. April, 1959.

WESTMAN, H. (1961). *The Springs of Creativity*. New York, Atheneum Publishers; London, Routledge & Kegan Paul.

# 15

# THE THERAPEUTIC FUNCTION OF THE HOMOSEXUAL TRANSFERENCE

G. STEWART PRINCE, *London*

This short clinical paper was presented at the First International Congress for Analytical Psychology in 1958. It should be emphasized that the analysis from which the thesis is drawn was concluded some years before and that I had no inkling of Layard's thinking on this subject, or he of mine, until the approach of the Congress led us to discuss the matter a few weeks before the meeting (Layard, 1959). This paper focuses upon the significance of the latent homosexual orientation for symptom-formation, its influence upon the transference, and in particular on the part it plays in the therapeutic process.

## CLINICAL MATERIAL

### *Historical*

The patient was in his late twenties when he first became overtly ill. He had been aware from his late teens of difficulty in relating to women, and had failed in his only attempt at sexual intercourse. For some months he had maintained a romantic interest in a woman who appeared to him as gifted, artistic, and pure, but on discovering that she was ill-content with this role and wanted a man and a lover, he fled from the relationship, became mildly depressed, and developed phobic symptoms. Soon these had increased until he was in a state of almost perpetual panic. He was referred to an outpatient clinic; as he sat in the waiting-room the psychiatrist he was due to see showed himself in the corridor —a large, masculine, and rather stern figure in appearance—and my patient fled from the hospital, afterwards writing a letter of abject apology, and consequently being admitted to a neurosis ward for a few months. It was his fear of returning to the outside world, although his panic had diminished, that led to his referral to me. Before his first visit he sent me an enormous manuscript, detailing his symptoms, life history, and somewhat intellectualized reflections upon his condition, the whole couched in turgid English.

His father, a conventional English gentleman, had succeeded in business in Poland. The patient had little contact with him in his early years, and had built up an idealized image of him. This he consciously maintained, although he had found out in his teens that the father had long had a mistress, whom he eventually married when divorced by the mother. She was Polish in origin, and had dominated the patient's life, being volatile, unpredictable, demanding, domineering, and often embarrassing, and had finally ended in a mental hospital with a diagnosis of paranoia about the time of his own collapse. His only sister, some years younger than he, had developed schizophrenia in late adolescence, and had remained for some years in a mental hospital apparently unresponsive to any form of treatment.

In spite of much unhappiness in childhood, and an awareness of considerable difficulty in making relationships, my patient did very well academically, distinguished himself scholastically at a premier public school, and was a fine student of languages at university. He identified strongly with the collective values of this milieu, developed his undoubted intellectual gifts, and acquired some less-well-integrated pretensions to artistic and aesthetic interest. He disliked sports, and his sole exercise was got from playing squash, while his attitude towards his body was in general almost stoical, in that he seemed to have turned away interest from it to a remarkable degree. On leaving the university he started a career in the diplomatic sphere, furthered this with considerable success during his war service, and found himself returned to civil life with good prospects and considerable status at the age of twenty-five.

### *Analytical*

At the first interview I found a tall, thin young man, polite, precise, and rather pedantic; he referred to the written history he had sent me, and indicated that he expected some solution of his problem as the result of my having read it. He talked of his fear of returning to his work, and his shame at having had a breakdown. I liked him, felt he was terrified of me, and came to the conclusion that analysis would be difficult because of his extreme intellectualism and manifest fear of the unconscious, taken in conjunction with the malign family history. After a few meetings, however, he came deeply impressed with the following dream:

> *Dream* 1. I am going to play squash. In the hall of the club I meet two dogs, copulating. One of them belongs to a middle-aged woman, who does not seem embarrassed. I try to separate them. I go to change. I overhear this woman talking to another; they are saying that it is useless to get their daughters to try to develop interests. I intervene and protest that there must be something to be done. I see the two daughters, aged about eight. They are pale and ill-looking. The woman says there is a burglar about. I feel he is in a cupboard. I feel very frightened, realizing that I am naked under a big towel.

It need hardly be said that, for a man of his psychological type, this dream, although impressive, was obscure; however, he reacted most markedly to the last scene, in which he was frightened about the burglar and felt exposed and defenceless in his nudity under the towel. He had no associations to the first part of the dream, except that he played squash regularly with male friends, out of a sense of need to take exercise, rather than with any real pleasure. To me this part seemed to give a graphic picture of his psychic state at the beginning of analysis. The situation is dominated by the mother archetype, shown in the negative elementary character (Neumann, 1955, Ch. 11) in her possession of the dog—Artemis-Hecate. The symbol of the copulating dogs is capable of more expansion than I can attempt here, but I will mention my original feeling that it contained the beginning of the therapeutic process. The conversation between the mothers tells of the state of the anima—the dreamer sees the daughters as pale and ill, but protests that there must be something to be done.

The burglar figure, felt by the dreamer as powerful, aggressive, and sexual, can be linked to his manifest anxiety, and seen as personal shadow. He is, however, in the cupboard, and appears functionally as part of the mother archetype, her phallic aspect.

A few days later another dream is reported:

> *Dream* 2. In a station. There is a beautiful, fair child about three years old in a train-carriage. I go to greet him. I am overwhelmed with affection and embrace the child. I ejaculate over him.

The dreamer could only say about this that the child reminded him of his godchild, and that he felt sure the dream was "not really sexual". This will be commented on later.

In the analysis the patient's homosexual problem came quickly to the fore, manifested in dreams, in his relationship to his superior at work (whom he began to see as a fat Satyr), to various other men of his present and past acquaintance, and most particularly in the transference. He came to regard me as a tutor, likened me to a favourite don at the University whom he felt to have made a powerful impression upon him, and treated me with admiring respect. Behind this, however, lay considerable hostility and anxiety, and this was catalysed by an occasion when it was necessary for me to take him down in the lift at the end of a session. This produced a dream in which he identified me with a senior in the Army, an avowed homosexual, who had made tentative approaches from which my patient had fled.

It need hardly be said that he was very resistant to analysis of this, but after a particularly stormy denial he had the following dream:

> *Dream* 3. I am at a table with friends. One of them draws attention to the fact that on my left foot and spreading up the leg I have a rash. It is a livid red thing of spots and sort of arrows. I notice that my right leg is like jelly, so that the bones can be seen.

His only association here was to a fungus infection suffered at school, which had produced a rash in his groin and occasioned him much shame. This led to further memories of his school and college days, in which, fundamentally lonely and incapable of warm relationships, he would build up elaborate fantasy relationships with senior boys and teachers, admired for their intellectual or artistic qualities. From his dreams in particular the repressed homo-erotic aspect of these clearly emerged.

A possibility of change in his attitude of horrified rejection of all this seemed to be contained in a further dream:

> *Dream* 4. I am on a journey. I fall in with a youth of my age, a vagabond. Hostility arises. We wrestle, like Jacob and the angel. I overcome him and stun him. I wonder if he is dead, and feel that I have already committed a murder. I decide not to flee. He revives, and we walk along in perfect amity.

This will remind us of what Neumann has aptly called "the long succession of fraternal feuds in mythology", which opens with the squabbles between Osiris and Set, Baal and Mot. Neumann also states (1954, p. 180), "Consciousness of the bond between the male opponents is the beginning of masculine self-consciousness". And later (p. 181), "... on one level the ego's assimilation of the earthly shadow-brother, i.e. its instinctual, destructive, and self-destroying side, is more evident, while on another it is the alliance of the earthly ego with its immortal twin brother, the self".

At this stage of the analysis two matters became of urgent importance. The patient's mother, released from hospital, was actively persecuting him in various ways, and he began to find an increasing inhibition in his capacity to work, in particular when called upon to interrogate important political suspects, or to lecture to large groups of relatively senior officials.

Psycho-analysis has long drawn attention to the fact that such inhibition is often based on inhibition of aggressiveness due to anxieties and guilt, and related to conflicts over dependence, duty, and obedience (Fenichel, 1945, pp. 178, 183). For my patient these conflicts were mobilized by his being torn in innumerable issues between his mother and father, and he was able gradually to find that under his conscious attitude of anxious appeasement toward the one and filial respect to the other there lay a great deal of resentment. Analysis of his feelings about paying fees, breaking appointments, and so on led him to be able also to hate me. Subsequently there was some improvement in his capacity to handle his mother and to cope with his work, but he felt stuck in the analysis, and became depressed. He wanted me to solve the impasse, to ask him questions, to probe, and in fact asked to be examined. I was reminded of the "thesis" he had sent me before our first interview, and of the important paper by the Kleinian psycho-analyst Thorner, "Examination Anxiety Without Examination" (Thorner, 1952).

In this paper Thorner extends the classical theory on examination anxiety, on the basis of the concept of internalized bad and good objects, and relates it to the symptom of impotence. The relevance for my patient was borne out by the fact that he began at this stage to revive a habit of anal masturbation; he had practised this as long as he could remember in childhood, but abandoned it abruptly at the onset of puberty, and he related it to his mother's early preoccupation with his bowel function and to her insistence on giving him frequent enemata. This also brought up the fact that he had introduced his sister to mutual anal play, and opened up his guilt about her serious illness. The link here with Layard's thesis is clear. After anal masturbation one night he had the following dream:

> *Dream* 5. I am sitting on a pot. There are people around but I do not worry. Suddenly there is a loud plop. I realize that a rat or mouse has dropped into the water in the pot and I am alarmed.

This was followed by the emergence of further anal material, including anal-aggressive fantasies directed towards me, to all of which the patient tended to react with horror and denial. Abenheimer has chided analytical psychologists for their neglect of anal symbolism, and emphasized its archetypal content (Abenheimer, 1952). He points out that (a) anal symbols are the earliest expression of ego power, of ego assertiveness, of self-reliance, of active self-expression; and (b) anal symbols represent the mother, later the complex of the great earth mother in its positive and negative aspects. He emphasizes the mythology of the creation of the world, or of man, from excreta, the use of faeces as prima materia, the placement of the first life centre in the bowels in Kundalini Yoga, and the use of excrement as a panacea, to balance the tendency to see only the negative aspects of anal symbolism. In relation to the dream, I also mention his opinion that it is often a sign of overcoming the utter regression signified by faecal symbols when they are replaced by living animals, instancing rats. Whitmont's recent contribution to the psychology of the obsessional state likewise draws our attention to the magical significance of anal symbols, and their function of assisting the ego to overcome the fear of the negative earth mother (Whitmont, 1957).

Emergence and analysis of such anal material led to a dramatic change in the patient. His work inhibition disappeared, and he became able to deal with his mother much more objectively. He then reported that he had fallen in love—significantly with an Indian woman of considerable beauty, divorced wife of an Englishman and mother of an eight-year-old child. To his delight he found himself sexually stirred by her, and was able to become her lover without difficulty. Some months later they were married, and in spite of many adventitious difficulties this relationship proved successful.

In the final phase of his analysis the homosexual problem and its reflection in the transference re-emerged. This was catalysed by his meeting the tutor whom he had idealized in his university days, and finding that he had married a much younger woman, whom the patient felt strongly to be intellectually inferior, frivolously feminine, and sensual. This revived memories and stimulated dreams of his student days which high-lighted the physical homosexual fantasies behind his artistic and intellectual activities, and re-awakened his feelings towards me, his jealousy of my wife, his fantasies about my sexual activities and so on. Then came a dream which seems to me to indicate a focal point in the analytical process:

> *Dream* 6. I am in a dimly-lit room with a religious atmosphere. A man approaches me from behind as I kneel in an attitude of prayer. He ejaculates on to my head and rubs my head as if anointing me with the sperm.

The dreamer added that his impression of the man was of a benign, wise, and powerful person, and that he associated him with me. Shortly after this he was called overseas by his duties for several months, during which time he assisted in carrying out a piece of work of international importance. As a result he was offered a higher post outside England, which he accepted with little hesitation, and after two months of further analysis of a more superficial sort the treatment was terminated by his departure.

### *Commentary*

It is striking that, although Jung in a lecture delivered in 1925 (cf. Jung, 1928) clearly outlined the unconscious meaning of homosexuality in a young man, Jungian writers have done little to take this further; Storr (1957) and Lambert (unpublished) in London have recently made contributions, as has Whitmont in New York. Storr in particular has emphasized the teleological implications of such symptoms as fetishism and transvestitism in men who are psychologically homosexual, and has shown how this widens the understanding of psycho-analytic and other psychopathological contributions to the field. In fact, the psycho-analyst Bychowski (1945) emphasized the comparative neglect of study of the ego of the homosexual, and its importance for treatment. Working forward from Freud's statement (Freud, 1930, p. 11, fn. 12) that its functioning is based on "archaic constitution and by primitive psychic mechanisms" he reaches some interesting conclusions which I can only hint at by quoting from his closing remarks: "Since the ego seems unable to realize virility within itself, for all these various reasons, it preserves the pattern of being fascinated by it in the outside world and begins to search for it in other men." This seems to me to come close to Storr's position.

From the first dream I have given we see the ego of my patient as terrified by and fascinated with the "burglar", whose significance I find most meaningfully elaborated in Whitmont's (1957) concept of the phallic magician and chthonic man, part of the mother complex. The symbol of the dogs copulating (from behind), which the dreamer mistakenly attempts to reject, stands in antithetical relationship to the atmosphere of Dream 2, in which the dreamer ejaculates over the fair child; here we have Layard's second man, the *puer aeternus*, hermaphroditic. The early appearance and recognition of the homosexual quality of his transference was of central importance, leading as it did to the dream of the livid rash on his leg. The idea of the wound or blemish from which healing can occur is familiar, and Onians (1951) takes us further with his material on birth taking place from the knees, and in particular with the legend of the king who pierced his swollen leg, from which sprang "a wonderfully beautiful maiden with all her body armed and carrying lance and helm". The dynamic significance of the wound from which healing can come has been amplified by Adler in his study of the dynamics of the self (Adler, 1951). The sequence of anal material is enlightened by a sentence from Abenheimer's paper already referred to. He states (1952, p. 6): "The fantasy that the male is head and phallus and that the body is female and identified with faeces is typical, particularly of the homosexual imagination". Once again confrontation with his primitive anal-aggressive impulses and fantasies in the transference situation enables the patient to continue with his task of facing and integrating the earth-mother complex.

In the final phase it is again his homosexual feelings, realized in the transference, which lead to the crucial dream, to which I would like to refer in more detail, and which seems to me to offer the closest of clinical parallels to Layard's thesis. The religious atmosphere of the dream, and the idea of being anointed with sperm, were obvious to the dreamer himself. I had expected to find further elucidation in liturgical sources, but have been disappointed. However, Onians in his *Origins of European Thought* devotes a chapter to "The Strength". He quotes from the *Zohar* of the Hebrew Kabbalah, for instance, that in the testes "are gathered all the oil, the dignity and the strength of the male from the whole body", amplifying on the equation between sperm and oil for inunction. With regard to inunction his passage on the anointing of the divine son of the Father-God is explicit, and confirms Layard's interpretation of "the symbolic semen fulfilling the same function as the Holy Spirit". That the symbol of sperm should be retained in this dream, with its patently spiritual atmosphere, I find best explained by Neumann (1954); following his discussion on lower (phallic, sexual) masculinity compared with higher masculinity as head and eye, he points out (p. 159), "Only the combination of both zones produces a whole masculinity", and it is such a combination that is achieved in the dream.

The possibility of union of the opposites and a development of masculinity and consciousness implicit in this dream seemed to me to have depended upon the emergence, acceptance, and transformation of the patient's latent homosexuality within the transference situation.

## REFERENCES

ABENHEIMER, K. M. (1952). "Re-assessment of the Theoretical and Therapeutic Meaning of Anal Symbolism", London, Guild of Pastoral Psychology Lecture No. 72.

ADLER, G. (1951). "Notes Regarding the Dynamics of the Self", *Brit. J. med. Psychol.*, **24**, 2.

BYCHOWSKI, G. (1945). "The Ego of Homosexuals", *Int. J. Psycho-anal.*, **26**, 3.

FENICHEL, O. (1945). *The Psychoanalytic Theory of Neurosis.* London, Routledge & Kegan Paul; New York, Norton.

FREUD, S. (1930). *Three Contributions to the Theory of Sex.* New York and Washington, Nervous and Mental Disease Publishing Co.

JUNG, C. G. (1928). "The Significance of the Unconscious in Individual Education". *Contributions to Analytical Psychology.* London, Routledge & Kegan Paul; New York, Harcourt Brace. Republished in *Coll. Wks.*, **17**.

LAYARD, J. (1959). "Homo-eroticism in Primitive Society as a Function of the Self", *J. analyt. Psychol.*, **4**, 2.

NEUMANN, E. (1954). *The Origins and History of Consciousness.* Bollingen Series 42. New York, Pantheon; London, Routledge & Kegan Paul.

NEUMANN, E. (1955). *The Great Mother.* Bollingen Series 47. New York, Pantheon; London, Routledge & Kegan Paul.

ONIANS, R. B. (1951). *The Origins of European Thought.* London, Cambridge University Press.

STORR, A. (1957), "The Psychopathology of Fetishism and Transvestitism", *J. analyt. Psychol.*, **2**, 2.

THORNER, H. A. (1952). "Examination Anxiety Without Examination", *Int. J. Psycho-anal.*, **33**, 2.

WHITMONT, E. (1957). "Magic and the Psychology of Compulsive States", *J. analyt. Psychol.*, **2**, 1.

# 16

## HOMO-EROTICISM IN PRIMITIVE SOCIETY AS A FUNCTION OF THE SELF

JOHN LAYARD, *Oxford*

THE title of this paper reflects a study that I have now been engaged on for many years, that of the organization of primitive society as an externalized form of what we think of as the self. In this paper I will deal with its homo-erotic aspect, but I must first give a few general explanations.

What is here meant by primitive society is *primitive kinship*, for as the reader doubtless knows the terms "society" and "kinship" are synonymous in primitive life, as they are still today in the infant's life. In primitive society, however, this is a fact of adult life as well as of infantile life. Though on a broader scale than that of the nuclear family, it remains true of the most primitive communities that there are no "people" who are not kinsmen. In an aboriginal Australian community, for instance, or what is called a "horde", which is an entirely self-sufficient community of between 40 and 200 men, women, and children living in a pre-agricultural state and depending on food-gathering and a little hunting for its very subsistence, those who belong to this community are thought of as human beings, but those outside it, whom they occasionally meet, are not. They are "not men", unless they can be recognized as some kind of putative distant or "totemic" kinsmen. The words for "human being" and "kinsman" are the same. Those who are not kinsmen are "outside the pale", that is to say outside the invisible fence that surrounds, or the living mandala of the kinship system that includes, all relatives and keeps out all those who are not relatives.

Just as we so quickly lose sight of our own personal origins, so also such primitive communities are on the point of disappearing altogether. We are, therefore, extremely fortunate in that, through the devoted labours of a certain school of anthropologists, we have succeeded in obtaining before it is too late records of at least some of the main lines of such primitive social organization, whereby we may catch glimpses of our own internal psychic organization and thus get some help in sorting ourselves out.

The concept of such primitive kinship organization as an externalized psychic mandala is based on the still broader concept that whatever happens externally also happens internally, that external and internal are mirrors of one another, and that, as with the hen and the egg, no one can say which came first. For they, the inner and the outer, are dual manifestations of the same all-embracing phenomenon of human development, which in this case has its external manifestation in the kinship system and its internal manifestation in the psychic organization of each individual composing it. There are exceptions, of course: those who fail to fit in with the accepted system, who either drop out (for instance may be killed for the too public breaking of incest taboos), or who by contrast may lead the way to new expansions of a system that once was necessary but is now felt as being too restrictive. We will not here, however, be concerned with these. Our present concern is with the basic pattern, and in particular the homo-erotic side of it: that which, so often unperceived, builds up society.

It may be said that it is marriage which builds up society. This is, of course, quite true. But marriage in primitive society is not an individual affair. All primitive marriages are arranged. They are arranged by parents for their children in accordance with the basic pattern that has arisen out of the fundamental human needs of, on the one hand, solidarity (endogamy) and, on the other, division and the union of opposites (exogamy). The most primitive communities in Australia are *externally endogamous* ("Those who do not belong to us just are not 'men' "), but they are *internally exogamous*, that is to say strictly divided into two sets of paired social groups which we call "moieties": two matrilineal moieties which are mutually exogamous; and two patrilineal moieties which are likewise mutually exogamous.

These, crossing one another, together divide society into four "kinship sections", as they are called, which resemble the basic four functions of the self structured in pairs, such as the *adept* and *anima, soror* and *animus*, which will be seen to correspond to the brother-sister pairs in the actual kinship system. Marriages are arranged in such a way that both patrilineal *and* matrilineal rules of exogamy are strictly observed, and that the children shall marry into the opposite section of each pair of moieties, that is to say their opposites both matrilineally and patrilineally.

This is exogamy in its extremest possible form from the kinship point of view. But it is combined also with the extremest possible form of endogamy outside actual incest with the mother, sister, or daughter. It results from what is called "sister-exchange marriage". This is a form of marriage which I have described more fully in my article on "The Incest Taboo and the Virgin Archetype" in *Eranos-Jahrbuch* (1945), which Jung elaborated on the following year in his *Psychology of the Transference* (1946), and which I explained still further in another Eranos lecture on *Identification with the Sacrificial Animal* (1956). Those wishing to study this subject more closely may refer to these works, and later to a small book on *Primitive Kinship for the Psychologist* which I am now preparing.

In such a society there are no individual marriages, but only double marriages between brother-sister pairs, who exchange sisters for wives in such a way that each man "gives" his sister to be married to the other, and takes this other man's sister to be his wife. This is as near-incestuous a relationship as possible, and I have therefore termed it "near-incest". If there is no actual sister, there are always sister substitutes, what are called parallel cousins, who rank as sisters in the kinship system. Marriages are arranged (and this is important) primarily by the fathers of the prospective bride and bridegroom who, as the males, are the makers of society, as opposed to the women, the bearers of the children who are the *prima materia* of society and carry it on. The two fathers have themselves married one another's sister, so that in a four-section system of this kind the marriages which they arrange between their children in fulfilment of the pattern are all first-cousin marriages on both sides, the matrilineal and the patrilineal. Such cousins are called "bilateral first cross-cousins".

Society, that is the kinship mandala, is thus so much more important than the individual that children, while free to make any temporary sexual unions they like so long as they do not publicly violate the framework of the incest taboos, have no say whatever in the choice of a marriage partner.

This being the case, the whole of the collective society, though implemented by the men, functions as a "male mother" demanding total obedience from her sons. It must be borne in mind in what follows with regard to the homo-erotic relationships that grow up under these conditions that, though these may appear on the surface to be "accidental" in the psychological meaning of the term, they are no more so than are the pathological homosexual relationships which grow up in our own society as a result of personal as well as of impersonal factors in contrast to the collectively dominating "male mother" constellated in the kinship system.

If the kinship system is an externalization of the inferred structure of the self, the self is at the same time an internalized mirror or imprint of the known structure of the kinship system. The two go hand in hand. One mirrors the other. Each has in it the same potentialities for expansion or for degeneration, which we will now examine in relation to the homo-erotic element which grows up under cover of, and with the assistance of, the heterosexual one. For whereas the marriages contracted by the two brothers-in-law in this four-section system take place with one another's sisters, the homo-erotic element, which later spreads to a far wider field, springs up originally between the two brothers-in-law themselves. It is these brothers-in-law, representing the two complementary opposite male elements in the kinship system, who contract the first own-generation homo-erotic relationship and are, in certain circumstances, the first socially recognized homosexual partners. This is psychologically speaking a mixed "shadow" and "anima" phenomenon, as may be seen in the following diagram (*Figure* 1) illustrating the structural features of every marriage contracted in the community.

In this diagram each brother-sister pair is bracketed, and each man marries the other man's sister.

This leads to a complex situation, very important to understand, of Ego's brother-in-law being at the same time his wife's brother *and* his sister's husband. These are *not two persons*, as they are in our social system. They are *one person*. I have thus called this brother-in-law relationship a "double" brother-in-law relationship, and the brother-in-law a "double" brother-in-law.

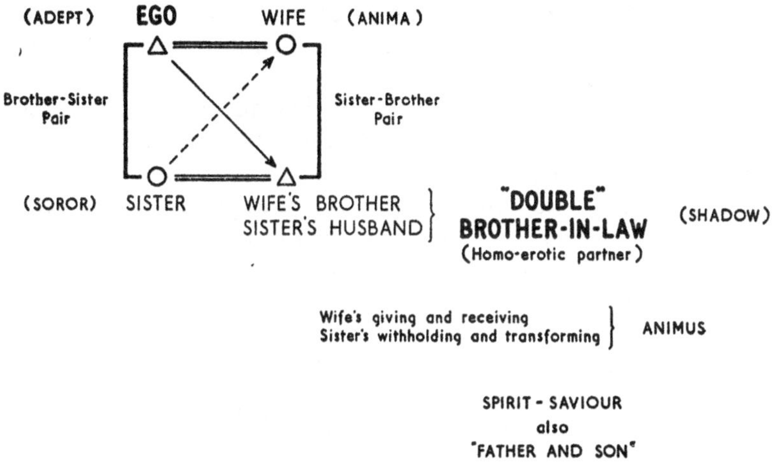


*Figure* 1

Before we pass on to consider what this implies I will present a second diagram (*Figure* 2) to show these same facts in circular

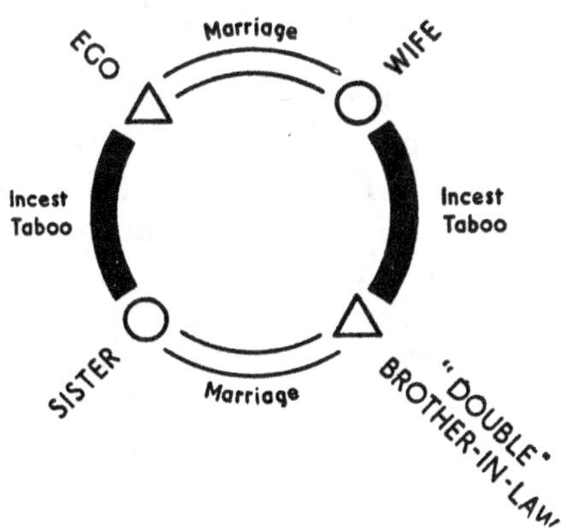


*Figure* 2

form, to demonstrate why all such systems are called "circular connubiums", and how in this way they closely resemble the self in its self-containedness and its uniting of the opposites. Both diagrams are perfect "symbols" in the original Greek sense of the word, which, as was shown by Stein (1957) and Fordham (1957), was founded on the concept of two halves of an original unity which have been parted and rejoined in a new and more creative synthesis.

It will be seen from this how brother and sister have been parted by the incest taboo, only to be rejoined in a more complex fourfold and subtle manner through the interposition of the brother-in-law, who marries Ego's sister and gives his own sister in exchange. The pattern of "2", which is incestuous, has given way to one of "4", which is not actually incestuous. The double-marriage appears here as a mandala, showing how the opposites interact so as to create a larger whole. Each sister-incest taboo leads to a marriage with the sister of the brother-in-law. In the next generation each such marriage leads in its turn to another incest taboo erected between the son and the daughter of that marriage, which results in the same pattern being repeated, so that the system reproduces itself endogamously and needs no outside blood in order to maintain its own internal exogamies.

To show how the two generations interact would need a third diagram, which it is beyond the scope of the present paper to present. What we are concerned with here is the own-generation relationship between the two brothers-in-law who are the homosexual partners.

Psychologists will in the first place not fail to see in this relationship a significant situation regarding what I have termed, on the sister-level, "near-incest". There is no actual incest, for a man does not marry his own sister, but it is near-incest in the very important respect that, of these two brothers-in-law, each fulfils the other's sister-incest desire. There is thus, apart from any other consideration, the closest bond between them of the greatest ambivalence. On the one hand they are affinal allies, each being the other's wife's brother. On the other hand (though this is of course repressed), as sisters' husbands, they are the intensest sex rivals, each having supplanted the other in the fulfilment of his own sister-incest desire.

This leads to the most complicated social situations, not excluding the fact that, since men in such societies are as a rule not even allowed to speak to their sisters and there is every kind of avoidance taboo, the mutual visits and ritual relationships between the brothers-in-law are fraught with difficulties and every kind of social subterfuge to hide this ambivalence and to keep society going, for society is based on it.

## II

This has by itself far-reaching results, which are still further complicated by another factor, that of polygamy, which in a mild form is practised by most primitive peoples, giving the parents yet further social hold over their children by creating a scarcity of wives for the younger men, with the result that they are yet more dependent on the parents to procure wives for them. One of the effects of this is infant betrothal, which in some cases reaches such a pitch that a father in search of a first wife for his growing son will betroth him to a not yet nubile girl or to a baby girl, or even, as is quite frequent, will arrange for him to be betrothed to a daughter as yet unborn of any of the wives of that particular brother-in-law with whom he is arranging the exchange.

The son is thus both married and not yet married. There is a Freudian concept here that may help us to understand something of what follows. Fenichel, in summarizing the findings of the psycho-analysts, says that, "in children the sex of the partner is far less important than it is in adults . . . Initially, everyone is able to develop sexual feelings indiscriminately, and the search for an object is less limited by the sex of the object than is commonly supposed" (Fenichel, 1945, p. 328). This statement is amply borne out, not only for the child but for the adolescent, by what has been reported by, for instance, Spencer and Gillen in their study of the Arunta of Central Australia, who have an eight-section circular connubium based on the same sister-exchanging principles as the four-section one and combined with polygamy. Speaking of the prospective young bridegroom, they write that in the case outlined above, "It frequently happens that the woman whose daughter is thus allotted to him may have a son and no daughter born, and in this case, without waiting on the chance of a girl being born, the man may agree to take the boy .... This establishes a relationship between the boy and the man, as a result of which the former has, until he (is circumcised), to give his hair to the man, who, on his part, has, in a certain way, to look after the boy ..." (Spencer and Gillen, 1927, Vol. II, p. 470).

It would take too long here to describe all the hair-giving customs having to do with marriage. The authors (*ibid.*, p. 486 and Index), first writing over sixty years ago in the hey-day of our own Victorian era, had more prudish delicacy than would be exercised today. According to verbal reports (regarding not only this area but also others in Australia), the "certain way" in which the frustrated bridegroom would "look after" this boy includes having physical relations with him as though he were a wife. The authors do bring themselves to say that one of the bridegroom's duties is to "grease" the boy's body occasionally. This is a good deal more important than these writers would imply, or possibly know of. Such customs, or shall we say symbolic acts, are not confined to Australia. We shall see later that in a New Guinea myth the "grease" envisaged is said to be semen. This comes near to what we would call "anointing". For it is male "stuff" that the boy is said to be anointed with, as opposed to the female blood-tinged fluid seen to flow out from the mother with him when he is born and with which he is presumed to be surrounded when in her womb.

We shall see shortly how this whole theme develops in initiation rites, how the entire homo-erotic development has two sides to it, physical and psychic, and how the homosexual act itself has in it at least one element of initiation in the replacing of female influence by male influence, of which this act is but a sign, as well as doubtless having its pleasurable side.

A similar relationship between the hopeful bridegroom and the prospective bride's brother may arise if the girl is born but not yet nubile. An elder brother of the girl may become the boy-lover of the man, and will return to his own people when the girl is ready to be married. In a year or two, the boy, now of an age to marry, will find himself taking the opposite role of bridegroom with a boy-lover of his own who is the brother of a prospective wife, who in turn is, or ranks as, the sister of his original man-lover. In this way it is not only sisters who are exchanged for wives, but it may be also their brothers. In each case the boy-lover and the man-lover are thus prospective "double" brothers-in-law.

We may now see the added complication in the relation between these brothers-in-law: that each, while *after* marriage fulfilling the other's sister-incest desire by marrying this other one's sister, *before* marriage fulfils it in his own person.

We thus find in this primitive kinship source external evidence of what has long been suspected psychologically regarding homosexual intercourse as an incest-substitute.

## III

I will now trace this relationship as it develops elsewhere in Oceania, taking as my examples parts of New Guinea and that part of Melanesia with which I am familiar, the island of Malekula and Small Islands off the north-east coast of it.

One of the best works so far published on the psychology of kinship, and what the author calls "identification between members of opposite sexes", is *Naven* by Gregory Bateson, who is now in America and was once closely associated with Margaret Mead in joint investigations on the Sepik River in New Guinea. In the course of discussing other kinship identifications he says: "I have a casual mention in mythology of a man who rubbed his buttocks on the leg of the man who was marrying his sister. If we bear in mind the identification of a man with his sister, this conduct is comprehensible—at least from the structural point of view. The man expressed his relationship to his sister's husband by ritually making a sexual gesture in which he identified himself with his sister" (Bateson, 1936, p. 81). He does not mention, I think, overt homosexuality, but this is near to it. What is to be noted is that it is the sister's husband who is thus acted towards by the wife's brother. This is the universal pattern all over this very wide area embracing three sub-continents.

## IV

We will return later to another part of New Guinea from which homosexual practices of a similar nature have been reported. Over the whole of the area that I have mentioned, from whatever part of it we have reports of homosexuality as a recognized social institution, the boy-lover is called the "wife" or by some equivalent term, and the man-lover is called by the kinship term otherwise used for "sister's husband". There can be no doubt whatever that this is basically connected with, and in part-compensation for, the sister-incest taboo resulting in an elementary split between sex and incest, the incestuous component of which, being denied heterosexual expression, develops partly along homo-erotic lines, whether these are expressed homosexually or not. This theme has been expanded in one of the articles already mentioned (Layard, 1956, pp. 360 ff.), in which it is suggested that all relationships between males who are not siblings, beginning with that between the brothers-in-law, are founded externally on kinship exogamy (which is certainly the case) but internally, as shadow-phenomena, on the incestuous element of man's desire transferred from women on to men, forming that psychic bond between men which is the foundation of society.

This may include overt sex relations, or it may not. In the areas under consideration it does. And there develops in many places, including Malekula, a love relationship between the man and his boy-lover that may be very far from negative, resembling that among the Greeks though not so martial in its character. "Love" is a word not lightly used by anthropologists, but there is little doubt that it begins in primitive society not heterosexually between men and women, but between men and men, in this case between the man-lover and the boy-lover who is his own sister-substitute and the man-lover's wife-substitute.

It is much later in the history of culture that such love (as opposed to purely sexual) relationship gets transferred back on to women as wives. But it begins in this wife's brother substitute relationship precisely on account of the repressed, because forbidden, female element through which it operates, that of the absent sister of the boy-lover and the absent bride-to-be of the man-lover, who thus looks after and cherishes the boy as though he were a wife, while the boy works for him.

In Malekula the boy works for him as a wife would work, but, as he cannot bear children, gives his affection instead. Either will mourn the other's death as primitive man rarely mourns that of a wife, but as all men's deaths are mourned. For these are men-admiring societies, not women-admiring ones, and men are only just beginning to win independence from their womenkind, their deep unconscious resentment of them being expressed in the mythology of devouring goddesses (see Layard, 1942, pp. 218 ff.; 1956, pp. 373 ff.). It is the men here who decorate themselves, not the women. For this is Malekula, not Polynesia, where the men have become free enough to cultivate women.

## V

In this relationship it is the elder man-lover who penetrates the younger boy-lover, and thus symbolically endows him with whatever measure of "psychic masculinity" he may have himself achieved by accepting the primary frustration that has been thrust on him in the first place by the incest taboo and secondly through the temporary deprivation of a wife; which, it should be noted, is not basically a sex deprivation, for he is not debarred from other heterosexual intercourse, but a social and therefore a psychic one.

We shall see now to what lengths this belief in injecting "masculinity" into the boy attains, in two quite opposite directions.

There is a widespread belief throughout all this area that homosexual intercourse, by which is meant anal intercourse, promotes bodily growth, not only of the male sex organ of the junior partner but of his whole body. There is a corresponding belief that psychic growth also results from it. It is an aspect of initiation, in this part of the world and at this level of culture, that what is held to be introjected into the boy novice, along with much other cultural influence, is "masculinity" in the form either of actual semen (considered as bodily "food") or of "symbolic semen" said, in initiation, to be introjected anally by the spirits of the ancestors who are the extensions in time (and psychic depth) of the initiating men.

This is an extremely complex subject, in which it is often difficult to know how far this part-initiating act is physical and how far it is referred to as a symbol for its psychic transformation. We have in Malekula, for instance, the most extreme contrasts. In the interior of North Malekula there are powerful chiefs who have a virtual monopoly of the women, so that there is a highly organized system of what psycho-analysts call an "accidental" type of homosexuality due to lack of access to women, in which the whole male population is involved, including even the chiefs themselves, who enjoy both kinds of sexual intercourse and for whom, therefore, the "accidental" has turned into a pleasure *sui generis*. As in its more primitive form in a four-section system, where it is restricted, so far as I know, to the circumstances of infant betrothal, this much more highly organized and graded form of homosexuality in North Malekula is still run on exogamous lines in exactly the same way as heterosexual intercourse, it being considered incestuous to have homosexual intercourse that would contravene any of the ordinary exogamous regulations.

The anthropologist who first recorded this socialization of homosexuality in North Malekula, but had no knowledge of its kinship history, thought that the boy-lover called his man-lover by the term used for "sister's husband" as a "jest" (Deacon, 1934, p. 261). It may have become so there, but comparative studies show us the reason why, even though the North Malekulans themselves may have forgotten its origin.

The practice there has become so far divorced from this origin that a boy-lover may be "sold", as wives are "sold", to other men-lovers, though he will be expected nevertheless to return to his "betrothed" man-lover, with whom he, theoretically at least, has a bond of love-friendship that transcends such purely physical infidelities. There are cases also of extreme homosexual jealousy, particularly when the man-lover is old and may in fact be a "grandfather" charged with "educating" and stimulating the growth of the boy-lover who is so much younger (Guiart, pp. 15 ff.). Such cases obviously verge on the pathological.

But there is another aspect to all this which has, in the Small Islands where I worked, the greatest educational significance. The boy-lover is in North Malekula called by a special term, *mugh vel*, in the Small Islands *mov ghal* (Layard, 1942, pp. 503 ff.) or *mohewal*. When the time comes for him to be initiated he is given a guardian, or "tutor" as I call him, who looks to his needs and helps him through all his initiatory crises. This man is called the "husband" (the same term as is used for "sister's husband") and the novice is called the "wife". In North Malekula they cohabit as such. The tutor possesses the novice as a man possesses his wife, apart from the short time—only a few weeks—which it takes for the boy to be circumcised and for his wound to heal. He will on the one hand be jealous if the boy is unfaithful to him. On the other hand he "mothers" and tends him as a mother would tend her child, and feeds him royally in the intervals between the many painful experiences (both physical and psychic) which every novice is made to undergo.

In the Small Islands, where there are no chiefs monopolizing the women and the society is altogether a more balanced one with little active homosexuality, novice and tutor call one another "husband" (that is to say "sister's husband") and "wife" (which means "woman"), and there is much banter to this effect, but it is doubtful whether this indicates a physical relationship. For this is in any case in line with the almost universal treatment of initiation novices as being "only women" or "like women" before initiation and being turned into "men" through initiation, whether there are any homosexual practices connected with this or not.

The concept of the novice's "femininity" and therefore potential (though psychic) pregnancy is however very evident in that the whole period of initiation lasts nine months—the period of a woman's pregnancy—and the intensive period during which the boy is super-incised (a modified form of circumcision consisting of slitting the foreskin but not removing it, making him bleed like a menstruating woman) and many other trials are undergone lasts precisely a month, which is the period of the menstrual cycle.

So does the symbolism of anal penetration persist, though on a totally new level. For, during the whole of the intensive month of trials following this operation, when the novices are more or less immobilized in their initiation lodge, they are, in one of the "hoaxes" constantly practised on them, frequently threatened with being anally penetrated by the spirits of the ancestors. To make this all the more realistic, the tutors and others previously initiated make scrabbling noises on the sloping roof of the initiation lodge which the novices are told are made by the ancestral spirits trying to "get in".

I have not heard of this threat of anal penetration by the

ancestral spirits outside of the Small Islands where I constantly heard of it from my informants, some of whom were at that time "tutors" themselves. This may appear to us to be somewhat ludicrous, but to the natives it is of the highest character-forming value. It is a case of the "lowest" turned into the "highest", for what is actually meant by the "ancestral spirits" (more popularly called "ancestral ghosts") is *the collective spirit of the ancestors* who are the guardians of tribal morality and of the highest cultural and psychic values that the natives know. This is the native expression for what we call "conscience", the inner voice that tells a man what is socially right and what he ought to do in spite of possible inclinations to do otherwise.

The main function of these "spirits" is to enforce incest taboos. That is to make them *appear* "natural" and therefore more easily observable, although they are in fact "unnatural" and therefore dependent on that "supernatural" sanction which the belief in ancestral spirits, or spirit in general, implies.

On the one hand the novices fear this psycho-physical threat (which the tutors make great play of, the tutors themselves being these ancestors' living cultural representatives and having themselves suffered in a like way), for the ancestors are thought to be up to every kind of trick. On the other hand it suggests symbolically the impregnation of the novices, not with physical children as the New Guinea natives, as we shall see later, suppose, but with the psychic and cultural values which the ancestral spirits uphold and which the ancestors themselves during their lifetimes helped to establish.

This influence comes in "from behind", that is by way of the unconscious, where man is female as well as male. As the natives put it: Where else can the ancestral spirits "come into" the novice's body to initiate him? They cannot come in through the mouth. That is where the mother penetrates with her breast during the boy's infancy. The male influence comes in anally where the man can penetrate, but the woman, who has no organ with which to do so, cannot penetrate.

The same motive is also represented in another part of Malekula by a dramatic performance in which all those previously initiated lie down on the ground, head to feet, in a long line leading from the "mother-drum" set up in the dancing-ground to the neighbouring initiation-lodge in which the novices are, with huge rolls of leaves symbolizing penises stretching from one man's genitals to the other's so as to form a continuous symbolic phallus reaching from the mother-drum to the novices. This is a male "umbilical cord" by means of which the female influence from the mother-drum is symbolically transmuted into a male one for the psychic benefit of the novices who are thought to be impregnated by it, so that they themselves become pregnant of psychic (male) matter, called *ta-mats*, that which has "died" to the mother-principle and has been reborn into a new male psychic one.

(For a preliminary account, to be expanded later, of initiation rites in the Small Islands, see Layard, 1942, Chapters XVIII, XIX; for the hoax just recounted see Deacon, 1934, pp. 233–4.)

## VI

Such symbolism is not confined to Malekula, nor are the initiating homosexual practices that go along with it. They are widespread, but have not always been recorded; very largely, I think, on account of prudery and of European misapprehension coupled with fear of what might be stirred up in the white man's unconscious were such practices and their associated fantasies fully realized.

The same pattern of behaviour between initiating tutors and their novices obtains in at least one other part of New Guinea (the Trans-Fly River area) from which there is no report of supposed anal penetration by the ancestors but, as in North Malekula, the tutors themselves fulfil this role.

Here the homosexual aspect of homo-eroticism seems to have run riot in a way that it has not done in the Small Islands, the novices being at the service not only of their own tutors but of all those male members of the opposite kinship moiety, whether fellow-villagers or visitors, "who wish to practise sodomy" (Williams, 1936, p. 199). There also the notion of the novices' psychic pregnancy has become confused with the idea of physical pregnancy to the extent that it is believed that through this act the boys may become physically pregnant, which is considered undesirable. The further confusion between oral penetration (by the woman's breast) and anal penetration (by the man's penis) is such that, in order to "neutralize the effects of the homosexual intercourse" the novices have lime emptied down their throats (*ibid.*, p. 201). This effort to prevent their pregnancy causes considerable agony with blistered mouths, and is in line in this respect with the many other physical and psychic trials which they have to undergo.

Williams recorded the names of five pot-bellied males (in a predominantly lean population), of whom it was thought that this anti-pregnancy operation had failed, so that they "were thought to be with child" (*ibid.*, p. 201). Psychologists will not miss here the identification between the male oral cavity and the female vaginal one.

For the most part neither the anal penetration nor the forced feeding with lime seem to have any permanent bad physical effect (as I have not heard of ill effects from anal penetration from any other source), but here Williams does say that he knew of one boy recently initiated who died owing, as he thought, to severe anal infection (*ibid.*, p. 199, note 1).

In this part of New Guinea, as elsewhere, the novices call their tutor men-lovers by the term locally used for "sister's husband", and, despite the obvious degeneracy of some of the practices, strict rules of homosexual exogamy still obtain.

## VII

To conclude, I will cite a myth from this same area of New Guinea concerning "The Origin of Sodomy". There was a male Originator or First Cause named *Kambel* who was identified with the moon, and his wife with the sun. This is a very frequent primitive concept—the sun symbolizing nature and the obvious, and the whole female world of the first creation thought of as "the mother" which never changes (for women have no "souls"). The moon on the other hand symbolizes the psychic agency working in the darkness to change all that. It is the "light in the darkness" (the psyche), and, as a phenomenon that changes with each change in phase, is the "thinker" and so the "transformer". It therefore comes from "the father" who symbolizes this male transforming influence. Being male, it is also "the son". These two, the father and the son, together are in this place "the moon".

> *Kambel* had a son named *Gufa* who "despite good feeding and attention, was a wretched undersized little boy, described as pot-bellied and constipated. He was the despair of his father until one day, ostensibly with the sole idea of promoting his growth, he conceived the idea of sodomizing him. He took him apart from his mother during the night and put his idea into effect". There are two versions of what he did. One has it that he bid his son stoop to drink at a pool and, as he did so, took this opportunity to penetrate him. The other is that he rubbed "semen over the child's body. The result was a miraculous increase in growth. The boy was instructed to keep this a dead secret from his mother, and when she next saw him she was delighted at the change but attributed it wrongly to the good food which *Kambel* must have given him, just as nowadays mothers are supposed to attribute the size of initiates to the special feeding they have had" (Williams, 1936, p. 309 and footnotes).

This myth is packed with symbolism which many may be pleased to analyse. But there is one feature in it that needs special anthropological knowledge to understand. This is the "reversal of external fact" contained in all myths of origin which is their special characteristic and without which there is and can be no myth of origin.

Among the people who relate this myth no father would sodomize his son, since they belong to the same clan and patrilineal moiety. Such an act would be patrilineally incestuous. The ultimate purpose of all incest taboo is not only to expand society, but to create within the psyche precisely that which has been tabooed externally. In the case of the matrilineal incest taboo this is the anima. The anima is for a man, however, mainly a go-between or mediating function for the realization of his own "shadow" or inner masculinity which is the ultimate goal of his own development.

The patrilineal incest taboo is in fact what all this homosexuality is concerned with, particularly on its fantasy side. *Kambel* and *Gufa* are not human father and son. They are what the natives conceive of as gods. "Gods" are not men. They symbolize not external life, but inner life. The "father", then, in this case is not the father in external life, with whom all such intercourse is forbidden. He is a god, in fact a "founder" god, founder and creator, that is, not of the body but of the spirit. *Kambel* and *Gufa* both symbolize psychic functions: the one all-wise and mature, "God the Father", Originator or First Cause; the other "God the Son", who is as yet in the making, having the characteristics of ignorant man combined with a divine receptivity to the wisdom of the Father who "knows", and who can inject what he knows if the recipient can receive it.

There are two versions of this myth which are not mutually exclusive. The tale is told with amusement of the boy being made to bend over the pool, so as to be taken unawares. The pool is symbolic, being a frequent primitive symbol for that which mirrors its opposite. Primitive myths are often an exquisite mixture of human humour and divine seriousness. Humans have always to be divinely "tricked" into self-realization. The incest taboo is such a world-wide divine "trick". So is the reversal that takes place in the psyche, in which incest turns into *hieros gamos*. This *hieros gamos* is not hetero-erotic, but is homo-erotic. *Gufa* is not only penetrated by the father-principle anally from behind, that is to say via the unconscious which took him by surprise, but he is also "anointed" in a way that he or anyone can see. He is "the sacrifice" and he is also "the anointed one".

The Son thus has the Father both inside him and without, so that we have here adumbrated in this very primitive myth the highest doctrine of "the Father in Me, and I in Him", with the symbolic semen fulfilling the same function as the Holy Spirit (the spirits of the ancestors) which is the carrier of the love between the Father and the Son. This impregnates and anoints the son, the shadow-figure that at first sight always appears so odd or bad or disappointing but that is known to show forth the figure of the potential Saviour under such disguise.

All this occurs in primitive mythology alongside the most flagrant misconceptions and abuses. This is a phenomenon not confined to New Guinea or to the "primitives". We have it flourishing among ourselves.

Turning to another "primitive", we find that St. Paul knew something about this when, in his diatribe against homosexuality, and clearly speaking from experience, he describes homosexuals as those "who hold the truth in unrighteousness, because *that which may be known of God is manifest in them*, for *God hath showed it unto them*" (Romans, 1, 19), but "even as they did not like to retain God in their knowledge, God gave them over to a reprobate mind" (*ibid.*, 1, 28).

Nevertheless he goes on, "Therefore thou art inexcusable, O man, whosoever thou art that judgest: for wherein thou judgest another, thou condemnest thyself; for thou that judgest doest the same things" (*ibid.*, 2, 1). Further, about the "resurrection of the dead", which psychologically means that which has been repressed, "it is sown in dishonour, it is raised in glory" ... "the first Adam was made a living soul; the second Adam was made a quickening spirit" ... "the first man is of the earth, earthy: the second man is the Lord from heaven" (I Cor. 42–47).

The second man is symbolized in the New Guinea myth by the boy-lover, the *puer aeternus*, hermaphrodite, appearing male but inwardly female. The man-lover, who both penetrates and surrounds, is complementarily hermaphrodite.

Dreams not unlike this myth are dreamt today by heterosexuals who are latent homosexuals. Once understood they may become the most healing symbols.

## REFERENCES

BATESON, G. (1936). *Naven*. London, Cambridge University Press.

DEACON, B. (1934). *Malekula: A Vanishing People in the New Hebrides*. London, Routledge.

FENICHEL, O. (1945). *The Psychoanalytic Theory of Neurosis*. London, Routledge & Kegan Paul; New York, Norton.

FORDHAM, M. (1957). "Reflections on Image and Symbol", *J. analyt. Psychol.* **2**, 1.

GUIART, J. (undated). *L'Organisation sociale et politique du Nord Malekula*. (Rapport général d'une Mission aux Nouvelles-Hébrides effectuée au cours de l'été 1950–1951). Issued in multigraphed typescript by the Office de la Recherche Scientifique Outre-Mer, Institut Français d'Océanie, Nouméa, New Caledonia.

JUNG, C. G. (1946). *Die Psychologie der Übertragung*. Zürich, Rascher. Trans. "Psychology of the Transference", *Coll. Wks.*, **16**.

LAYARD, J. (1942). *Stone Men of Malekula*. London, Chatto & Windus.

LAYARD, J. (1945). "The Incest Taboo and the Virgin Archetype", *Eran-Jb.*, **12**.

LAYARD, J. (1956). "Identification with the Sacrificial Animal", *Eran-Jb.*, **24**
SPENCER, Sir B. and GILLEN, F. J. (1927). *The Arunta*. London, Macmillan.
STEIN, L. (1957). "What is a Symbol Supposed to Be?" *J. analyt. Psychol.*, **2**, 1
WILLIAMS, F. E. (1936). *Papuans of the Trans-Fly*. Oxford, Clarendon Press

# 17

## THE PROBLEM OF DICTATORSHIP AS REPRESENTED IN MOBY-DICK

JAMES KIRSCH, *Los Angeles*

LITERARY historians have had great difficulty in classifying *Moby-Dick* (1851) since its character has many features unusual in the classical form of the novel. Its vastness and its poetic rhythm undoubtedly give it the grandeur of an epic. Its monologues, dialogues, mass-scenes and the inclusion of whales, ships, sea and sky as participating actors lend it an intensely dramatic quality. Thus the unavoidable conclusion was that *Moby-Dick* could not be classified among any of the known forms of literature—that it was a unique work of art. In approaching it from the psychological point-of-view it appears to me that *Moby-Dick* has the greatest similarity to a fairy-tale or, rather, a myth. However, a fairy-tale or myth generally describes the psychological and spiritual situation of a particular age or people; it is stripped of individual characteristics and frequently reveals in great detail the collective psychic condition of the people who produced it.

*Moby-Dick* is the work of *one* man and yet it has all the earmarks of a great myth. In a fascinating and at the same time exasperating manner it shows a blending of the most personal attributes and inclinations of its author, Herman Melville, together with collective problems of his time. It was C. G. Jung (1933, p. 178) who first pointed out that *Moby-Dick* was born out of the collective unconscious. Certainly it is the personal myth of its author and as such determined Melville's development and fate, and beyond that it is a myth which gives us magnificent insight into the psychological status of the nineteenth-century man. I have dealt with the biographical aspect of *Moby-Dick* in another paper (Kirsch, 1958). Here I would like to go more deeply into the historical and generally human aspect of this work since I believe that Melville anticipated in a detailed and poetic way aspects of universal modern psychology which still have full sway over us. It is no coincidence that here in *Moby-Dick* a modern myth is presented to us which describes the objective psyche as experienced by an individual human being. It is an indication of the modern trend in history which places man in the centre of the universe and involves the ego in the processes of the psyche. In contrast to Shakespeare—Melville's mentor and model who disappears as it were behind his work and about whose personality development we can make out very little—Melville is very much in his work and is profoundly affected by everything that happens and by every character who acts in his story. While it is impossible for us to say to what extent Shakespeare was Macbeth, Hamlet or Prospero, we can clearly state to what extent Melville was Ishmael or Ahab or even the whale or the sea. It is obvious that all the figures in Melville's works were components of his personality since he had an experience of the total psyche and since his artistic work is determined by just this experience.

Since he gave us such a full description of his psychic processes we gain an insight into the collective psychology of our time. He describes changes in the relationship between ego and self which have since played a destructive role in the conduct of human affairs everywhere. I refer to the figure of the *dictator* which in *Moby-Dick* is represented by Ahab. In a technical sense we could speak of the development of the power-complex of the ego as it occurs in the nineteenth century. The choice of this biblical name already establishes Ahab as a tyrant and as a rebel against God. I Kings XVI 30–33 characterizes Ahab as one who "did evil in the sight of the Lord above all that were before him". Ahab usurped Naboth's paternal inheritance. Just as the biblical king has an opponent in the prophet Elijah, so does Melville's Ahab have a prophet of the same name as antagonist. The Bible gives a great deal of attention to the relationship between Ahab and Elijah, but in *Moby-Dick* their relationship is only darkly hinted at (Melville, 1851, Ch. 19). Elijah tries, however, to give Ishmael full information about Captain Ahab as a dictator on board the Pequod and as a man who reviled and cursed the name of God and who somehow had lost his leg in an unequal battle with God. In Elijah's short and concise statements about Ahab ("Old Thunder", "He gives the order and you must jump") he connects the fact of Ahab's dictatorship with his blasphemous and destructive attitude in his relationship to God. Ishmael, of course, does not yet understand anything that this Christ-like prophet tries to convey to him, and thus the journey has to be undertaken and a full unfoldment of this vital conflict has to occur. The quest for consciousness, the violent desire for ultimate truth and the battle against God make up the drama of the epic. The conflict between man and God in the image of the Leviathan is painted in the grandest colours. It is developed in the form of a night-sea journey across all oceans and ends in the region of the equator in a momentous three-day battle. The opponents are Ahab and the enormous white whale.

In *Moby-Dick* we find a comprehensive description of all sorts of whales and even a classification of all those sea-animals which Melville, against much better scientific knowledge, prefers to call "fish" (*ibid.*, p. 132) and frequently names "Leviathans" (*ibid*, p. 131), which at once makes us think of the biblical animals of God. There are many references to the book of Job and the direct quotation of the 41st chapter. The sermon by Father Mapple (*ibid.*, Ch. 9) is a fascinating and highly controversial exegesis of the book of Jonah. All these things make it clear beyond the shadow of a doubt that Ahab's journey is meant by Melville as another *Answer to Job*, i.e. a search for God. The quest of this seeker, however, is not for the redemption of the human being nor for a reconciliation between man and God. This journey, across all oceans of this planet into the furthest reaches of the unconscious, rather serves first of all the purpose of showing that the man of today can do all the things that God, appearing in the whirlwind, told Job he could never hope to achieve. "Canst thou fill his skin with barbed irons? or his head with fish-spears? . . . darts are counted as stubble" (*ibid*, p. 334). Oh, of course I-man, Ahab, can do that. Melville ironically dismisses the biblical statement with a short sentence: "Oh! that unfulfilments should follow the prophets" (*ibid.*, p. 335).

While large parts of the epic are devoted to the hunting of

whales and to demonstrating man's undoubted superiority and dominance over all nature, there is *one* specimen who is unique among all the sperm whales. He is "not only ubiquitous, but immortal" (*ibid.*, p. 179); he possesses "unwonted magnitude", "infernal aforethought of ferocity", uncanny intelligence, cunning and malice. The whalehunters come upon him in the ordinary business of whaling, abysmally ignorant of his specific individualizing features. In attacking him with the usual method of line harpoon they always meet with some untoward accident: boats are splintered; a man is lost; a captain loses his arm. It is even told that occasionally he staves a big ship. Therefore this monster has received an individual name: Moby-Dick. These occurrences breed a particular terror in the whaling community and they avoid any further encounter with this monster.

Ahab, the captain of the Pequod, originally came upon Moby-Dick in the same way as all the other whalemen, that is: most ignorantly. In the wild battle with Moby-Dick, Ahab lost one leg but in contrast to all the other captains he decided to go after Moby-Dick and destroy him. And so the second and all-consuming intention of this journey was to destroy God himself or that image of God which clearly has all the attributes of the Old Testament God. In fact, as Jung shows in *Aion*, the Leviathan is the unredeemed part of the God-image, the human aspect of it.

The sea is the element in which the whales and Moby-Dick move. It comprises all oceans which are all interconnected and which to Melville form one great whole. Like everything else in this epic, the ocean is a symbol and as such expresses all moods and mystical powers of nature. The particular fascination which the whale exerts on Ahab is due to the fact that "of all divers" he, the sperm whale, "dives the deepest" (*ibid.*, pp. 309–10), has "moved amid this world's foundations", has his "most familiar home" in "that awful water-land". "The sun hides not the ocean which is the dark side of this earth" (*ibid*, p. 422). The ocean and the human psyche are very close to each other—they are almost the same. Ahab exclaims: "O Nature, and O soul of man! how far beyond all utterance are your linked analogies! not the smallest atom stirs or lives on matter, but has its cunning duplicate in mind" (*ibid.*, p. 310). Because of these "linked analogies" the attack against nature becomes also an attack against the human mind and against the self. Thus the seeker of knowledge is transformed into a hunter, conqueror and killer.

The *participation mystique* between the sea with its whales and the unconscious with its dominant contents, the archetypes, creates in Melville a psychological situation similar to that of the alchemists. To the alchemists matter was the great unknown and therefore became the receptacle of the unconscious. Owing to this projection matter and psyche were to them indistinguishable from each other. While the ocean and the objective psyche, the whale and the Leviathan, are often not differentiated from each other there is often an awareness that affects, moods or other contents of the unconscious are projected on the ocean and its living contents, the whales; for example, when he writes that Ahab "piled upon the whale's white hump the sum of all the general rage and hate felt by his whole race from Adam down" (*ibid.*, p. 182); or speaking of a special behaviour of the whales, he says they have "mystic gestures . . . akin to Freemason signs and symbols". And with clear reference to Exod. XXXIII, 33, he continues: "I know him not, and never will . . . Thou shalt see my back parts, my tail, he seems to say, but my face shall not be seen. But I cannot completely make out his back parts; and hint what he will about his face, I say again he has no face" (*ibid.*, p. 376). Thus it is left ambiguous whether Melville means the whale or God.

I believe I have given enough quotations to show that Melville describes here the unconscious and its contents, the archetypes, that to a considerable extent he is aware of this fact, and that there is a particular whale or archetype which though it shares many characteristics of all the other archetypes is something very different, quite specific and unique. In Melville's language it is either God himself or an agent of God (*ibid.*, p. 162)—or as he says in the chapter, *First Day of the Chase*: ". . . the grand god revealed himself, sounded and went out of sight. . . . Not the white bull Jupiter. . . not Jove, not that great majesty Supreme! did surpass the glorified White Whale as he so divinely swam" (*ibid.*, p. 539). It is clearly an image of the Old Testament God but it is also obvious that a new image of God is emerging from the unconscious and blending with the old one. It has strongly psychological qualities. Melville does not yet have any conscious equipment to conceive or integrate it. In our modern psychological language we call it the "self".

We can now draw the conclusion that in *Moby-Dick* Melville is depicting the journey of modern man into the unconscious where he meets with contents which were constellated in his time. They are the archetypes and among them the outstanding archetype of the self in the image of a god with old and new qualities. An *Auseinandersetzung* between the ego and the self is sought which assumes the fateful and fatal aspect of a power struggle and battle for supremacy. The ego becomes a dictator, the self a destructive agent. *In the end, as could only be expected, the ego is destroyed by the self.*

How did it come about? I prefer this formulation to the simply casual question: what caused it? It is impossible to answer it in all of its implications. In a *personal* way we can state however that obviously Melville had an experience of the unconscious in his childhood—an experience he describes in Chapter 4 where he fell "into a troubled nightmare of a doze . . . half steeped in dreams" he "opened his eyes . . . a supernatural hand seemed placed in his . . . he lay there frozen with the most awful fears. The nameless unimaginable silent form or phantom . . . seemed seated by his bed. It was a horrid spell. To this very hour he puzzled himself with this mystery" (*ibid.*, p. 26). His meeting with Queequeg is felt as a continuation and unfoldment of this great mystery. In other words, Melville the child has been touched by the unconscious. It never left him alone and sooner or later he had to meet its terror again.

In a *collective* way we can say that the middle of the nineteenth century was a time in which collective contents entered consciousness in a most intensive way—as Aniela Jaffé magnificently describes in her article on "Der Goldene Topf", the fairy tale by E. T. A. Hoffmann (Jung, 1950). On the American continent the United States was in a state of fermentation. Prophets of all kinds made their appearance, new religions were born and social conflicts arose which ultimately led to the Civil War. These events were expressions of an activated unconscious. Behind all of them stood the powerful emergence of a new image of God and with it a new image of man and the problem of their mutual relationship. These tendencies and movements took hold of Melville's fertile imagination. It was a time in which man became aware of his suddenly growing knowledge and power over nature and became drunk with them. The unconscious acted and reacted correspondingly. It would be true to a certain extent to say that Melville is the prophet of the ego and its doom just as Nietzsche was some thirty years later in his Zarathustra. It would be equally true to say that Melville discovered the unconscious and even certain aspects of the way of individuation. But Melville could not accept himself as a prophet and therefore felt himself "a greater sinner" than ordinary man.

The particular reason for this deeply-felt guilt and failure to achieve individuation, the tragedy is the intentional bypassing, ridiculing and outright repression of the anima as a factor to be taken seriously. This fact is described in the very first few lines of the book. The result of this repression is a most intense affect-laden hostility between ego and self. No attempt at co-existence, relationship or coming to terms with the self is ever made. Only occasionally does Ahab retain a "considerating touch of humanity". Mostly, Moody Ahab, as he is often termed, is filled with a monomaniac hatred against the White Whale. The self cannot be seen as anything else but the Leviathan who must be destroyed. Those few other symbols of the self like the squid (Melville, 1851, Ch. 59) and the spirit-spout (*ibid.*, Ch. 51) are received with negative numinous feelings—and also bypassed.

It is therefore no wonder that a development or maturing in the proper sense of the word does not take place in Ahab. He emerges step by step out of Ishmael's unconscious. In the course of the story his full portrait is painted. Many incidents serve only to depict in full detail the stiffening of the stubborn, mad ego. The further the journey develops the more he rejects all support offered by human beings, the more arrogantly he discards all instruments for conscious orientation like the compass and the quadrant. Events and people try to persuade him to go back to the ordinary pursuits of man, to return to human society and to be human among humans, but he refuses to listen. The result is a fatal contraction of the human personality and synchronistically a sinister change of wind, weather and sea-life against the 'Pequod'. Toward the end, as it is stated in Chapter 130, "all humour, forced or natural, vanished . . . Alike joy and sorrow, hope and fear, seemed ground to finest dust, and powdered, for the time, in the clamped mortar of Ahab's iron soul" (*ibid.*, p. 527).

Ishmael, through whose eyes we see the whole journey, receives from the beginning a good deal of information, from strange incidents and rather directly from Elijah, which tell him that conditions on this ship are very strange and that unknown dangers lurk in the whole enterprise. Ishmael is aware that Ahab is to be the absolute dictator of the whalehunt but, as he continues: "When a man suspects any wrong, it sometimes happens that... he insensibly strives to cover up his suspicions even from himself... I said nothing, and tried to think nothing" (*ibid*, p. 96). During the whole journey there is never an individual meeting between Ishmael and Ahab. Only once does Ishmael confront Ahab in the great scene on "The Quarter-Deck" (*ibid.*, Ch. 36)—a sort of black mass in which the whole crew commit themselves to help in the vengeful pursuit of Moby-Dick. The collective situation sweeps Ishmael away into the tremendous collective emotion and he agrees with all the others to the change of the purpose of this journey from a profitable whaling enterprise to the illegitimate pursuit of the captain's personal vengeance. Ahab gains ascendancy over his crew by staging a great, emotion-charged ritual. It is here first shown that Ahab himself is possessed —possessed by the one thought: to meet and to kill Moby-Dick. It has such exclusive power over him "you could almost see that thought turn in him as he turned, and pace in him as he paced; so completely possessing him, indeed, that it all but seemed the inward mould of every outer movement". Toward evening "he looked not unlike the weather horizon when a storm is coming up" (*ibid.*, p. 158).

In other words this murderous thought, coupled with extraordinary rage and hatred, has become an autonomous complex and possesses Ahab to the exclusion of everything else. It becomes personified in the figure of the Parsee, Fedallah: "a figure tall and swart, with one white tooth evilly protruding from its steel-like lips... funereally invested with a Chinese jacket of black cotton ... crowned with a glistening, white turban", who seems to be "one of the paid spies and secret confidential agents on the water of the *devil*" (*ibid.*, p. 215). Coming up from the "unknown nooks and ash-holes of the earth", he seems to be "Beelzebub himself". What he really is "remained a muffled mystery to the last"; how he was linked with Ahab remained "half-hinted". He had influence on Ahab, even authority over him, but still Fedallah is a figure "civilized people only see in their dreams and that but dimly". He comes from the "Oriental isles to the east of the continent, which even in the semodern days still preserve much of the ghostly aboriginalness of earth's primal generations". In other words, Fedallah springs up from the deepest and most original layer of the primitive psyche. It is that stratum where "the memory of the first man was a distinct recollection, and all men his descendants" (*ibid.*, p. 229). As Jung (1951, trans. pp. 132, 249 f.) has stated, the primitive psyche contains as its most important content the image of the primal man, the Adam Kadmon, the anthropos, the four-aspected fire as a numinous expression of the self. In the same way Ishmael experiences numinous emotions toward this figure of the first man, but significantly enough realizes them only as negative and can evaluate the emerging of the self into consciousness only as a sinister and destructive event. That is why he associates the appearance of this "phantom", as he calls Fedallah, with the idea that in the same way "according to Genesis the angels indeed consorted with the daughters of men, the devils also, add the uncanonical Rabbins, indulged in mundane amours" (Melville, 1952, p. 230). Psychologically speaking, according to Jung (1952, trans. pp. 421 f.) this marriage of the angels—actually the sons of God (Genesis VI)—with real women represents an inflation, a psychological condition in which consciousness is filled with archetypal contents. Correspondingly, the indulgence of the devils in mundane amours also represents an inflation. It appears that in the process of becoming conscious the emergence of archetypal contents into consciousness almost unavoidably brings about an inflation and as such is an unfavourable psychic condition. It is imperative for the individual so affected to make a clear distinction between himself and the archetypal accruements. As we psychotherapists know, this is a labour which requires tremendous effort, patience, intelligence and many other virtues. In Ahab's case the inflation symbolized by devils indulging in mundane amours has an ominous portent. The association between Ahab and Fedallah is very close. For example it is stated in Chapter 73: "Ahab chanced so to stand that the Parsee occupied his shadow while if the Parsee's shadow was there at all it seemed only to blend with, and lengthen Ahab's" (Melville, p. 1952, 327). The conclusion is therefore compelling that Fedallah represents the self—the idea of totality as contained and intuited in the ego (Jung, 1955, Vol. I, pp. 118 ff.). The identity between ego and self is almost complete. The autonomous complex which possesses Ahab is so powerful and all-embracing just because it contains the archetype of the self with all its libido and numinosity.

For this reason an uncanny magical power radiates from Ahab, makes the whole crew willingly obey every order, forego every material advantage and adopt their commander's vengeance as their own. They bow to indignities and as the chapter "Queen Mab" demonstrates, the unconscious helps to fortify Ahab's dictatorship. In Stubb's dream Ahab seemed a pyramid and a badger-haired old merman argues that "it's an honour to be kicked by Ahab", an honour worth boasting of. It is interesting to see that the unconscious itself states the identification of Ahab with the self.

Ahab deliberately uses his magical power over individuals as well as over the crew. He "shocks them into the game" (Melville, 1851, p. 164) including Starbuck, the one member who at all times is aware of his own humanity and his human limitations in general, and who again and again attempts to bring Ahab back to the ordinary business of whaling, to human values, to love and friendship. It is only in Starbuck, the first mate, that Ahab finds any resistance against the mad enterprise. Starbuck, representing the ordinary man, is willing to face any danger "if it fairly comes in the way of the business we follow; but I came here to hunt whales, not my commander's vengeance" (*ibid.*, p. 161). This reply evokes only contempt from Ahab but it forces him to reveal what is so exasperating to him in the White Whale: "He (the whale) tasks me; he heaps me; I see in him outrageous strength, with an inscrutable malice sinewing it. That inscrutable thing is chiefly what I hate . . . Talk not to me of blasphemy, man; I'd strike the sun if it insulted me . . . Who's over me? Truth has no confines . . . my heat has melted thee to anger-glow" (*ibid.*, p. 162).

Here it is said in classical terms that he, the human ego, wants to pierce through the walls of unconsciousness by power, violence and hatred. He is aware that God is in it; he objects to the charge of blasphemy because what he is seeking is truth: "Truth has no confines" and stands above all gods. But can we ever know ultimate truth? Hating the self and "seeing nothing but malice sinewing it" is an attitude which makes it impossible to find oneself and renders the search for God hopeless. In assuming this attitude he frankly expresses the hybris of the human ego: "I'd strike the sun if it insulted me". Such a shocking statement shows how far Ahab has gone in his identification with the self and demonstrates that to Ahab the sun is a symbol of the self or, as Melville puts it, a "linked analogy". It also shows that the ego is fully aware of the superior power, outrageous strength, intelligence and purposefulness of his antagonist, but he does not submit in Christian humility and attempt to come to terms with it. Instead this unconscious identification with the self begets in him the idea that to maintain his own identity he must destroy the self, because if the sun can insult him he will strike it.

This is clearly madness. Ahab far overestimates the power and capacity of the ego: "What I've dared, I've willed; and what I've willed, I'll do!" (*ibid.*, p. 164). He has met the self once before in the shape of the White Whale. Though ego and self are usually far apart and most men anxiously avoid any approach to the self, the very fact of having met it once before kindles the desire in Ahab to search for it and to find it. But the injury, psychic as well as physical, has transformed this natural desire into the demoniac conviction that he can also destroy it. The change in Ahab's personality is such that we today must agree with Ishmael's term "monomaniacal Ahab" and apply the clinical term of insanity to him. We know that such a psychotic state is frequently quite contagious. The fact that even Starbuck succumbs to Ahab's spell is seen by Melville as a "complete abasement of his fortitude . . . the fall of valor in the soul". Starbuck is otherwise the one human being in his company who approaches Melville's ideal of man: "Man, in the ideal, is so noble and so sparkling, such a grand and glowing creature, that over any ignominious blemish in him all his fellows should run to throw their costliest robes. That immaculate manliness we feel within ourselves, so far within us, that it remains intact though all the outer character seem gone, bleeds with keenest anguish at the undraped spectacle of a valor-ruined man.. Thou shalt see it... that democratic dignity which, on all hands, radiates without end from God; Himself! The great God absolute! The centre and circumference of all democracy! His omnipresence, our divine equality!" (*ibid.*, pp. 113–14).

Starbuck is also the only man on board who until the last keeps a cool head and clearly realizes that continuing the journey under Ahab's command means certain death for him and the whole crew. He therefore decides to kill Ahab. Such an intention naturally throws this decent man into a terrible conflict: "Shall this crazed old man be tamely suffered to drag a whole ship's company down to doom with him?... Not reasoning; not remonstrance; not entreaty wilt thou hearken to; all this thou scornest. Flat obedience to thy own flat commands, this is all thou breathest... and say'st the men have vow'd thy vow; say'st all of us are Ahabs. Great God forbid!" (*ibid.*, p. 507). But there is no lawful way for Starbuck to remove Ahab from the command of the ship. He could not endure the sight of the old man caged as a prisoner nor is he able to murder him. And so he retires from the conflict and allows the journey to continue in full knowledge that it means death for him and the thirty other men on board.

Have we not frequently seen such a conflict in our time when, owing to lack of valour in the soul, a perfectly decent man avoids action in a horrible situation into which a dictator or his henchmen have thrown him? Have we not seen it millions of times in our day that the ordinary human being is despoiled by a dictator and made a willing collaborator in the most heinous crimes?

We may now draw the following conclusions about the figure of the dictator as described by Melville in *Moby-Dick:*

(1) A close contact between ego and self is established in childhood.

(2) In later life a collision between ego and self occurs which injures the ego, resulting in the development of an explosive affectivity.

(3) Still later an identification between ego and self develops. This is the most powerful inflation to which the ego can fall

victim. Such a condition (*Gott-Aehnlichkeit*) produces a remarkable increase of the intellect and of power over other human beings but dehumanizes it. Thus demonized the ego subjects individuals and groups to its own wishes and goals, assimilates them into its own system and estranges them from themselves morally and in every other way.

(4) Such a *Gott-Aehnlichkeit* ultimately leads to the destruction of the ego and of all who willingly accept this power. Individually this means psychosis, collectively a violent breakdown of the social order.

Though Melville did not want to be a prophet he nevertheless became one. He perceived in himself processes of the objective psyche which came to the surface in the twentieth century. He is one of the discoverers of the collective unconscious and of the self as the unique archetype among all other contents of the psyche. In Ahab, the hero of his "wicked book" (Melville's own expression for it), Melville describes the dangerous possibilities of the closeness between man and God. The figure of the modern dictator, the tragic condition of the inflated ego and the catastrophe necessarily resulting from its hybris (for himself and his followers) are shockingly painted in dark but true colours. But Melville is also a prophet of a new vision of man, of the ordinary man who has "that democratic dignity which, on all hands, radiates without end from God; Himself! The Great God absolute! The center and the circumference of all democracy! His omnipresence our equality".

In Ahab's case the closeness between man and God is misunderstood and misused. There is little comfort left in the fact that Ishmael is saved by the devious-cruising Rachel since he is an orphan.

The quest has to begin again and with a totally different attitude if man wants to find totality. The irresistible currents of time have constellated the image of the anthropos, of the total man again and again since Melville's time and now enforce its realization in many individuals. Unavoidably this trend creates dictatorship, the God-man in the ego, and thus dictatorship makes its appearance in small and large groups today.

The analytical relationship is such a group. The self is always constellated in every analysis in which the collective unconscious manifests itself with all its numinosity, with all its promises and all its dangers. The possibility is always given that "the sea drowns the infinite of the analyst's soul", that he becomes an Ahab and that he responds to the challenge of his life with Freud's "Flectere si nequeo superos, Acheronta movebo". But there is also the possibility that he is "carried down alive to wondrous depths, where strange shapes of the unwarped primal world glide to and fro before his passive eyes; and the misermerman, Wisdom, reveals his hoarded heaps; and where man, wandering from all mortal reason, comes at last to that celestial thought, which, to reason, is absurd and frantic".

It is Jung's merit that he avoided the mortal danger of dictatorship, that he responded with totality to the challenge of totality, thus discovering the soul and bringing the lux moderna, the light of psychological cognition, into the darkness and dissociation of our conflicted psyche. As he has shown in his life and in his opus, the result of this attitude is not dictatorship but a whole human being and a further realization of the anthropos.

## REFERENCES

JUNG, C. G. (1933). *Modern Man in Search of a Soul.* London: Kegan Paul; New York, Harcourt, Brace.

JUNG, C. G. (1950). *Gestaltungen des Unbewussten.* Zürich, Rascher.

JUNG, C. G. (1951). *Aion.* Zürich, Rascher. Trans. *Coll. Wks.*, **9**, 2.

JUNG, C. G. (1952). *Antwort auf Hiob.* Zürich, Rascher. Trans. "Answer to Job", in *Coll. Wks.*, **11**.

JUNG, C. G. (1955). *Mysterium Coniunctionis.* Zürich, Rascher.

KIRSCH, J. (1958). "The Enigma of Moby Dick", *J. analyt. Psychol.* **3**, No. 2.

MELVILLE, H. (1851). *Moby-Dick or The Whale* (quot. from 1952 edition). New York, Hendricks House.

# 18

## AN APPROACH TO GROUP ANALYSIS

ROBERT F. HOBSON, *London*

The term "group analysis" is distasteful to many analytical psychologists. Underlying their attitude is an assumption that the group is synonymous with an organization of collective standards, incompatible with the development of unique individuality, which is the goal of analysis. Jung, however, has stressed that individuation has two essential aspects, "an internal and subjective process of integration" and "an equally indispensable process of objective relationship" (Jung, 1946, *Coll. Wks.*, **16**, p. 234). His statements that "individuation does not shut one out from the world, but gathers the world to oneself" (Jung, 1947, trans. p. 435), and that "relationship to the self is at once relationship to our fellowman" (Jung, 1946, *Coll. Wks.*, **16**, p. 233) suggest that the concept of the self must include modes of integration which operate in interpersonal relationships. The importance of the study of transference relationships has been underlined by Jung and others, but it has been assumed, all too often, that, by extension from the material of personal analyses, valid pronouncements can be made about larger groups and about society in general.

Psychological development at any age occurs in, and is dependent upon, complex patterns of group relationships and it is vital that these should be studied directly. Knowledge of group psychology can come, only, from observation of groups in action and, as in every scientific project, this entails a limitation of variables by a more or less structured situation. Whatever the therapeutic significance of group analysis, there can be no doubt of its importance for research.

*Robert F. Hobson*

In view of the comparative lack of interest in group analysis shown by analytical psychologists, a discussion of general attitudes and approaches is a necessary preliminary to more detailed studies. This paper has such an aim: to intimate, in broad outline, some methods of investigation of, and a few tentative formulations about, the structure and dynamics of analytic groups. It is based upon my personal observation of various types of group over several years, during which time, by design, I remained quite unacquainted with other work in this field.

## METHODS OF DESCRIPTION

A group can be described and understood in two different ways, either in terms of the psychological mechanisms of each of its members or in terms of the dynamic patterns observed in the group as a whole. These can be termed "personal" and "group" descriptions, respectively.

In personal descriptions, formulations can be made of how a member, as subject, perceives and adapts to the others, as objects, in accordance with his constitution, psychological type, and experience. For example, events can be interpreted in terms of his attempt to manipulate others in conformity with his inner images and personal needs; and development can be described as the modification of his personal attitudes in particular relationships.

A group description does not involve a summation of a number of personal formulations, but intimates the changing patterns of the total group. The members are not considered as subject or object, but as contingent parts in a dynamic whole. For example, I shall suggest that a group can be regarded as a system with self-regulatory homeostatic mechanisms which, by a process involving splitting and recombination, can develop towards a state of integration.

In my view, these two categories apply also to what is called "individual analysis" but what I prefer to regard as analysis in a "two-group", to use Sullivan's term. It seems to me that in his developed work on the transference Jung is attempting to describe a total situation which is not the same as the sum of transference and countertransference considered in relation to separate psychic systems.

It must be stressed that this differentiation does not imply the existence of a "group mind" and an "individual mind". The distinction is between two ways of thinking which are in different logical categories; both are valuable and neither is more "true" than the other. It is no mere logical nicety, but refers to essential, practical operations. In analysis it is important to see the same events in two contexts, constantly conceiving of the group both as a multiplicity and as a unity. Interpretations are made in personal and group terms and it is necessary, in my view, repeatedly to supplement one by the other, maintaining a creative tension between two images of the group—as a collection of separate units and as one body with differentiated members.

## OBSERVATION OF GROUP DYNAMICS

The succeeding formulations are based upon observations with many groups of various sizes but, in order to make illustration easier, all examples will be given from a small group of four. The members, Mr. W., Mr. X., Mrs. Y., and Mrs. Z., were all married, with children, and their ages ranged from 32 to 50. All had been ill for some years; other treatments had failed, and, being unfit for work, they were patients in a day hospital. Hence they met each day, apart from analytic sessions, a fact which meant special difficulties in analysis, owing to leakage, but which allowed observation of the behaviour of members when out of the analytic chairs. Sessions lasting one and a half hours were held twice weekly for over two years.

In following the fascinating, and often bewildering, changes in the patterns of relationships, such mundane facts as choice of seats, bodily movements, and amount and direction of talk were often more revealing than the content of dream, fantasy, and thought.

Five chairs were placed ready in a circle and the four members of the group entered the room together. They chose their seats, leaving one for me. In this way, it could be observed how the positions of the members varied from session to session, and the changes, or absence of changes, revealed in a striking way tensions, alignments, barriers, and communications. Affects, attitudes, and lines of communication were indicated by breaks in the circle, by movements of chairs, by changes in posture, by gestures, by glances, and by the amount and direction of talk.

From such observations, diagrams were constructed of the communications network in the group. These diagrams could be made reliable by using rigid numerical methods, such as recording the number of times each person spoke, to whom. For example, *Figure* 1 represents a record obtained in 30 minutes, each arrow representing 3 communications (A = analyst).

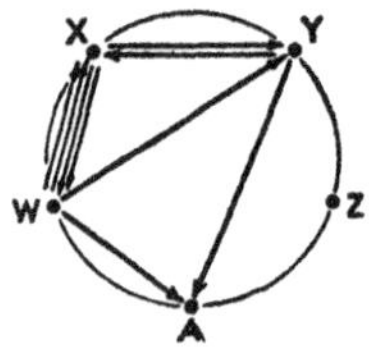


*Figure 1*

This diagram suggests that Z is isolated and that there is a strong bond between W and X. It neglects, however, the variations in type and content of talk. This might be associative or directed; it might be in the nature of personal confession or of reactions to others; it might be defensive questioning of "tea-table talk", which communicates less than a meaningful silence. Furthermore, all other non-verbal communications are ignored.

In constructing the diagrams which illustrate the text of this paper, I have sacrificed reliability in an attempt to cover as many observations as possible. They represent, then, observation plus a certain amount of interpretation. The lines represent degrees of communications between members (intense ●—●, free ●—●, little or absent ● ●, or a barrier ● ] ● ). They are based upon my assessments and do not indicate the degree of awareness of the state of affairs by the group. Nor do they imply what is communicated, e.g. negative or positive feelings. This will be hinted at in some of the examples, but the differentiation of cohesive and disruptive forces, of positive and negative valencies, and of conscious and unconscious situations, will not yet be made.

PATTERNS OF COMMUNICATION

(a) *Free Intercommunication*

This is a representation of a state which is never completely achieved, but which intimates the main aim of analysis—the interpretation and removal of splits and barriers. The chairs are kept in a circle, seats are changed freely at each session, and talk is relatively unrestricted in direction and content. The group tends to function as a whole (*Figure* 2).

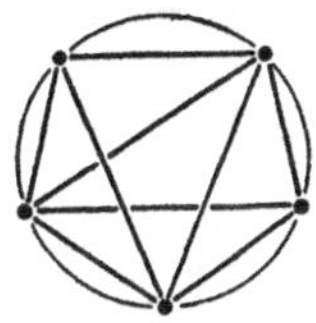

*Figure* 2

(b) *Isolation of One Member*

One chair might be moved out of the circle, often done unconsciously by the member who might later object to his position. In isolation, he may be separated by a barrier, showing no evidence of influence by the others in talk or movement (Y in *Figure* 3).

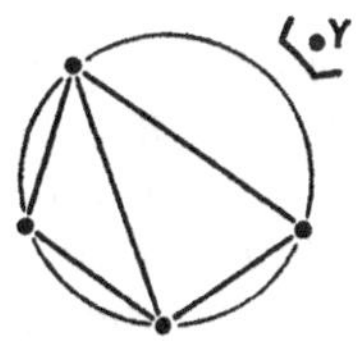


*Figure* 3

Often, however, when one member takes little part in the group, and yet continues to attend, there is communication with the analyst. Mrs. Y. and I shared an important secret, the sort of secret that is the most potent hindrance to free communication in a group. I had seen her alone when she was in a very disturbed state. She then confessed to me, with great guilt, that she had once smacked a neighbour's child without cause and had enjoyed doing so. She felt that she could never divulge this to the group and I did not urge her to do so. For some months she sat immediately on my right with her chair pushed out of the circle and nearer to me. She was very silent but often looked at me and listened attentively to all I said. Whenever she spoke her remarks were addressed directly to me. At times she became tense, this state being made evident by a quick tapping of her foot. The situation could be represented by *Figure* 4.

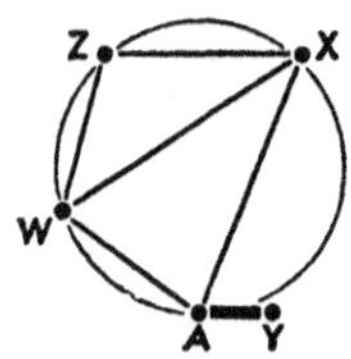


*Figure* 4

From time to time, others remarked with sympathy or resentment that she took little part. One day, the group was discussing aggression but the talk became intellectualized and finally dried up. Mrs. Y. began to tap with her feet and constantly stole glances at me. The other members began to wonder why things were not going well. Eventually all turned to Mrs. Y., at first saying that they needed her in the group and then going on to attack her for being selfish and obstinate. One of them said that she was afraid of speaking in the group because she feared her own deeper self. The rate of Mrs. Y.'s foot-tapping increased and she suddenly held out her hand and took mine, making evident the bond which was obstructing the group dialectic. This was discussed by the group and Mrs. Y. confessed her guilty secret. Thereafter, she ceased to sit by me every session and became a much more active member, and the group went on to analyse some aspects of aggression which will be outlined later.

(c) *Major Split*

A strong bond between two members with a shared emotionally loaded secret, conscious or unconscious, can lead to a major split. This situation is a common consequence of members meeting apart from analytic sessions.

Mr. X. had been feeling isolated and, as evidence of his rejection by the group, he pointed out how, often, his chair was pushed out of the circle, making him the stem of a letter Y. One day he related a dream in which he had to make a difficult and terrifying journey around the edge of a cliff, but felt unable to face it until a strange and fascinating woman appeared and led the way. Subsequently, it became clear to me that he had developed a strong emotional relationship with Mrs. Z. They sat close together, exchanged glances, and spoke usually to each other. It transpired later that they had been meeting frequently outside the group. *Figure* 5 represents the situation.

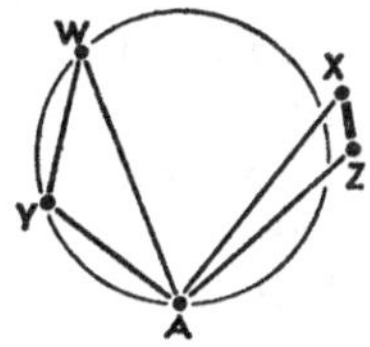


*Figure* 5

Mr. W. and Mrs. Y. did not remark on the situation but, as was usual in states of anxiety, turned more and more towards me and had less contact with each other (*Figure* 6). They utilized the typical defensive techniques, asking questions, seeking reassurance, and repeating my words in order to please me.

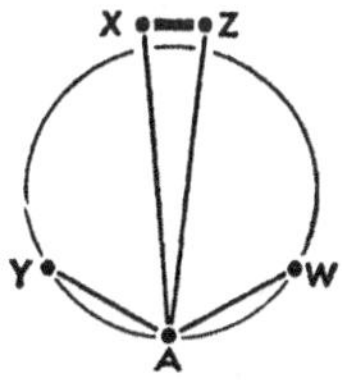


*Figure* 6

There was now a threatened disruption into the sub-group X–Z and the members W & Y. I pointed out the X–Z alliance and suggested that these two had secrets from the group. This was denied, at the time, but Mrs. Y. violently attacked Mrs. Z. for not expressing her feelings openly in the group. At the next session seats were changed and Mrs. Z. and Mr. X. were separated. Mrs. Y. and Mrs. Z. sat together and discussed their quarrel, with the help of the group, in terms of rivalry, of finding one's own faults in the other person, and of the resentment that Mrs. Y. and Mr. W. felt about the X–Z axis. Mr. X. now felt rejected once more, and he regressed into a childlike hysterical state, missing one session and trying in various ways to see me apart from the group. The members reacted in different ways. Mr. W. was practical and realistic and pointed out the ineffectiveness of such behaviour, Mrs. Y. was resentful of his conduct and regarded it as an attack upon the group, while Mrs. Z. recognized the importance of the childlike cry for love. I reminded them of Mr. X.'s dream, and this and his relationship with Mrs. Z. were understood in terms of a mother-anima situation. His efforts to manipulate the group on the basis of infantile needs were analysed and related by others to their own attitudes, and free intercommunication was re-established.

(d) *Total Defensive Patterns*

When anxiety is extreme, especially when it is not appreciated consciously, there ceases to be dynamic interaction. This state may be evident in two different types of pattern.

(i) Communication between each member and the analyst becomes paramount. Questions are frequent, seeking reassurance often about personal topics with little reference to what others are doing or saying (*Figure* 7).

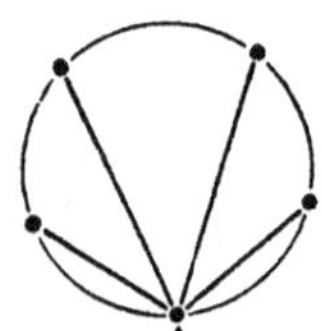


*Figure* 7

(ii) The group sometimes takes up a collective attitude in which all agree, with little or no variation, and clichés and platitudes abound. The attitude is usually adopted by the group towards the analyst either in agreement or disagreement with what they imagine to be his views, e.g. by rejection of psychology or by repetition of "respectable" psychological talk. Often the chairs are adjusted as a row in front of the teacher or as a hostile battle line (*Figure* 8).

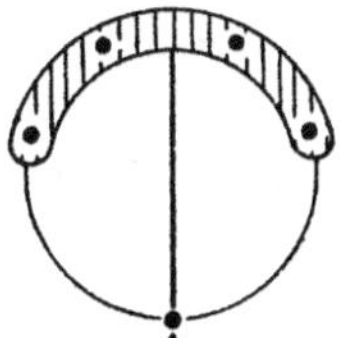


*Figure* 8

(e) *Centrally Directed Activity*

A rare state, which I hesitate to interpret, is one in which all, including myself, look and talk towards the centre, the talk becoming associative, with a good deal of fantasy. I suppose it is a state of collective identity in which I too am involved. My own fantasy at these times has, often, been of waiting for something new to be born from the centre.

These patterns apply also to silences, to which a whole paper could be devoted. From observations of movements and from preceding and succeeding material and events, silences can be described corresponding to the general patterns of relationship outlined above. The commonest are isolated, "dentist's waiting-room" silences, anxious dependent silences, collective, "hostile audience" silences, and centrally directed, creative, "good Quaker Meeting" silences.

## THEMES OF DEVELOPMENT

There are those who state that analysis, as commonly understood, cannot occur in a group setting. Much hangs upon the meaning of words, and definition is called for. By "analysis" I mean the modification of conscious attitudes by the assimilation of hitherto unconscious elements, achieved by experience and understanding of a relationship with one or more people. The main feature of analysis is the recognition, elucidation, and solution of resistances, resulting in more complete relationships, correction of defects in the apprehension of the external and social environment, and the release of healing (wholing) processes in the psyche.

All these conditions are satisfied in an analytic group such as I have been describing. I do not propose to devote any time to discussion of the analysis of associations, fantasy, dream, or personal resistance, except to note the importance of the fact that interpretations are given by all members of the group as well as by the analyst. In making such interpretations, it is important for the analyst to relate them constantly to the state of the group at the time, and it is his task to be concerned, constantly, with this state and to promote functioning of the group as a whole.

The diagram of this holistic ideal, given above (*Figure* 2), does not portray my fiction adequately. Each line should be taken to represent the action of opposing forces of attraction (A) and repulsion (R) (Hobson, 1955) and hence it should be conceived as a working model in which the whole constantly contracts and dilates with all parts in constant movement. The operation of disruptive and cohesive forces leads to constant development of new forms and more secure integration. Although not expressed in quite the same terms, this concept is similar to, and influenced by, that described by Fordham as "deintegration" (Fordham, 1957).

If defences and splits are analysed, the system works as a whole and disturbances or excesses in any part are corrected and compensated for by the reactions of other parts. It is striking how disturbance in any one member of a group is dealt with by the rest, often in an unconscious way, and how each becomes disturbed at different times. The remedy often comes from dreams or fantasies of other members. The analyst's task is to recognize and interpret resistances and to facilitate communication between all parts of the group, conscious and unconscious, allowing the action of these opposing forces and compensatory mechanisms.

The interests and activities of a group can be characterized as inwardly or outwardly directed, and it is interesting to compare these trends with the exogamous universalizing process and the endogamous "kinship libido" which Jung, following Layard, sees as opposing tendencies in society (Jung, 1946, *Coll. Wks.*, **16**, p. 224). When inwardly turned, topics relate wholly to the group, its functioning, values, and solidarity *vis-à-vis* the hostile external world. The members express attitudes which bring them nearer together and intense emotional bonds are expressed which, on analysis, are revealed as being incestuous. Such periods alternate with others in which work and home are discussed and the differences between members are emphasized. The "endogamous" periods are often characterized by a closer circle of chairs, which are more scattered in the "exogamous" ones. In my example, the day hospital formed an intermediate group, a wider circle than the analytic group but not so dispersed as the external world. The behaviour of the members of the group could be observed apart from analytic sessions and it was seen how they kept together at some times but, at others, made outside relationships. These phenomena corresponded to the inwardly and outwardly turned periods evident in the group.

Analysis, then, involves facilitating the holistic functioning of the group by recognizing and interpreting defences against the operation of the forces of attraction and repulsion. The analyst must be aware of, and treat, disruptions of the group by molar and molecular dissociations, or undue cohesion leading to collective identity, always attending to evidence of the unconscious forces opposing and compensating the conscious situation. Both splitting and coming together are important but, if there is to be a state of creative conflict and co-operation, both contact and distance must be maintained.

A general account, such as this, does not permit of a full discussion of transference. This can be considered in terms of personal projections or of dialectical encounters between one member and another, between members and the analyst, or involving the group as a whole. The attraction of the group is a potent one and, in the analysis quoted, there were only two absences in two and a half years, in spite of many upheavals. The analyst can represent many figures but, often, he clearly embodies the cohesion of the total group. The group as a whole can mean the comfort and protection of the mother, the authority of the father, but, also, a superordinate state which creates and nourishes the individual, in which he is included but to which he can also relate.

Nor can much be said about the subsidiary archetypal themes which express the fundamental pattern of cohesion and disruption.

The appearance of the leader, the hero, the scapegoat, the anima, and the shadow, and the working out of themes of death and rebirth, the night journey and the dragon fight, are evident at different times, as responses of the group to the problems of different members and to situations affecting the whole group. By study of groups it should be possible to formulate the archetypes in terms of patterns of relationship. Indeed, it seems to me that this is how archetypes must be described, and I suggest that "archetypal images" in dream and fantasy should be regarded as intimations of disturbed adaptation, i.e. the archetypal themes are not being developed satisfactorily in concrete relationships.

Special mention must be made of the significance of collective attitudes, since it has often been said that group therapy can lead only to "collectivism". Each member of the group brings the mores of his particular social group. Some standards (e.g. religious and political) vary from member to member but some are accepted ready-made by the whole group. Other collective attitudes are developed by the group. Some, such as to help and understand other members, to attend regularly, and to learn from the analyst, are early adopted in a conventional way. But, as time goes on, new ones arise, e.g. to speak one's mind and show one's feelings. These are, at first, foci of conflict but later can harden into conventions or even rules.

Modification of, and adaptation to, collective standards, with the development of a well-fitting persona, are features of group analysis and such attitudes need to be analysed constantly. In the face of anxiety, standards are used defensively, especially in a regressive way, but as analysis proceeds there is a development away from uniformity and unanimity towards the interaction of individual standards, a constant creation and recreation of patterns of values.

## ILLUSTRATIVE EXAMPLE OF A GROUP ANALYSIS

The following condensed fragment from the initial stages of an analysis is intended as an illustration of a phase in the development of the holistic functioning of the group, with alternating inwardly and outwardly turned activity, and to hint at how defences are analysed. In such an example it is not possible to do justice to the complexity of the situation, to the influences of life in the hospital and the outside world, to the details of analysis of personal factors, to the many ways in which members take up and interchange roles in response to local and group disturbances, or to demonstrate adequately the increasing individuality of the members. In the subsequent analysis the general themes were repeated again and again with differing content as new experiences, personal and group, arose and were analysed. But this extract might serve to underline my opinion that analysis in such a group of four or five members has some advantages over the usual "two-group". I cannot make a sharp distinction between individual and group analysis. I now speak only of analysis in groups, which must be sufficiently small to allow analysis of personal mechanisms, and yet large enough to permit the full play of healing group processes. The optimum size has yet to be worked out for different personalities and states, but it is far from certain that the traditional two-group is, always, the ideal.

When a group first meets each member tends to be orientated towards the analyst. For many sessions, the group of four expressed attitudes to me as to the teacher with authority, who was going to do something to each of them separately and, with this, some hostility about having to talk in the presence of others, i.e. the positive valences between each member and the analyst and the negative ones between each other.

The hostility was covered by conventional attitudes, e.g. "There doesn't seem to be much point in this but the doctor knows best". Questions directed to me about the treatment and about personal problems were frequent and, as these were thrown back for discussion by the group, anxiety increased. Silences became frequent, and were interpreted as anxious retreats into isolation or as shared resentment of me.

Later, resentment began to be expressed more openly, sometimes about the group being a complete waste of time, but often as a shared hostility on the part of Mr. W., Mrs. Y., and Mrs. Z. towards Mr. X., who now talked a great deal in intellectualized psychological jargon. The others felt that he was trying to be clever and currying favour with me. I pointed out the sibling rivalry, but also that they were disturbed by Mr. X.'s talk about violence.

Interpretations of underlying aggression led to increasing personal confessions and relief at discovering shared problems. With freer discussion the group began to change seats which, up till then, had been rigidly kept. Mrs. Y., however, remained on my immediate right until this situation was understood, as described earlier (p. 280).

The group now became more and more closely knit, sharing current problems, gaining security by the expression of forbidden and frightening material, and beginning to understand something of underlying motives. At this stage the situation was that of a safe family circle with me as a parent figure representing the security.

After some months the circle of chairs began to widen. The talk was still of immediate problems of the group, experienced as a special situation not understood by the world at large, which was usually spoken of as being hostile. But, in spite of the apparent wishes of the members, discussion of outside relationships came in more and more, and Mrs. Y. had a dream of eight people in a bus which was related to the unseen presence of the spouses of the members.

At this point, I interpreted the situation in terms of the anxiety of the group when faced with differences between members which threatened the solidarity of the group and, in particular, the fear of aggressive explosions. There was a silence, and later Mr. X. told of a dream in which the world had been blown into bits but he found himself in a plane making a landing on a new earth. As usual, this dream was discussed in relation not only to Mr. X.'s personal problems but also to the group situation—its need to be able to split up in order to come together again in a new form.

The next session began with some rather anxious joking and then there was silence of the isolated type. When the silence was broken, Mr. W. explained it as having been due to obstinacy, no one being willing to give in to the others, and Mr. X. said, "We split up in the hospital after lunch". Mrs. Y. remembered a dream of her father having died and went on to talk about her fear of what might happen while I was on holiday. Uneasy discussion followed in which phobias were related to fears of inability to control anger unless someone strong was present. Mrs. Y. became disturbed, feeling that I had laughed at her and pushed her off, and the session ended with a general sense of insecurity. For some sessions the seating positions of the group remained the same.

The theme of the anxiety of separation was repeated in terms of cows and calves, mothers and children, and the attempt to find solution in sexual union, infantile and adult. A striking commentary was provided by Mrs. Y.'s son aged 5, who, one day, banged on the door and demanded to be let in, holding a bag of sweets in one hand and a large gun in the other! As aggressive fantasies were produced Mr. W., who always advocated self-control and duty, became more and more isolated and silent.

The group, aware of his state, interpreted his fear of his aggression, but Mr. W. denied this. Then Mr. X. told of two dreams, the first of being in the R.A.F. and transferring from a fighter to a bomber squadron and the second of getting a job. He was struck by the fact that in the first dream he could see only one half of people. To everyone's surprise Mr. W., who seldom made interpretations, said the dream showed that Mr. X. was not so much on the defensive (fighter protection) and was now able to attack (bomber) but that he could really only relate to half the group. The others remarked on Mr. W.'s sudden interest in psychology, but he retreated and stated that he never dreamed himself although he thought perhaps he had once had a "sort of dream" about his wife, on whom he was dependent, going away. Mrs. Y. said, "You just want to get rid of the subconscious". I said, "It looks as if we are trying to get at the other half of the group that we don't see". Mr. W., who always put doctors on a pedestal, then went on to make an indirect attack on a psychiatrist he had seen on T.V. I suggested that he had difficulty in seeing his violent half. Mr. W. became more depressed in subsequent sessions and finally had an outburst of rage in which he said that all his talk about helping others was all nonsense, he didn't care about anybody and was going to leave the group and the hospital and get a job. He attacked the rest of the group for many actions over the past months. I interpreted his wish to smash up the group in a positive sense of breaking down rigid obstructions to development.

In subsequent sessions places changed freely, the group was less closely associated in the hospital, and topics of work and of social life became more common. Talk was free and there was intercommunication with expression of open conflict and co-operation, and analysis of separation anxiety and incestuous togetherness, relating childhood memories to the current group situation. An important theme was the transition from defensive isolation to creative aloneness.

## SUMMARY AND CONCLUSIONS

1. It is suggested that the direct study of group dynamics is a neglected, but vital, part of analytical psychology.

2. An outline is given of a general approach to group analysis, illustrated by case material.

3. A methodological and practical distinction is made between "personal descriptions" and "group descriptions", according to whether the group is conceived as a multiplicity or as a unity. It is suggested that both descriptions are necessary but are in different logical categories.

4. Some basic patterns of communication in groups are described.

5. The changes observed in these patterns are generalized in a heuristic fiction of a group as a self-regulating system of opposing, interacting forces of cohesion and disruption. The important work of analysis is described and illustrated as the recognition and solution of resistances to the operation of integrating processes occurring in the group as a whole. Development occurs which leads not to collectivism but to a state which can be described either as a more harmonious interaction of individuals or as an increasing differentiation within one body.

6. It is concluded that analysis is a term which can be applied to group situations and that similar principles can be applied to group analysis and classical analysis. The latter can, indeed, be regarded as analysis in a two-group.

The formations and models in this paper are first order generalizations of observation records, and further clinical studies, critical assessment of the literature, and logical analysis are necessary before more general theories can be formulated. It is apparent, however, that the image of the group, as a superordinate, self-compensating system which regulates opposing forces, conscious and unconscious, closely resembles Jung's description of the self.

It has been pointed out how the dynamics are described in terms similar to those used in Jung's conception of "the original social order", in which there is an interaction of endogenous and exogenous libido. He compares this "original and primitive order of human society" to the archetype of the self which refers both to an inner order of the psyche and to external relationships. The dynamic relation between ego and self in formulation of individual psychology is, in many respects, similar to that of the relation of a member to the group which creates, transcends, and yet includes him.

This paper is the outcome of work done at the Middlesex and at the Bethlem Royal and Maudsley Hospitals.

## REFERENCES

FORDHAM, M. (1957). *New Developments in Analytical Psychology*. London, Routledge & Kegan Paul.

HOBSON, R. F. (1955). "Archetypal Themes in Depression", *J. analyt. Psychol.*, **1**, 1.

JUNG, C. G. (1946). *Die Psychologie der Übertragung*. Zürich, Rascher. Trans. "Psychology of the Transference". *Coll. Wks.*, **16**.

JUNG, C. G. (1947). "Der Geist der Psychologie", *Eran-Jb.* **14**. Trans. "On the Nature of the Psyche", in *The Structure and Dynamics of the Psyche. Coll. Wks.* **8**.

# 19

## *SELBSTVERWIRKLICHUNG*

ALBERT JUNG, *Freiburg, Schweiz*

SELBSTVERWIRKLICHUNG beginnt bekanntlich in erster Linie mit *Selbsterkenntnis* und diese dort, wo wir Ressentiments entdecken, dem nachgehen, was uns ärgert, aufregt, uns verstimmt, uns so beherrscht, dass wir damit einfach nicht fertig werden. Sehr oft sind es Erlebnisse aus der Vergangenheit, unerfüllte Wünsche, ungelebtes Leben, grosse Enttäuschungen, "entthronte Götter", anerzogene Hemmungen, die seinerzeit einen Sinn hatten, ihn aber vielleicht heute verloren haben. Wir müssen neu Stellung beziehen dazu, Vernachlässigtes, so weit dies möglich ist, aufholen, Verdrängtes ans Licht ziehen, nochmals erleben und dann "abreagieren". Wir müssen erkennen, inwiefern wir ab-norm sind, von der allgemeinen Norm abweichen und müssen unsere Konsequenzen daraus ziehen. Wir müssen aber auch unsere Grenzen kennen lernen und merken, wieweit der Körper uns befiehlt und uns in Stimmungen versetzen kann, die unser Verhalten bestimmen. Dies kann soweit gehen, dass wir die Freiheit zur Entscheidung verlieren, ganz in den Bann einer somatisch bedingten "Verhexung", Verzauberung gelangen und zuerst dieser Bann gelöst werden muss, bevor der Geist wieder aus der "Flasche" hinaus kann. Wenn man viel mit vegetativdystonen Patienten zu tun hat, so sieht man, wie grundlegend eine somatische Behandlung sein kann um überhaupt den Weg zur Selbstverwirklichung frei zu machen. Im Banne der somatopsychischen "Verhexung", in der sehr leicht wirkliche "Hexenschüsse" auftreten, wie der Volksmund absolut richtig sagt, spielt die grosse Mutter als Sinnbild des absoluten Schutzes oder der Vater in allen seinen Abwandlungen als Beschützer,

Autorität, eine sehr grosse Rolle. Religion wird vorwiegend als Sicherung, als Schutz angesehen und mit Gott ein Vertragsverhältnis gesucht, das uns bis in alle Ewigkeit vor allem "Bösen" beschützen soll.

Jeder von uns trägt in sich ein Ziel-Bild, das ihn animiert, ein Ideal zu sehen, dem er nachjagen kann. Wenn einer glaubt, kein Ideal zu haben, dann fühlt er sich als "Realist", vergisst aber meist, dass jede Wirklichkeit ganz wesentlich subjektiv gefärbt ist, auch wenn wir nicht bis zur Mâjâ-Vorstellung hin alles subjektivieren wollen. Die meisten haben die eigene Wohlfahrt, die Wohlfahrt ihrer Familie, ihres Klans, ihres Betriebes, ihrer staatlichen Gemeinschaft, ja manche womöglich das der ganzen Menschheit im Auge. Wir sprechen von Entwicklung und Niedergang unserer Kultur, Fortschritten von Technik und Zivilisation, freuen uns, dass wir mehr und mehr die Natur beherrschen, ihr die innersten Geheimnisse abhorchen und uns von ihr emanzipiert haben.

Wer recht tief in *dieses* Stadium der Selbstverwirklichung eingedrungen ist, kommt zu dem Punkt, bei dem *er* der Masstab aller Dinge ist. Er entdeckt, dass er dei Wirklichkeit in sich selber trägt und seine Freiheit darin bestehe, dass er diese Wirklichkeit verwirkliche. Damit ist er beim *existentialistischen Subjektivismus und "Humanismus"* angelangt, den der Rationalismus ganz wesentlich unterstützt. Denn vernünftig, rational, ist von diesem Erleben aus das, was man als Subjekt so beurteilt, so erlebt. Ideale, die nicht der eigenen subjektiven Wirklichkeit, den eigenen Bedürfnissen, den eigenen Zielen entsprechen, werden verworfen, mit einem negativen Vorzeichen versehen und verurteilt, bekämpft. Dieser subjektivistische Individualismus ist tief im Menschen verankert und kommt immer dann zum Vorschein, wenn die Allgemeinverbindlichkeit von Werten und Normen zu schwanken beginnt oder die Machtverhältnisse seine Entwicklung bei einzelnen erlauben.

Es passt ganz in den Rahmen dieses Subjektivismus, dass man psychische Phänomene auch nur rein subjektiv ansieht und alles "Psychische" eingebildet ist, einem subjektiven "Mâjâ-Bild" entspricht und eine objektive Psyche unvorstellbar ist. Weil sie unvorstellbar ist, wird sie geleugnet und derjenige, der für sie eintritt, wird als Phantast angesehen.

Dieses Erleben, welches die Gefahr der Aufblähung des Ich-Subjektes in sich trägt, wird durchkreuzt durch das Erleben der Abhängigkeit, des Endlich-Seins, des Teil-Seins, der Unfreiheit. Daraus kann einerseits die Angst wachsen, dass das Ich-Subjekt ausgelöscht werde, anderseits der Wunsch entstehen, dass es als Teil im Ganzen aufgehen möge, jeder Gegensatz aufhöre, jedes eigene Streben erlösche im Aufgehen im All oder in der Gottheit, oder dass der Sohn-Geliebte in den Armen der Mutter, von ihr betrauert, sterbe. Nur zu leicht kommt es beim Platzen des aufgeblähten Ich-Ballons, der sich die ganze Wirklichkeit zum Objekt machte, zu einem Aufgehen im All, das dann als Nichts erlebt wird, weil keine Wirklichkeit und Objekt mehr da ist. Statt im All oder in der Natur, kann man auch in der Masse untergehen. Es kann sein, dass uns der Weg zur Selbstverwirklichung wirklich da hindurch führt, dass wir lernen *namenlos* zu sein. Dies hat Edgar Schaper einmal dargestellt und Heidegger erwähnt. Der Name ist von jeher das, was uns von anderen unterscheidet, mit dem man uns anrufen kann. Wir können dann, wenn wir namenlos geworden sind, nicht mehr individuell angerufen werden, haben jeden individuellen Wert verloren, können aber auch im dionysischen Rausch alle ethischen Bindungen fallen lassen. Anderseits können wir aber, weil wir wertlos geworden sind, die ganze Wirklichkeit, die ausserhalb unserer subjektiven Wertung steht, auf uns wirken lassen; wir können von der wirklichen Wahrheit erleuchtet werden und damit ins "Offene" gelangen, auf das Rilke in den Duineser Elegien so grossen Wert legt. Die Strahlen werden dann parallel, wie er sagt. Sie können dann aber auch nicht mehr auf ein göttliches Individuum, einen persönlichen Gott, gerichtet werden, weil dies eine konzentrische Strahlenrichtung verlangen würde.

Diese Kehrseite des subjektiven Existentialismus, dieses Hinausgehalten-, Hinausgeworfen-Sein ins Nichts, dieses Namenloswerden, ist schaurig, führt in tiefste Depression und Verzweiflung. Es trifft nicht nur diejenigen, die heimatlos wurden, weil sie fliehen mussten, oder diejenigen, die adynamisch, kraftlos wurden, deren Energien anderweitig gebunden sind, sondern im Durchgang auch die, welche in ihrer Umgebung, in der bisherigen Gemeinschaft, der bisherigen Weltanschauung heimatlos wurden und vor das Nichts gerieten, in die Nigredo kamen.

So ist auch nicht die Masse an sich gefährlich, sondern die "heimatlose" Masse, die Entwurzelten. Da verliert der einzelne den Halt an einer persönlichkeitsbildenden, kollektiven Tradition, die allerdings nur so lange Halt bietet, als sie echt, wirklichkeitsnahe und nicht verlogen, nur noch eine Hülle ist, die den Zerfall verdeckt, wie ein Patient kürzlich träumte: ein märchenhafter Palast, in dem es innen fürchterlich aussah. Diese heimatlose, wurzellose, formlose Masse, die nur noch materiell-biologische Werte kennt und in einem geistigen Sinne "wertlos" geworden ist, ist auf einem tiefen geistigen Niveau und lässt sich durch geschickte Demagogen in vorbereitete Kanäle leiten, in denen sie dem Gesetz der Schwerkraft folgend fliesst und dann, wenn die Kanäle aufhören, sich weiterwälzt und nur noch zerstört oder nur durch Terror beherrscht werden kann. Diese heimatlose Masse strebt nun nach allen Seiten nach kollektiver Sicherung, Versicherung, Schutz durch die absolute Planung mit Hilfe der Technik, Rationalisierung und Normung. Sie erwartet dies von ihren Führern und "vergöttert" sie, stürzt sie aber erbarmungslos, wenn ein anderer "Gott" erscheint.

Diese beiden Tendenzen: *Subjektivismus*, auch wenn er sich als Humanismus oder als Positivismus bezeichnet und die Wirklichkeit glaubt erfasst zu haben, und die Auflösung des Ichs im *Nihilismus*, sind Gegensätze, die auf der gleichen Ebene liegen und gerne in einander übergehen. Je mehr wir uns vom biologischen Geschehen aus, d.h. von den somatischen, evt. rhythmischen Stimmungsschwankungen, bestimmen lassen oder, ohne uns dagegen anstemmen zu können, bestimmt werden, umso ungehemmter, aber gefährlicher stürzen wir von einem Extrem ins andere, schwanken wir hin und her oder besser: werden wir hin und hergeworfen. Aber das ist nicht Selbstverwirklichung, nicht Menschwerdung. Das ist die Ebene, in der das Ich und sein Erleben allein massgebend sind, dasjenige gut ist, was mir nützt, mir zusagt, von mir als gut angenommen und anerkannt wird, auch wenn es anscheinend ein sehr hoch gestecktes, ideales Ziel ist, das ich mir steckte und das ich erreichen möchte oder glaube unbedingt erreichen zu müssen. Man streitet sich auf dieser Ebene, weil man sich mit dem identifiziert, was uns treibt und dadurch alles, was dem widerstrebt, affektiv erlebt als Gegensatz zu sich selber, als Gefahr für sein Ich und dessen Streben. Man kann sich auch mit einer offiziellen oder inoffiziellen Norm identifizieren und diese durch dick und dünn verteidigen und zwar umso heftiger, je mehr sie eigenen Zweifeln begegnet.

Die Selbstverwirklichung des heutigen und zukünftigen Menschen gipfelt nicht mehr im Helden, der, wie Herkules, grosse Taten verrichtet hat und im Sieg über andere zum stärksten Mann wurde, noch im Asketen, der seinen Leib verachtet um zum Geist zu gelangen, sondern sie beginnt damit, dass wir die Grenze dieser Gegensatzebene überschreiten, sie transzendieren, nicht aber überspringen. Wir müssen durch sie hindurchschreiten, an ihre Grenze kommen und versuchen, diese zu überschreiten. Der Held und der Asket, die beide es sehr weit brachten in der Selbstbeherrschung, müssen über sich hinauswachsen. Die Erkenntnis von Galilei, dass sich nicht das ganze Weltall um die Erde drehe, sondern diese nur einen Teil des Sonnensystems darstelle, muss auch für den Mikrokosmos eine neue Stellung im Makrokosmos schaffen.

Dichter wie Hölderlin und Rainer Maria Rilke, Denker wie Martin Heidegger, Frau Conrad-Martius und Leopold Ziegler, Mystiker wie Meister Eckehardt, Jakob Böhme und Franz v. Baader und Forscher wie C. G. Jung haben uns Wege gezeigt, wie wir Heutigen in einer Synthese von Glauben und Wissen zu diesem Uebergreifenden, für das Ich kaum und nur zum Teil Fassbaren gelangen können oder, besser gesagt, wie wir das, was uns von diesem Unfassbaren zustösst, bewusst erleben und uns aneignen können.

Im Geistesleben des Osten nennen die Chinesen das Uebergreifende bekanntlich Tao, gewisse Budhisten das Zen, die Inder das Atman. Im Westen hätten wir es wahrscheinlich mit der Technik und der Naturerkenntnis nicht so weit gebracht, wenn wir nicht den Gegensatz von Natur und Geist bis zu einer beinahe völligen Objekt-Subjekt-Spaltung getrieben und des Transzendente ins geistig-göttliche Jenseits verlegt hätten. Die Rückkehr zum einigenden Einbeziehen des Transzendenten in unseren Bereich oder der bewusste Uebersteig in die andere Dimension des "Seins" nach Heidegger, das Frau Conrad-Martius noch stark vertieft hat bis zur philosophisch-phänomenologischen Annäherung an die Begriffe der Zeitlosigkeit und Raumlosigkeit, die Erkenntnis und Annäherung an das "Selbst" im Sinne von

C. G. Jung ist zwar heute eine unbedingte Notwendigkeit, nachdem die Atombomben platzen und die Menschheit vernichten können, sie fällt uns aber ausserordentlich schwer und nur allzuoft fühlen wir und unsere Patienten an dieser Grenze ein Unvermögen, weiter zu gehen und zu führen. Wir müssen dann abwarten, was weiter geschieht. Aber gerade das kann mehr Reife und Ruhe verlangen, als in der betreffenden Situation, in der die Zeit weiterläuft, erträglich ist.

Dieser westliche, stark nach vorwärts drängende und im Christentum vorgezeichnete Weg ist in der Endstrecke dem östlichen entgegengesetzt. Die östliche Weisheit strebt *vor* die Trennung von Subjekt und Objekt, vor das Wegstreben des Ich von der Natur zurück und auch Heidegger geht in dieser Richtung. Der östliche Weise sagt am Ende seines Weges: "Ich bin Buddha" und "Buddha zieht seinen Durst zurück", er gibt das eigene Streben auf um das Unfassliche durch ihn hindurch wirken zu lassen. Eugen Herriegel hat das sehr aufschlussreich beschrieben in seinem Büchlein: "Zen in der Kunst des Bogenschiessens" (Herrigel). Der Zen-Meister im Bogenschiessen spannt den schweren Bogen ohne jegliche sichtbare Kraftanstrengung und der Pfeil fliegt ins Schwarze, auch wenn das Ziel im Dunkeln liegt. Der Bogen wird ihm gespannt und der Pfeil wird von ihm ins Schwarze weggetragen. Er bereitet sich so lange vor, bis eine Wirkung durch ihn hindurch zustande kommt, an der sein Ich unbeteiligt ist.

Der Westen ging aber in der Bewusstseinsentwicklung seinen eigenen Weg und zwar seit Plato und Aristoteles. Es besteht auch im Westen eine starke Tendenz *vor* die Entwicklung der Differenzierung und damit vor die Spezialisierung mit ihrem Vollkommenheitsanspruch zurückzugehen. Heidegger bezeichnet die Entwicklung der Philosophie seit Plato und Aristoteles als "Holzweg". Seine Fundamentalontologie führt auch tatsächlich zu einem ganzheitlichen Monismus, wie wir dies bei Boss sehen. Frau Conrad-Martius geht hier neue Wege und zeigt, dass dieser Monismus überwunden werden kann. Ich verweise auf ihre Werke über "die Zeit", "das Sein" und "den Raum".

Martin Buber geht zurück zum Prophetischen und Sakralen des ursprünglichen Judentums und lehnt die Differenzierung, sowie die Abspaltung des Jenseits im Spätjudentum und Christentum ab. (Siehe Hans-Urs Balthasar "Einsame Zwiesprache"). Eine ähnliche Tendenz finden wir bei Nietzsche, wie dies Jaspers in seinem Buch "Nietzsche und das Christentum" dargestellt hat.

Riwkah Schärf-Kluger zeigte in ihrer Arbeit über die Gestalt des Satans im alten Testament (Schärf, 1948) die sukzessive Ausschaltung Satans aus dem göttlichen Hof. Das Christentum hat diese Differenzierung aufgenommen und selber intensiv weiter entwickelt. Daher wird von all denen, die zu den Ursprüngen zurückkehren wollen und müssen das Christentum mit abgelehnt. Jung hat nun umgekehrt einen Weg gewählt der vorwärts führt. Wenn wir uns vermehrt mit Heraklit, ja mit der griechischen Mythologie, mit den vorderasiatischen Religionen, mit der östlichen Weisheit, mit der im Osten wie im Westen im Grunde übereinstimmenden Alchemie, zu der uns C. G. Jung den Zugang ganz wesentlich erleichterte, und mit der Gnosis in jeder echten Form beschäftigen, dann tun wir dies um unsere Lebensbasis zu erweitern und den Weg nach Innen, zu unserem Wesen, zu einer Einheit auf anderer Ebene zu finden und zwar den Weg, der unserer heutigen Situation als westliche Menschen entspricht. Im Unterschied zum östlichen Menschen neigen wir dazu mit Paulus zu sagen: "Christus lebt in mir" und damit nehmen wir das Kreuz der Gegensatzspannung auf uns. Das Ich behält seine Gestalt, behält Persönlichkeitscharakter, ist im "Selbst" im Sinne Jung's enthalten wie in analoger Weise in der göttlichen Trinität Christus und der hl. Geist selbständigen Persönlichkeitscharakter haben. In 1. Joh. 5, 7–10 steht u.a.: ... tres sunt, qui testimonium dant in caelo: Pater, Verbum et Spiritus sanctus: et hi tres unum sunt. Et tres sunt, qui testimonium dant in terra: spiritus et aqua et sanguis: et hi tres unum sunt ..."

Jung drängt auf Ergänzung der Trinität zur Quaternität, der Vollkommenheit zur Vollständigkeit, die aber auch erreicht wird, wenn zur oberen Trinität die untere tritt:

Pater ———————— Verbum
\ Spiritus sanctus /

————————————————

/ Spiritus (vegetativus) \
Sanguis ———————— Aqua

Bindeglied und Spannungszentrum sind der hl. Geist und der spiritus vegetativus der Erde, der Schöpfung, Offenbarung und Gnosis, letztere als "Naturweisheit", "Schlangenweisheit" verstanden.

Ebenso besteht in uns die Spannung zwischen der Uebermacht des "Selbst" (homo creatus est) und der Hybris, dem Uebermut des Bewusstseins (homo creator est) wie Jung ausführt in der Arbeit über "Das Wandlungssymbol in der Messe" (Jung, 1954, S. 294 ff.). Beide können Feinde sein, feindliche Brüder. Wir versuchen aber den Feind in uns und um uns zu erkennen, ihn ins Auge zu fassen und im Auge zu behalten, uns mit ihm zu messen, ihn aber nicht zu verurteilen, sondern als unseren notwendigen Gegensatz, als notwendige Opposition, als Antipoden, anzuerkennen. Wenn es uns gelingt einen Feind oder einen Antipoden in seinem Wesen anzunehmen, dann geben wir ihm die Würde des Menschseins und nicht blossen Objektseins. Je besser uns dies gelingt, umso weniger springt unsere Affektivität, Emotionalität, unser schlecht entwickeltes Gefühl als Schutz- und Abwehrfunktion ein und umso eher kann unsere Diskussion zum "liebenden Streit der Sache werden" wie dies Heidegger im Brief über den Humanismus ausdrückte. Dass dies ausserordentlich schwer ist, weiss jeder von uns. Aber dadurch gewännen wir die Freiheit, könnten wir so frei und ungebunden um uns blicken, die Wahrheit auf uns wirken lassen, wie dies Plato im "Höhlengleichnis" darstellt. Dies ist schon ein Teil dieses Ueberschrittes in eine andere Dimension, in der die Gegensatzspannungen erhalten bleiben, aber ein Punkt besteht, von dem aus auch das Ich wie das Du zum Objekt werden können.

Aber an diesem Punkt kommt neben der Gefahr der Hybris die mindestens ebenso bedeutsame Gefahr, dass der höhere Standpunkt nicht der des "Selbst", sondern des "Ueber-Ichs" ist, der Unterordnung unter ein Gesetz, eine Autorität weltlicher oder geistlicher Art, einen Codex. Dies ist für das Leben in der Gemeinschaft unbedingt nötig und sehr viele Konflikte, besonders jüngerer Leute, liegen auf der Ebene politischer oder moralischer Freiheit. Die erste Stufe dieses Kampfes haben wir schon erwähnt, das ist die Stufe der Ichfestigung, wo die Macht der Autorität des Vaters, der Lehrer, der Tradition, der kirchlichen Autorität überwunden werden muss, damit ein Ich festwerden kann. Die zweite Stufe besteht dann in einer gewissen Rückkehr zur Autorität, zur Tradition, zur Konfession als kodifizierte religiöse Gemeinschaft, die Versöhnung mit dem Ueber-Ich, das als gleichwertig anerkannt wird.

Dies ist aber nicht *die* Transzendenz, der Ueberschritt in die so schwer erreichbare neue Dimension, die erst die wahre Würde des Menschen heraufführt und uns den Sinn unseres Lebens erhellen kann und von dem alle Völkerüberlieferungen sprechen. Die Schwierigkeit liegt in dem, dass mit der Einführung einer neuen Dimension die Anschaulichkeit und leichte Fassbarkeit verloren geht wie in der Mathematik durch die Einführung der vierten Dimension. Auf physiologisch-medizinischem Gebiet wird es unanschaulich und schwer, wenn wir zu den Regulationen und Korrelationen übergehen (wie dies W. R. Hess meisterhaft entwickelte). Ich versuchte von da aus den Zugang zu den Archetypen als Ordnern und Anordnern ebenso zu finden wie über die Philosophie Heideggers im Beitrag zur Festschrift zum 80 Geburtstag von C. G. Jung.

Der Uebergang zu einer neuen Dimension geht nicht ohne Opfer und darüber hat Jung eingehend und mehrfach geschrieben. Am Schluss der Ausführungen über das Opfer schreibt er: "Solange das Selbst unbewusst ist, entspricht es dem Ueber-Ich Freuds und bildet eine Quelle beständiger moralischer Konflikte. Wird es aber aus der Projektion zurückgezogen, d.h. ist es nicht mehr die Meinung der anderen, der Gemeinschaft, der Norm, dann weiss man, dass man sein eigenes Ja und Nein ist. Dann wirkt das Selbst als eine unio oppositorum und bildet damit die unmittelbarste Offenbarung des Göttlichen, welche psychologisch überhaupt fassbar ist". Leopold Ziegler führt eine jüdische Legende an, in der ein Rabbi vor eine ausweglose Situation gerät und nach den Gesetzen diese zu lösen versucht. Elia ist damit nicht einverstanden, erscheint ihm im Traum und sagt: "Was warst Du eingedenk der Mischna des Gesetzes? Nicht eingedenk jedoch der Mischna aller wahrhaft Frommen, die sich in die Herzen der Gerechten einschreibt? Wo die Not am höchsten, helfen Dir die Meister nicht, weder die gewesenen, noch die zukünftigen. Da bist Du allein mit Gott. Da muss Du menschliche Nichtigkeit bis auf den Grund vor ihm erleiden. Weh Dir, dass Du zu irdischer Hilfe Deine Zuflucht nahmst und Gottes

Angesicht nicht aushieltst". Der Rabbi war damit eingeklemmt zwischen Schuld und Schuld. Wie er sich auch entschied, musste er schuldig werden. Homo non potest non peccare: das Schuldigwerden ist unentrinnbar. Leopold Ziegler schreibt in der "Menschwerdung": "Und eben der Einzelne darf gewiss sein—der Herr wird ihm eines Tages die Larve seiner eigensüchtigen und darum falschen Unschuld vom Antlitz reissen und ihm aufs klärlichste beweisen, wie ich will und nicht wie Du willst. Bei diesem Aufeinanderprall des stärksten, besten Motivs mit dem höchsten Willen wird es dann letzterem vielleicht sogar belieben, dem eigenständig Einzelnen selbst seine Unschuld abzufordern". Da steht man dann evt. unmittelbar vor dem furchtbaren Gott, der uns als deus absconditus ganz allein lässt, wie Christus am Kreuz sagte: "Mein Gott, mein Gott, warum hast Du mich verlassen? . . ." Wenn Sonderung-Sünde ist, dann ahnt uns, was es heisst, dass Christus diese Sonderung-Sünde auf sich genommen und erlitten hat, wo der letzte Anspruch auf Anerkennung, Rechtfertigung, Ich-verwirklichung, der letzte Hauch eines egoistischen Anspruches geopfert werden muss, eine wirkliche Nacht, eine wirkliche Nigredo anbricht, aber auch *die* Antwort auf Hiob gegeben wird, die Jung meint: dass auch Gott Mensch werden und das qualvolle Ausgespanntsein zwischen Himmel und Erde, angeheftet an das Kreuz, an die "Mutter" erleiden will. Der Selbstopferer-Gott will das Selbstopfer, zu dem er uns treibt, vorerleben. Jung schreibt: "*Wir* gewinen aus dem Selbstopfer uns selbst, *das* Selbst; denn nur was wir geben, das haben wir. Was aber gewinnt das Selbst? Wir sehen, dass es in Erscheinung tritt, dass es sich aus der unbewussten Projektion löst, dass es, indem es uns ergreift, auch in uns selber eintritt und damit aus dem dissoluten Zustand des Unbewusstseins in den des Bewusstseins und aus dem potentiellen in den aktuellen Zustand übergeht. Was es im unbewussten Zustand ist, wissen wir nicht; jetzt aber wissen wir, dass es *Mensch*, ja *uns selber geworden ist* . . . Einesteils ist die Bewusstwerdung, als eine Zusammenführung abgesplitterter Teile, eine bewusste Willensleistung des Ich, anderenteils aber bedeutet sie auch ein spontanes Hervortreten des Selbst, das von jeher war ["allein durch die Gnade"]. Einerseits erscheint die Individuation als Synthese einer neuen Einheit, die zuvor aus zerstreuten Teilen bestand, andererseits aber als das Offenbar-werden eines Wesens, das dem Ich präexistent, ja dessen Vater oder Schöpfer und dessen Ganzheit ist. Wir erschaffen gewissermassen das Selbst durch das Bewusstmachen unbewusster Inhalte und insofern ist es unser *Sohn* ... Wir werden zu dieser Bemühung aber veranlasst durch das unbewusste Vorhandensein des Selbst, von dem stärkste Bestimmungen zur Ueberwindung der Unbewusstheit ausgehen. In dieser Beziehung ist das Selbst der *Vater*" (Jung, 1954, 302–304).

Wenn die Ursünde die Sonderung aus der unbewussten Einheit ist mit der Entwicklung eines Ichs, mit dem Essen vom Baum der Erkenntnis des Guten und des Bösen, mit dem Treubruch an den Göttern, an Gott, mit dem listigen Stehlen des Feuers und anderen Listen und Zaubermitteln mit denen z.B. Medea als Priesterin der Hekate dem Jason zum goldenen Vliess verhilft, was ausser dem Treubuch am Vater einen Brudermord zur Folge hat, wenn wir all diese Verfehlungen, Sünden, dieses Schuldigwerden psychologisch verstehen als unentrinnbare Verstrickungen im Gespinst der Nornen, die eine Verfolgung durch die Erinnyen, die Harpyien unmittelbar nach sich zieht, bis ein Opfer die Schuld tilgt, dann müssen wir wirklich gestehen, dass auch von dieser Sicht aus das einzige Opfer, das völlig entsühnen kann, das Selbstopfer ist. Aber dieses Selbstopfer verlangt ein stark entwickeltes Ich und das ist, psychologisch und religiös gesehen, nicht nur der grösste Gegensatz zum Ueber-Ich, sondern auch zum unbewussten Urgrund. Die Erlösung besteht darin, dass dies nicht mehr als Schuld, als Ursünde angesehen wird, sondern dass die Menschwerdung eben darin gipfelt, dass ein stark entwickeltes Ich, ein seiner selbst bewusst gewordenes Ich nicht in der Hybris erstarrt, sondern sich opfern lässt und sich selber opfert, um in die Transzendenz hinüberzuschreiten, in die neue Dimension des "Selbst", das die Gegensatzspannungen umgreift, umspannt und daher aus einer feindlichen Trennung in polare Gegensätzlichkeit hinüberholt.

Die Menschwerdung ist eine dem Menschen gestellte Aufgabe, eine Entwicklung und als solche verstrickt sie unweigerlich in Schuld, Treubruch, Verrat, Scheubarkeitsfrevel.

Wenn man das alles überdenkt und erlebt, dann möchte man bitten: "Führe uns nicht in Versuchung und lass den Kelch, wirklich Mensch werden zu müssen, an uns vorbeigehen".

In der analytischen Psychologie müssen wir beide Seiten sehen und entwickeln, die starke Ich-Persönlichkeit, die möglichst viele Projektionen zurückzieht, aber auch das Selbstopfer, das die Verbindung mit dem Urgrund wieder holt, wieder pflegt und die Grenzen anerkennt, die uns in der Zurückziehung der Projektionen gegeben sind. In dieser niemals ganz erfüllbaren Dimension unseres Menschseins, im Wohnen im Stand des "Selbst", wäre erst eigentlich der wahre Gottesdienst, die ständige Religion, der hieros gamos möglich. Vorher müssen wir uns mit den erreichbaren Teillösungen abfinden, aber doch versuchen, dem Ziel der Menschwerdung so nahe als möglich zu kommen.

## REFERENCES

BALTHASAR, HANS-URS (1958). *Einsame Zwiesprache. Martin Buber und das Christentum.* Köln und Olten: Verlag Jakob Hegner.

CONRAD-MARTIUS, HEDWIG (1949). *Bios und Psyche.* München, Kösel-Verlag.

CONRAD-MARTIUS, HEDWIG (1954). *Die Zeit.* München, Kösel-Verlag.

CONRAD-MARTIUS, HEDWIG (1957). *Das Sein.* München, Kösel-Verlag.

CONRAD-MARTIUS, HEDWIG (1958). *Der Raum.* München, Kösel-Verlag.

HEIDEGGER, MARTIN (1927). *Sein und Zeit.* Halle a.d. Saale, M. Niemeyer.

HEIDEGGER, MARTIN (1947). Im "Brief über den Humanismus", enthalten in *Platons Lehre von der Wahrheit, mit einem Brief über den Humanismus.* Bern, Verlag A. Francke A. G.

HERRIGEL, E. (1953). *Zen in the Art of Archery.* London, Routledge.

HESS, W. R. (1950). "Symposium über das Zwischenhirn." *Helv. Physiol. et Pharmacol. Acta.* Supp. IV. Basel, Benno Schwabe.

JASPERS, K. (1950). *Nietzsche.* 3. Aufl. Berlin, Walter de Gruyter.

JASPERS, K. (1952). *Nietzsche und das Christentum.* München, R. Piper und Co. Verlag.

JUNG, A. (1954). "Grundsätzliches zur psychosomatischen Medizin im Lichte der komplexen Psychologie von C. G. Jung". In *Studien zur analytischen Psychologie C. G. Jungs* (Festschrift zum 80. Geburtstag) Bd. I, S. 170-204. Zürich, Rascher.

JUNG, C. G. (1954) "Das Wandlungssymbol in der Messe". In: *Von den Wurzeln des Bewusstseins.* Zürich, Rascher. Trans. "Transformation Symbolism in the Mass", in *Psychology and Religion: West and East. Coll. Wks.*, **11**, 1958.

SCHAPER, E. (1951). *Die Macht der Ohnmächtigen, Roman,* Olten und Köln, Jakob Hegner.

SCHÄRF, R. (1948). *Die Gestalt des Satans im Alten Testament.* Glarus, Tschudi.

ZIEGLER, L. (1948). *Menschwerdung.* Bd. I und II. Olten, Summa-Verlag.

## *SELF-REALIZATION*

We all know that self-realization, in the sense of becoming oneself, starts in the first place with *self-knowledge*, and the latter begins with the discovery of resentments and with inquiring into things that annoy us, disturb us, put us in a bad humour, and so dominate our life that we cannot get rid of them. Very often such things are experiences from the past, unfulfilled wishes, unlived life, great disappointments, "fallen idols", inhibitions that once had a meaning but have become meaningless. We have to adopt a new attitude towards this: as far as is possible catch up with what has been neglected, undo repressions, re-experience and abreact what was repressed. We must recognize how far we are ab-normal, how far we deviate from the general norm, and draw the relevant consequences. We must also learn to know our limitations and observe how far we are controlled by our own body, with its capacity to create moods that determine our behaviour. This may go so far as to deprive us of freedom of choice and we fall "bewitched" under a somatically induced spell which has to be broken before the genie can get out of the bottle again. If one has a great deal to do with vegetatively dystonic patients, one sees how extremely important somatic treatment can be, in order to give the patient any chance at all of self-realization. Under the influence of this psychosomatic "bewitchment"[1], a very important role is played by the great mother, symbol of complete protection, or the father, in all his manifestations as protection and authority. Religion is mainly seen as security and protection, and God as the possible partner in a contract that will protect us for all time from everything "evil".

Each one of us carries in himself the image of a goal inspiring him as an ideal that he can pursue. Anyone who believes that he has no ideal may consider himself a "realist", but usually forgets

[1]The author also refers to the attacks of lumbago that so often occur in this condition, and which popular wisdom describes, in German, as *Hexenschüsse*, or "witch-shots" (Trans.).

that every reality has an essentially subjective colouring, even if we do not subjectivize everything as *maya*. Most people have their own well-being in mind, or the well-being of their family, their clan, their business, their national community, or even the well-being of the human race. We talk of the rise and decline of our culture, the progress of science and civilization, congratulate ourselves on an ever-increasing mastery of nature, on the way we are emancipating ourselves by wresting from nature its ultimate secrets.

Whoever is deeply involved in *this* stage of self-realization comes to the point at which *he* becomes the sole yardstick of measurement. He discovers that he carries reality in himself and that his freedom consists in realizing this reality. This means he has reached a stage of *existentialist subjectivism and "humanism"*, strongly supported by rationalism. From this point of view the sensible and rational is that which we, as subjects, deem to be so on the basis of our own experience. Ideals that do not conform to one's own subjective reality or needs or aims are rejected, depreciated, condemned, and attacked. This subjectivistic individualism is deeply ingrained in humanity and always comes to the surface when the binding forces of common values and norms begin to weaken, or the circumstances of power relationships allow it to develop in individuals.

It is quite in keeping with this subjectivism to consider all psychological phenomena as purely subjective, everything "psychic" imaginary, corresponding to a subjective concept of *maya*. An objective psyche is inconceivable and since it is inconceivable, its existence is denied and anyone who maintains its existence is treated as a visionary.

This attitude to life, which entails the danger of an inflation of the ego-subject, is countered by the experience of dependence, of temporality, of being only a particle, and unfree. This may, on the one hand, lead to anxiety lest the ego-subject be extinguished, on the other, to the wish to be absorbed in the whole, with every contradiction stilled, every individual effort absorbed in the All, or in the deity, or that the son-lover may die in the arms of his sorrowing mother. When the inflated ego-balloon is pricked, it is all too easy to come to this absorption in the All, which is then experienced as Nothing, since there is no longer reality and no longer an object. Instead of being submerged in the All, or in nature, the individual may also disappear into the mass. The way to self-realization may indeed lead one through the state of learning to be *nameless*. This notion has already been expounded by Edgar Schaper, and mentioned by Heidegger. One's name has always been that which distinguishes one from others, that by which one can be called. When we have become nameless we can no longer be spoken to as individuals, have lost all individual value, and can let all ethical restrictions slide in a Dionysiac intoxication. But again, since we have become valueless we can allow all that reality which is beyond our subjective evaluation to work upon us, we can be enlightened by real truth and come out into that "openness" on which Rilke placed so much value in his *Duino Elegies*. There the beams of light are parallel, he says. They cannot be directed, or can no longer be directed, towards a divine individual, a personal God, since this would mean that the rays were convergent.

This obverse side of subjective existentialism, this sense of being cast out, thrown out into the void, this namelessness, is terrible and leads into deepest depression and despair. It strikes not only those who became homeless because they had to flee, or those who are weak, adynamic, or whose energies are elsewhere engaged, but also, as a transitional phase, those who have become homeless in their usual surroundings, in their former community, in their former opinions, and who have tumbled into the void, into the *nigredo*.

The mass as such is not dangerous, but only the "homeless" mass of the uprooted. In such a mass the individual loses all hold on a collective tradition, in which personality can develop, although such a tradition can offer guidance only so long as it is authentic and related to reality, and not a sham, an empty shell cloaking decay—as a patient recently dreamt: a fabulously beautiful palace, with an interior that was terrible. This homeless, rootless, formless mass, recognizing only material and biological standards, has lost all spiritual values, is on a very low spiritual level, and can easily be guided by skilful demagogues into prearranged channels down which they can swim with the stream of power. If the channel comes to an end, they sweep on of their own accord, and can only be destroyed, or brought under control by terror. This homeless mass is striving in every direction to find collective security, reassurance, and protection through total planning, with its techniques, rationalization, and norms. The mass expects this from its leaders, and idolizes them, only to overthrow them ruthlessly when another idol appears.

These two tendencies, *subjectivism*, whether described as humanism or positivism, which considers itself to have laid hold on reality, and the dissolution of the ego in *nihilism*, are opposites that lie on the same plane and can easily slip over into the other. The more we are determined by biological events, that is, by somatic, perhaps cyclical, changes of mood, without being able to regulate them, the more uninhibitedly yet dangerously we stumble from one extreme to another, swaying or, more accurately, being thrown hither and thither. This is not self-realization or becoming fully human. It is the plane on which the ego and its experience alone have significance; the criteria employed in evaluating what is good relate purely to personal advantage, preference, and aspiration, even though the chosen aim may show an apparent correspondence with exalted ideals. One comes into conflict on this plane, because one identifies with whatever moves one; anything striving in a different direction is experienced affectively as the opposite of oneself, as a danger to the ego and its own striving. One may be identified with an official or an unofficial norm, defending it through thick and thin, and all the more strongly the more one may have one's own doubts about it.

The self-realization of modern or future man can no longer find its highest example in the hero who, like Hercules, accomplishes great feats and proves himself the strongest by subduing others; or in the ascetic, who despises his body in order to become spirit. Self-realization begins with transcending the frontiers of this plane of opposites, not with jumping over them. We have to become acquainted with the whole plane, reach its frontiers, and try to cross them. The hero and the ascetic, who have both travelled far in self-mastery, have to outgrow themselves. Galileo's discovery that the universe did not revolve around the earth, but that the earth was part of the solar system, must also help the microcosm to find a new relationship to the macrocosm.

Poets like Hölderlin and Rainer Maria Rilke, thinkers like

Martin Heidegger, Mme Conrad-Martius and Leopold Ziegler, mystics like Miester Eckhart, Jacob Boehme, and Franz von Baader, and pioneers like C. G. Jung have shown us the way in which we moderns can, by a synthesis of faith and knowledge, attain to a transcendence, which is scarcely and only partially conceivable by the ego; or rather, how we can consciously experience and integrate whatever happens to reach us from this indefinable transcendence.

In the East the Chinese, as we know, call this transcendence Tao; some Buddhists call it Zen; the Hindus, Atman. In the West we should probably not have progressed so far in technics and the natural sciences if we had not forced the opposites, mind and nature, into an almost complete dissociation of object and subject and had not projected the transcendent into some spiritual or religious hereafter. We must needs return to the realization of this transcendence as part of our existence and to a conscious contact with a higher dimension of being, as Heidegger has put it, or in the still deeper sense developed by Mme Conrad-Martius, who has enlarged the concept until it approaches, philosophically and phenomenologically, the idea of timelessness and spacelessness; we need, further, an understanding of and approach to the self, as shown by C. G. Jung. This is by no means easy, now that nuclear explosions carry the threat of annihilation to mankind, and all too often we and our patients reach this boundary and cannot cross it. We must then wait and see what happens. But this is something that sets higher demands on maturity and tranquillity than is tolerable in our historical situation.

The final objective of the Western, forward-driving, basically Christian path, is the opposite of the Eastern. Eastern wisdom strives towards a state *before* the separation of subject and object, of ego and nature, and even Heidegger moves in this direction. The Eastern sage, at the end of his path, says: "I am Buddha", and "Buddha takes back his thirst"; he gives up his own striving in order to let the inconceivable work in and through him. Eugen Herrigel has given a highly instructive description of this attitude in his little book—*Zen in the Art of Archery* (Herrigel, 1953). The Zen master of archery strings his heavy bow without any apparent effort and the arrow flies into the centre even when the target lies in darkness. The bow is strung for him, the arrow carried away from him into the centre. To achieve this he has to get into a state of preparedness beforehand, until he is ready for something to happen through him without any ego participation.

In the West, however, the development of consciousness has followed its own way ever since Plato and Aristotle. In the West too there is a strong tendency back *towards* a state *before* differentiation and away from specialization with its demand for perfection. Heidegger has said that philosophy since Plato and Aristotle has followed a false trail. His fundamental ontology does in fact lead to a holistic monism, as we find it in Boss. Here Mme Conrad-Martius opens up new horizons and shows how this monism can be overcome. I would draw your attention to her works on "Time", "Being" and "Space" (Conrad-Martius, 1954, 1957, 1958).

Martin Buber goes back to the prophetic and sacral aspects of original Judaism and rejects differentiation and the divorce of the secular from the eternal that occurred in Christianity and late Judaism (see Hans-Urs Balthasar, *Einsame Zwiesprache*, 1958). A similar tendency is to be found in Nietzsche, as Jaspers has shown in his book *Nietzsche and Christianity* (1952).

In her study of the figure of Satan in the Old Testament, Riwkah Schärf-Kluger (1948) has shown the stages by which Satan was banished from Heaven. Christianity has followed up this differentiation and developed it intensively. Thus all those who wish to return to the original source must and will thereby discard Christianity. Jung, on the other hand, has chosen a way that leads forward. If we are more and more concerned with Heraclitus, with Greek mythology, with Middle-eastern religions, with Eastern wisdom, with the gnosis, with alchemy, which C. G. Jung has made so much more accessible to us, and which is more or less common ground in East and West, if we are concerned with all these, in any of their authentic forms, we are so in order to broaden the basis of our existence and to find the way inward, to our own nature, to a unity on another plane, and a way that corresponds to our present situation as Westerners. Unlike the East, we are inclined to say with Paul: "Christ lives in us", and we thereby take the cross of the tension of opposites upon ourselves. The ego retains its form, retains its personality, yet is contained in the self, in Jung's sense of the word as, by analogy, Christ and the Holy Ghost have independent personalities within the Holy Trinity. In I John v. 17–18[1] it is said: "...tres sunt, qui testimonium dant in caelo: Pater, Verbum et Spiritus sanctus: et hi tres unum sunt. Et tres sunt, qui testimonium dant in terra: spiritus et aqua et sanguis: et hi tres unum sunt..."

Jung has made clear the importance of the completion of the Trinity to the Quaternity, of perfection to completeness; that can, however, only be achieved when the higher Trinity is joined by the lower:

Pater ——— Verbum
Spiritus Sanctus

---

Spiritus (vegetativus)
Sanguis ——— Aqua

The connecting link and the centre of tension are the Holy Ghost and the *spiritus vegetativus* of the earth, creation, revelation and gnosis, the latter understood as "the wisdom of nature", "the wisdom of the serpent".

Similarly there is in us a tension between the preponderance of the self (*homo creatus est*) and *hybris*, the arrogance of consciousness (*homo creator est*), as Jung has explained in his essay "Transformation Symbolism in the Mass" (Jung, 1954, *Coll. Wks.*, **11**, pp. 256 ff.). Both can be enemies, hostile brothers. We try, however, to know the enemy within and without, to look him in the eye and measure ourselves against him. Yet we must not condemn him, but recognize him as our necessary opposite, as a necessary opposite, our antagonist. If we succeed in accepting our enemy, our antagonist, if we succeed in accepting our enemy, our antagonist, as himself, then we value him as a human being, not merely as an object. The more we succeed in this, the less our affectivity, our emotionality, and our undifferentiated feeling spring to our defence and protection, and our discussion is all the more likely to become "a loving contention about the matter", as Heidegger (1947) in his *Letter on Humanism*

[1] "For there are three that bear record in heaven, the Father, the Word, and the Holy Ghost: and these three are one. And there are three that bear witness in earth, the spirit, and the water, and the blood: and these three agree in one."

expresses it. We all know how difficult that is. But if we are able to turn a free, unfettered gaze upon ourselves, we thereby gain the freedom to let truth work upon us, as Plato showed in his simile of the cave. This is already a step in the transition to another dimension in which the tension of opposites still exists, but where a point arises from which both the "I" and the "Thou" can become an object.

At this point, however, in addition to the danger of *hybris*, there arises another and at least equally important danger, that this higher standpoint may be, not that of the self, but of the superego, entailing submission to a law, a temporal or spiritual authority, a code of behaviour. This is essential to life in a community, and many conflicts, particularly in younger people, occur on the plane of political or moral freedom. We have already mentioned the first stage of this conflict, it is the stage of ego consolidation, when the power of authority vested in father, teacher, tradition, or the Church has to be overcome so that the ego can be consolidated. The second stage consists of a certain return to authority, to tradition, to a denomination as the expression of an organized religious community, and reconciliation with the superego, which is recognized as an equal.

This, however, is not *the* transcendence, the transition, so difficult to achieve, into that new dimension, mentioned in the tradition of all peoples, which can alone bring true dignity to human life and show us its meaning. The difficulty lies in the fact that with the introduction of a new dimension there is a loss of representability and clarity, as happens in mathematics with the introduction of the fourth dimension. In the medico-physiological sphere there arises a similar difficulty when we come to the regulating and coordinating functions (a point developed in a masterly way by W. R. Hess, 1950). From here I tried to find an approach to the archetypes as regulators and coordinators, as I did in relation to Heidegger's philosophy in my contribution to the *Festschrift* for C. G. Jung's 80th birthday (Jung, A., 1954).

The transition to a new dimension is not possible without sacrifice, as Jung has so often pointed out. At the end of his comments on the nature of the sacrifice, he writes (Jung, 1954, *Coll. Wks.*, **11**, p. 261): "So long as the self is unconscious, it corresponds to Freud's superego and is a source of perpetual moral conflict. If, however, it is withdrawn from projection and is no longer identical with public opinion, then one is truly one's own yea and nay. The self then functions as a union of opposites and thus constitutes the most immediate experience of the Divine which it is psychologically possible to imagine." Leopold Ziegler quotes a Jewish legend in which a Rabbi is faced with an insoluble problem and tries to solve it according to the Law. Elijah is dissatisfied, and appears to him in a dream, saying: "Why are you thinking of the Mishnah of the Law? Why didn't you think of the Mishnah of all truly pious ones, which is written in the heart of the just ones? When the need is greatest none of the masters can help, neither those of the past nor those of the future. Then you are alone with God. Then you must suffer the full knowledge of human nothingness before Him. Woe to you, that you took refuge in human help and could not hold out before the face of God." The Rabbi was in a cleft stick, between guilt and guilt. Whichever way he decided, he would be guilty. *Homo non potest non peccare*: to become guilty is inevitable. Leopold Ziegler writes in *Menschwerden* ("Becoming Human") "And so the individual can be certain . . . one day the Lord will snatch the mask of selfish and therefore false innocence from his face, and show him unmistakably, as I will and not as Thou wilt. In this clash between the strongest, best motive and the highest Will it may please the latter to require of the self-sufficient individual even his innocence". Here perhaps one is standing directly in the presence of the terrible God who, as *deus absconditus*, leaves us alone. Here Christ speaks on the Cross: "My God, My God, why hast Thou forsaken me?" When separation is identical with sin, we begin to apprehend the meaning of the Crucifixion. On the one hand Christ's passion on the Cross involved the sacrifice of every claim to recognition, self-justification, and ego-realization, the last trace of egoistical demand, and the journey into the true night, the true *nigredo*; on the other hand it also implies *the* answer to Job, as Jung has it in mind: that even God wishes to become man and, nailed to the Cross, the 'mother', to suffer that bitter suspension between heaven and earth. God, the self-sacrificer, will first experience in Himself the sacrifice to which He calls us. Jung writes: "From that sacrifice we gain ourselves—our 'self'—for we have only what we give. But what does the self gain? We see it entering into manifestation, freeing itself from unconscious projection, and, as it grips us, entering into our lives and so passing from unconsciousness into consciousness, from potentiality into actuality. What it is in the diffuse unconscious state we do not know; we only know that in becoming ourself it has become man . . . Conscious realization or the bringing together of the scattered parts is in one sense an act of the ego's will, but in another sense it is a spontaneous manifestation of the self, which was always there" ("alone through Grace"). "Individuation appears, on the one hand, as the synthesis of a new unity which previously consisted of scattered particles, and on the other hand, as the revelation of something which existed before the ego and is in fact its father or creator and also its totality. Up to a point we create the self by making ourselves conscious of our unconscious contents, and to that extent it is our son . . . But we are forced to make this effort by the unconscious presence of the self, which is all the time urging us to overcome our unconsciousness. From that point of view the self is the father". (Jung, 1954, *Coll. Wks.*, **11**, pp. 262 f.).

It may be said that original sin was separation from the unconscious unity, through the development of the ego, through eating from the tree of the knowledge of good and evil, through disloyalty to the gods, to God, through the cunning theft of fire, and other tricks and sorceries, such as those by which Medea helped Jason to win the Golden Fleece (this disloyalty to the father being followed by fratricide). We must therefore take all these failures, these sins, this guilt, in their psychological significance, as threads spun by the Norns, inescapable, leading directly to persecution by the Erinyes, or the Harpies, until a sacrifice purges the guilt. When we really understand all this, then we see that from this aspect the only sacrifice that can give full expiation is the self-sacrifice. But this self-sacrifice requires an integrated ego and that, both psychologically and in the religious sense, is not only the greatest opposite to the superego but also to the primal unconscious. Redemption lies, not in seeing the ego as guilt, as original sin, but in realizing that the climax of becoming fully human lies in the self-sacrifice of the differentiated ego. Then an ego that has become conscious of itself does not become petrified in its *hybris*, but self-sacrifice passes over into the transcendence, into the new dimension of the self, embracing the opposites in all their tension and transforming hostile separation into polar opposition.

To become fully human is a duty laid upon man, a development that inevitably involves guilt, disloyalty, treachery, sacrilege.

On consideration, we might well say: "Lead us not into temptation, and let this cup, of having to be truly human, pass from me".

In analytical psychology we must see and develop both sides, the strong ego-personality that can withdraw the greatest number of projections, and also the self-sacrifice that restores and cultivates the relationship to the primal source. We must also recognize the limits that are set to the withdrawal of projection. In this never completely realized dimension of being, this living in the orbit of the self, lies the only possibility of true worship, of lasting religion, and of the *hieros gamos*. Until then we must content ourselves with partial solutions, while endeavouring to approach as closely as possible to our goal of becoming fully human.

(*For References see p. 303*)

# Index

*This Index covers the papers written originally in English, and the translations of those written originally in French and German.*

# Plates

WALTER ZÜBLIN

The Mother Figure in the Fantasies of a Boy suffering from Early Deprivation



ROBERT MOODY

A Contribution to the Psychology of the Mother-Child Relationship



HEINZ WESTMAN

From Schizophrenia to Art: Excerpts from a Case-History

1

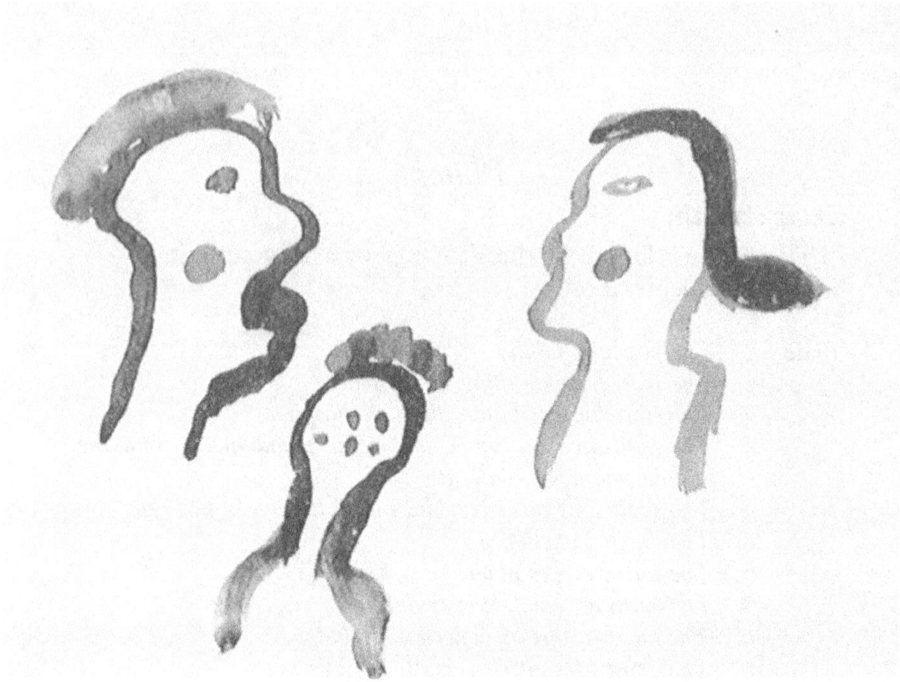

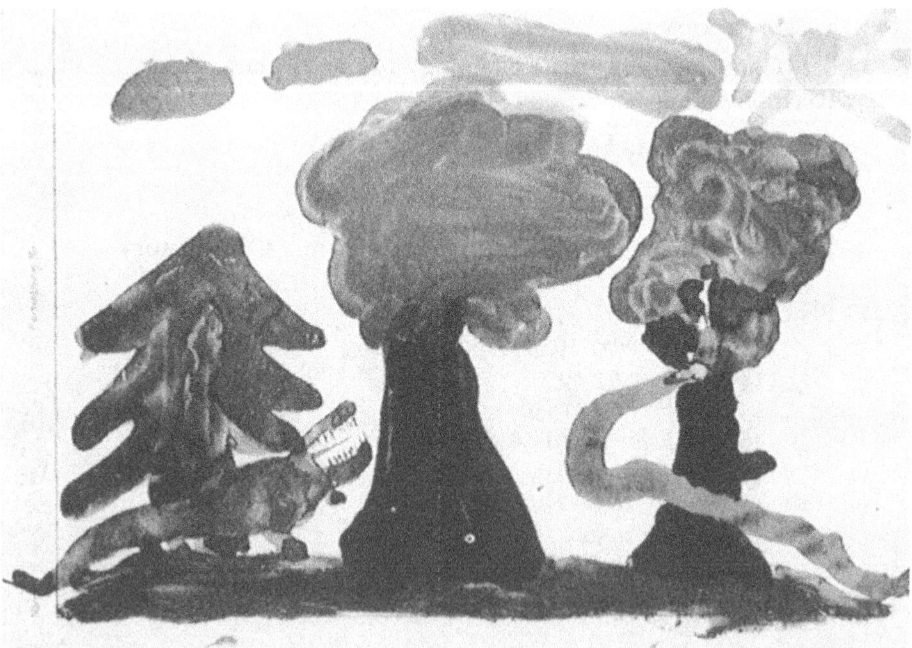

2

3

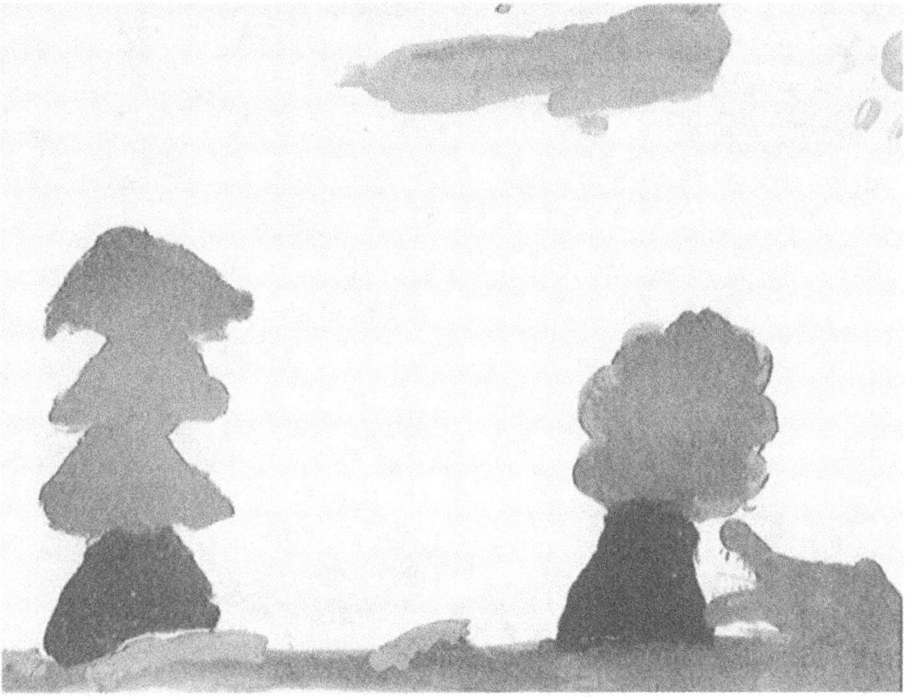

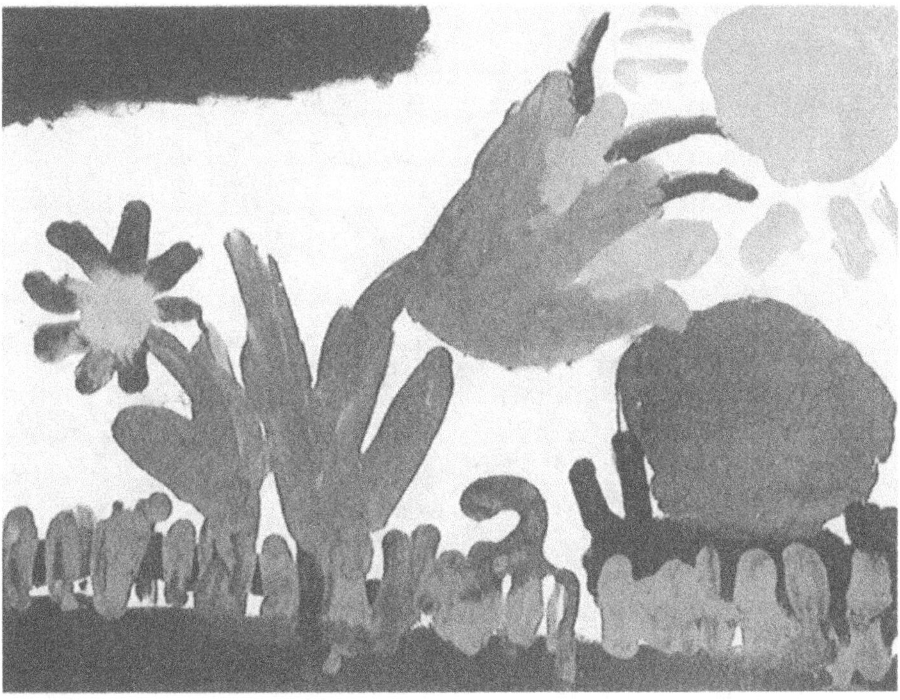

4

5

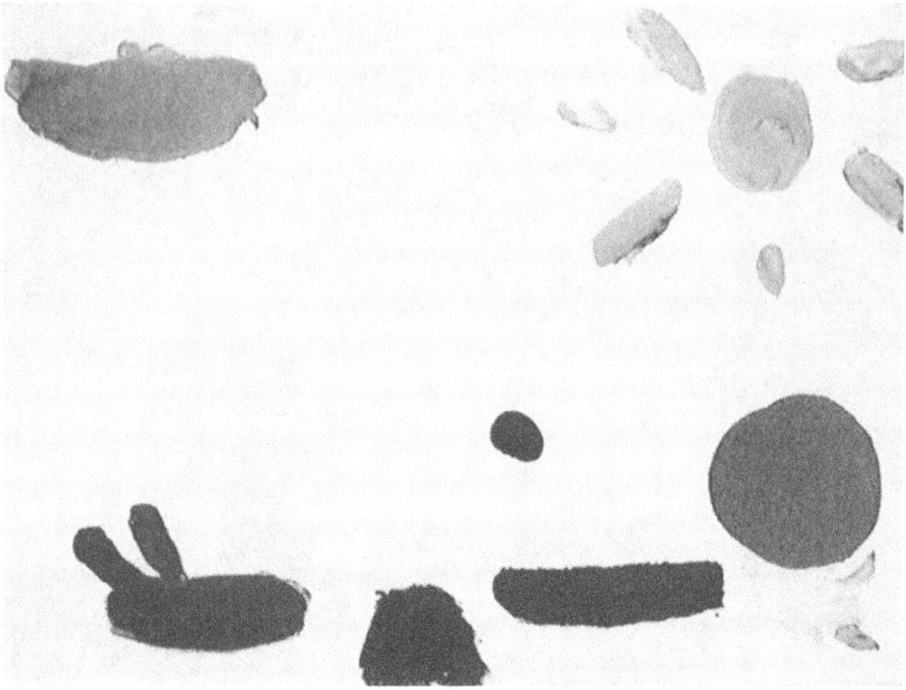

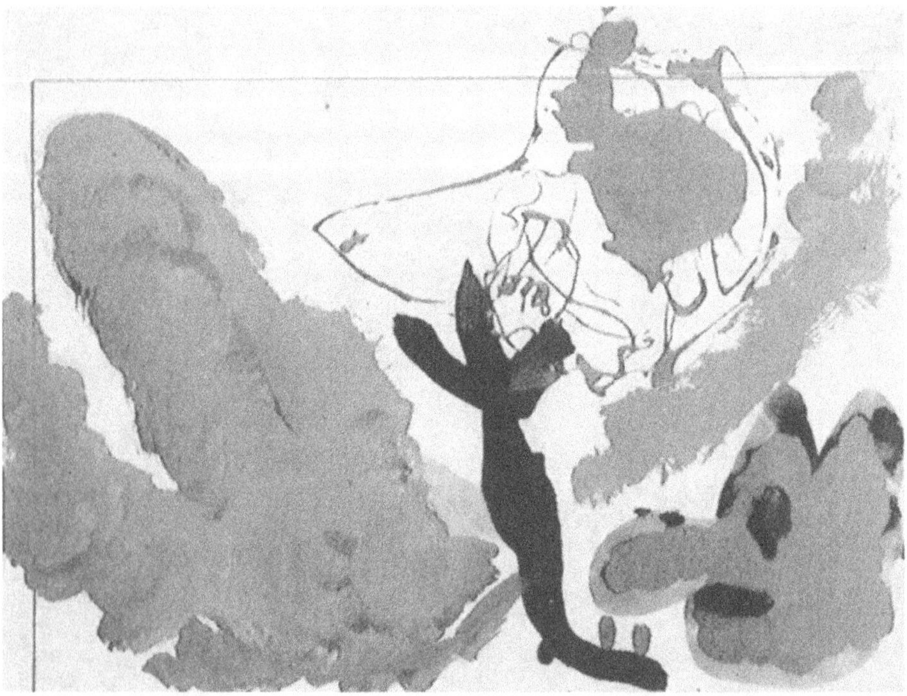

6

7

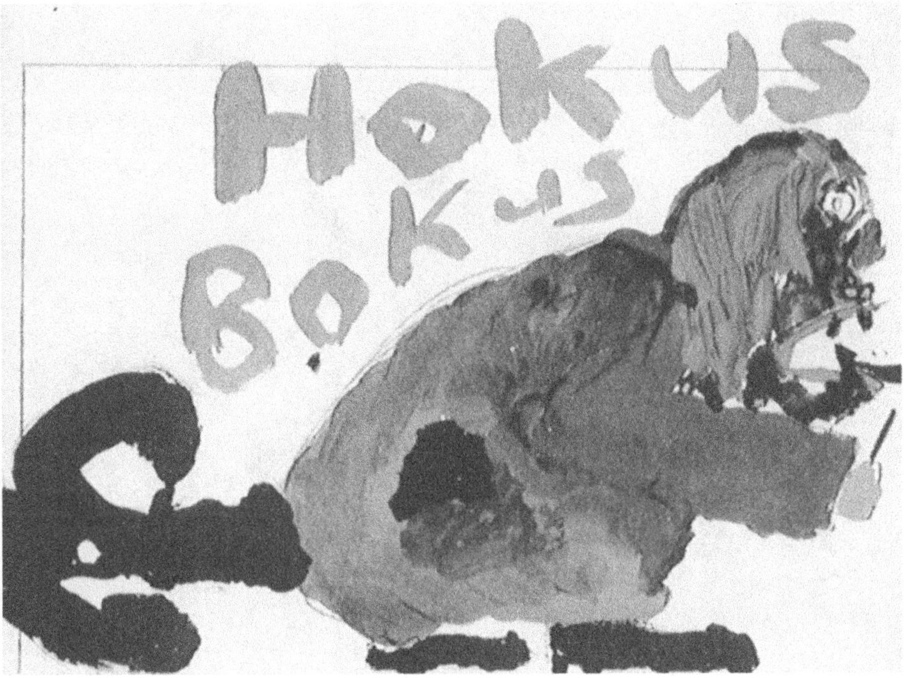


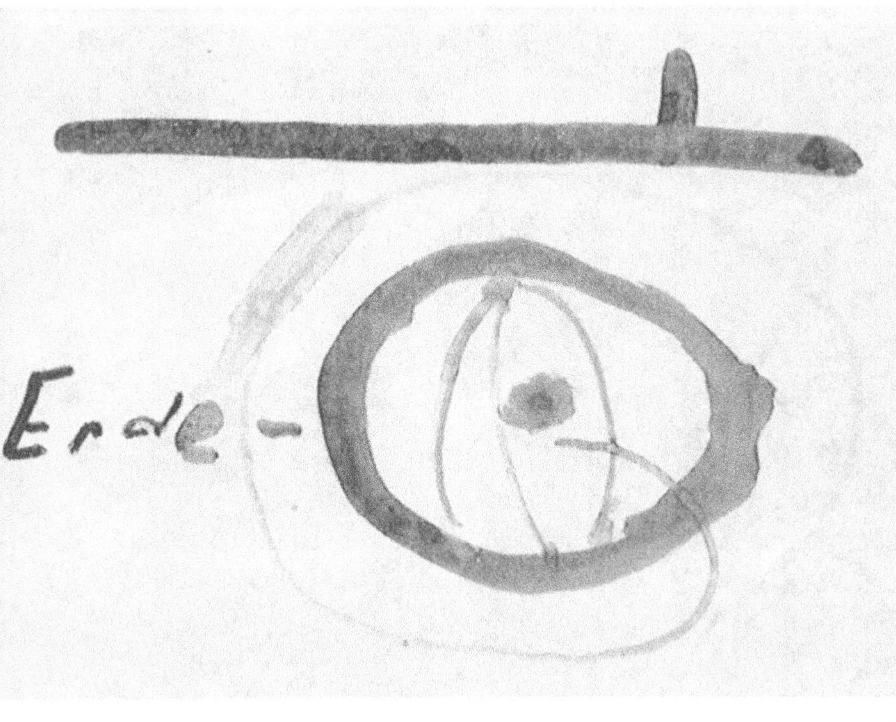


8

9

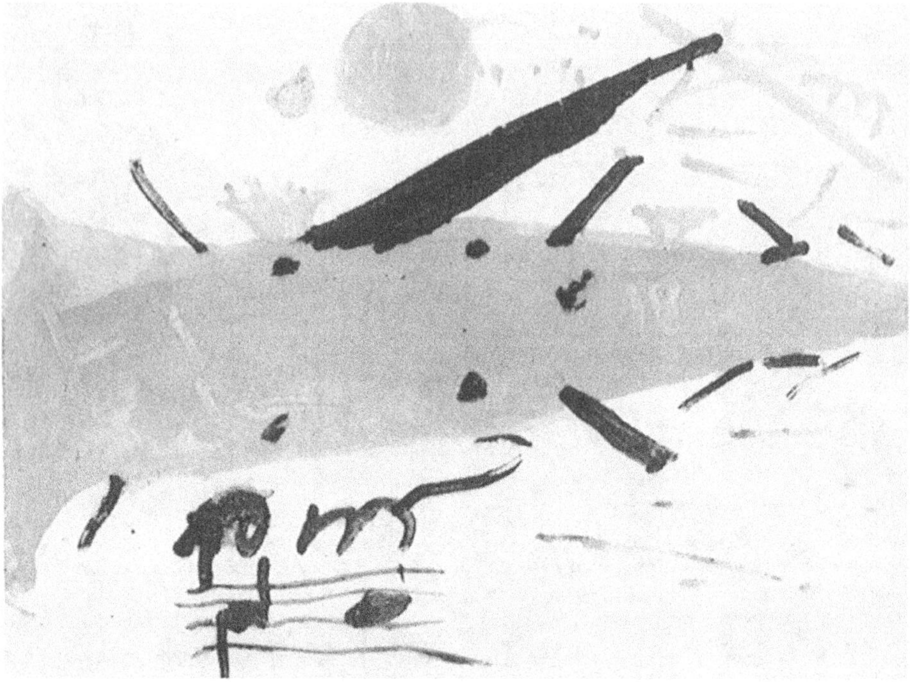

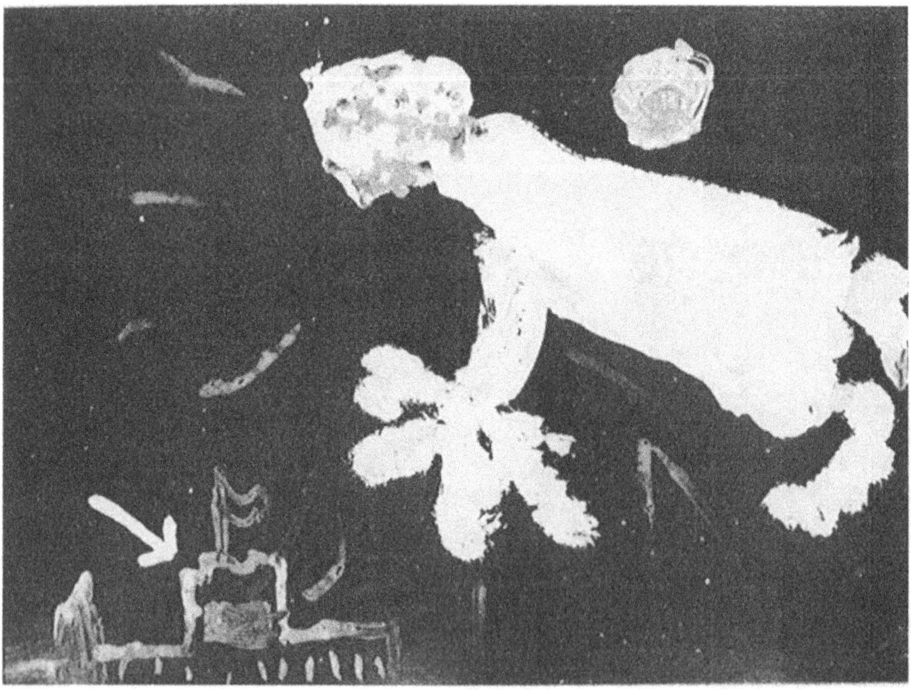

10

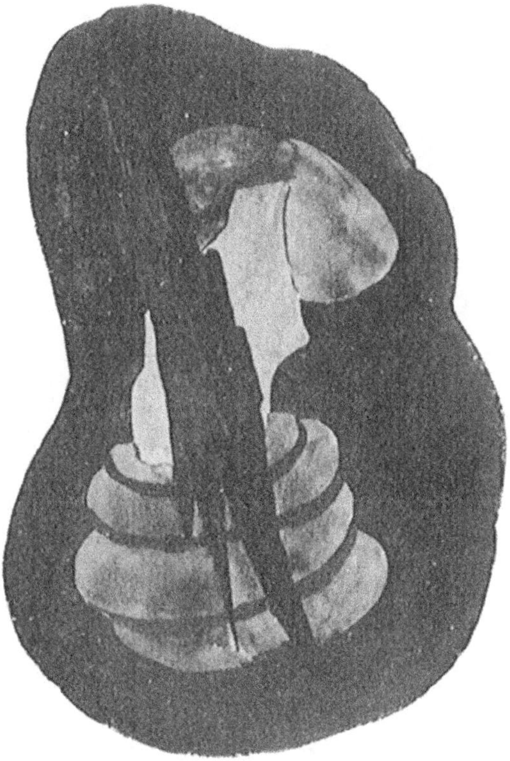

11

12

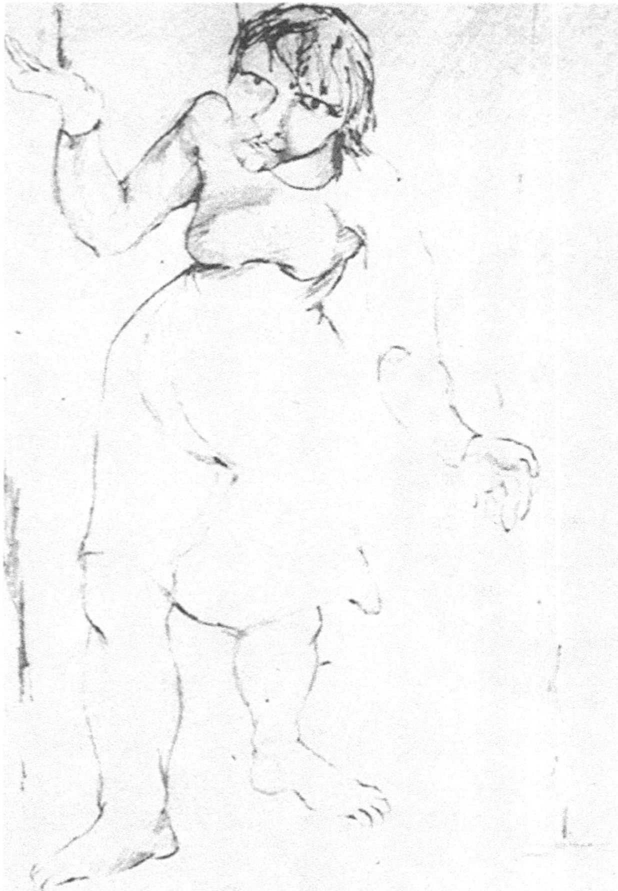

13

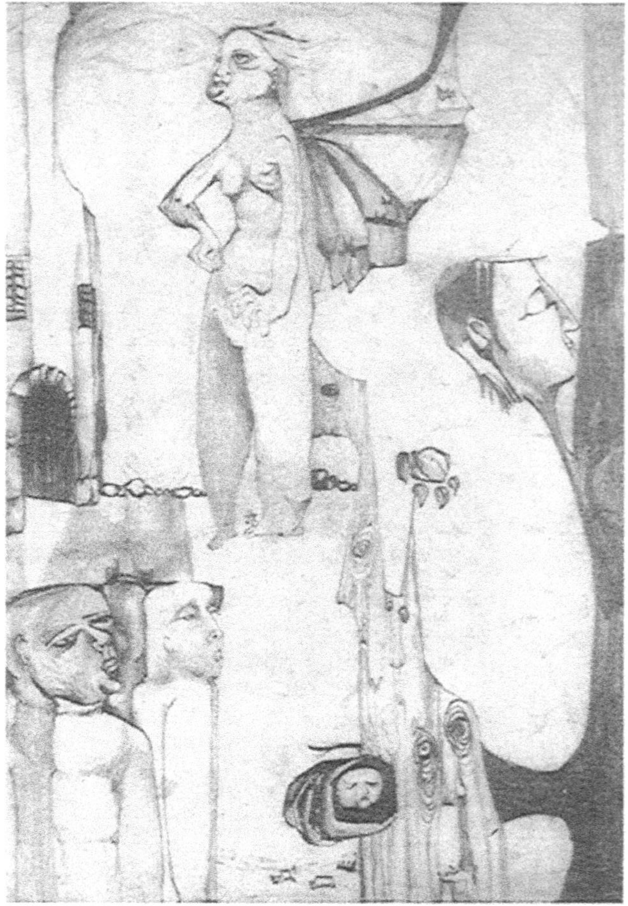

14

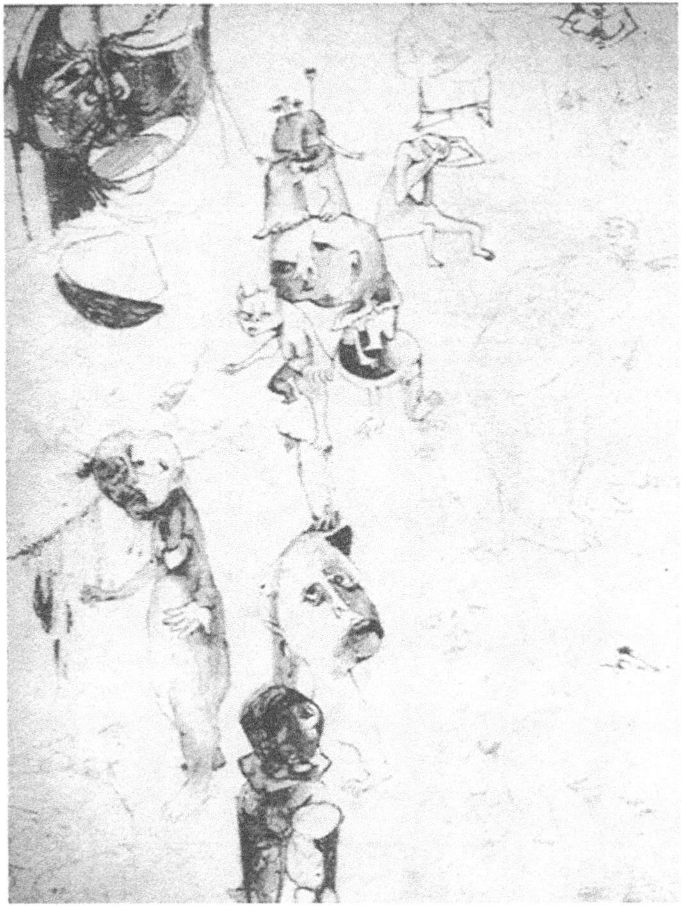

15

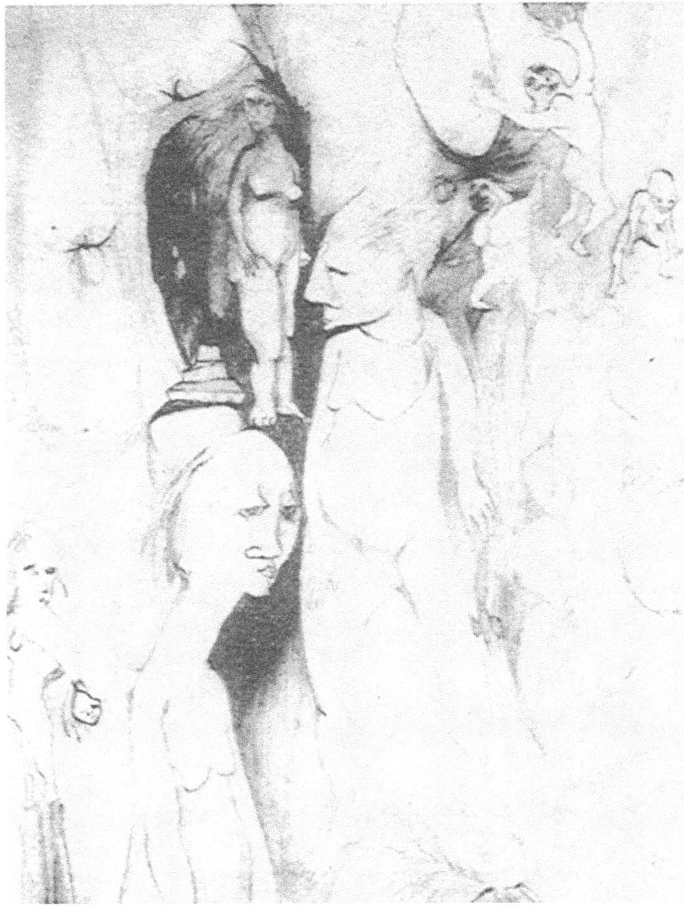

16

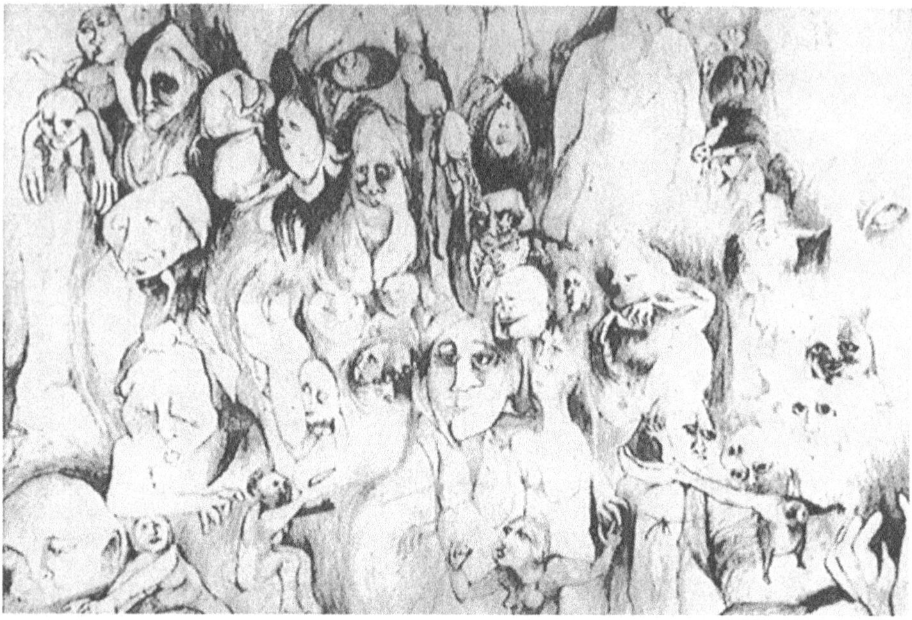

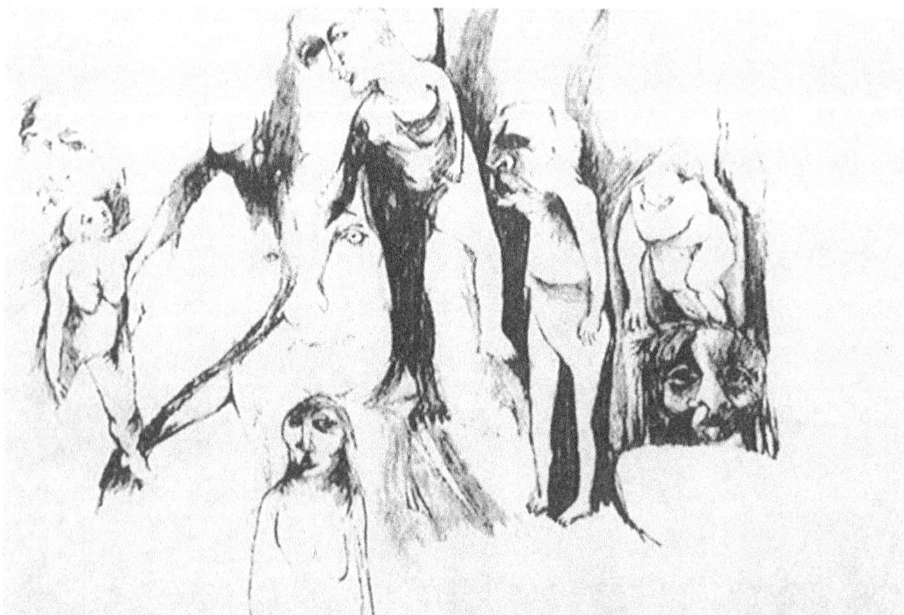

17

18

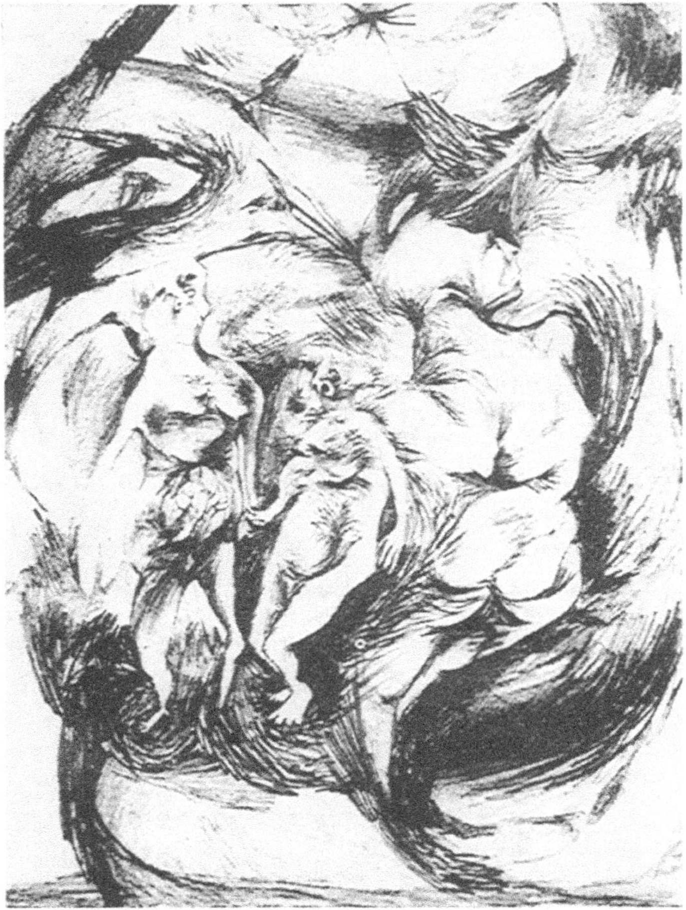

19

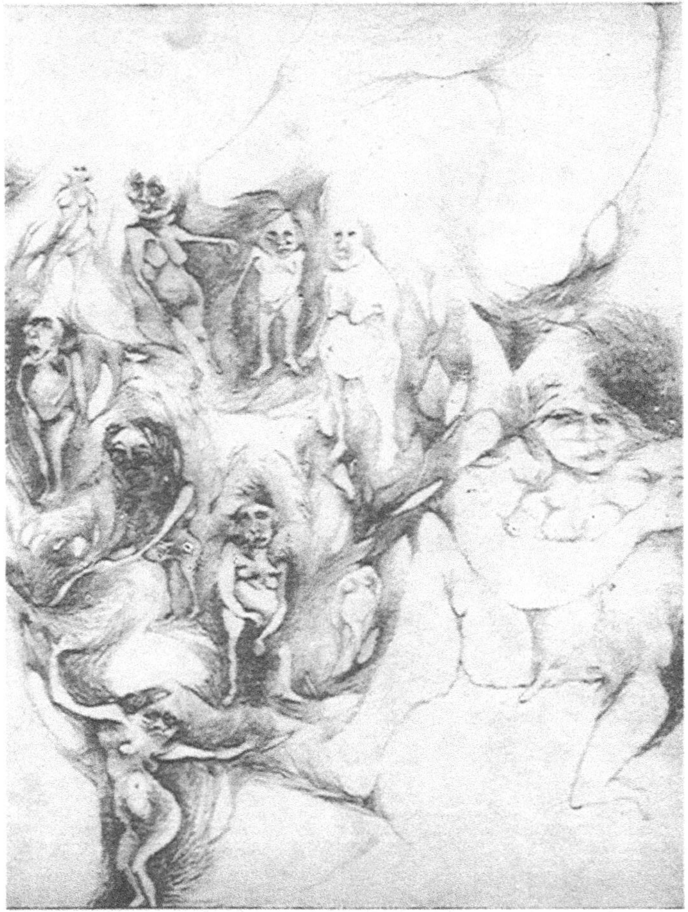

20

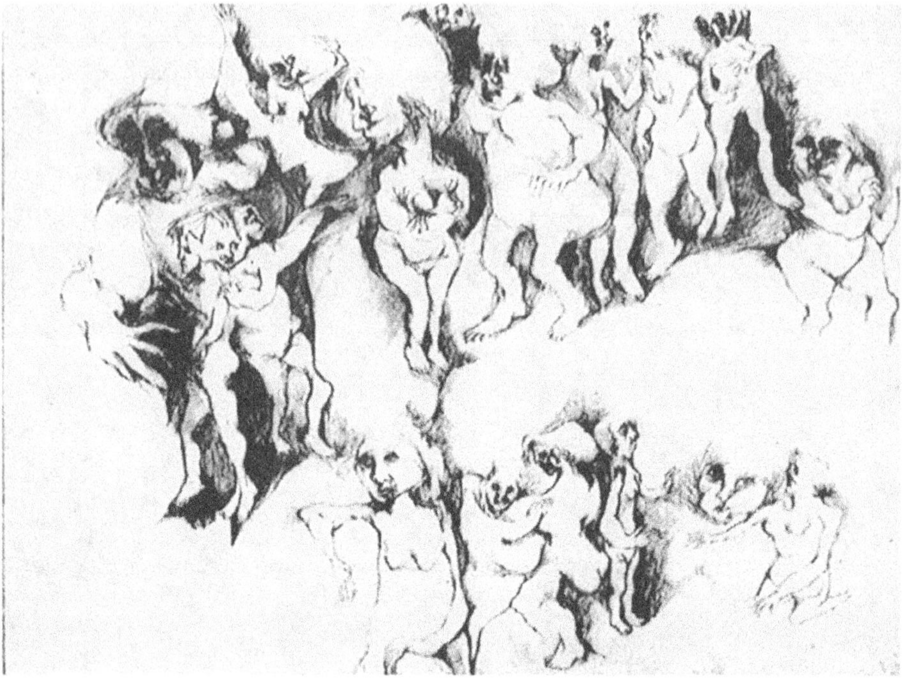

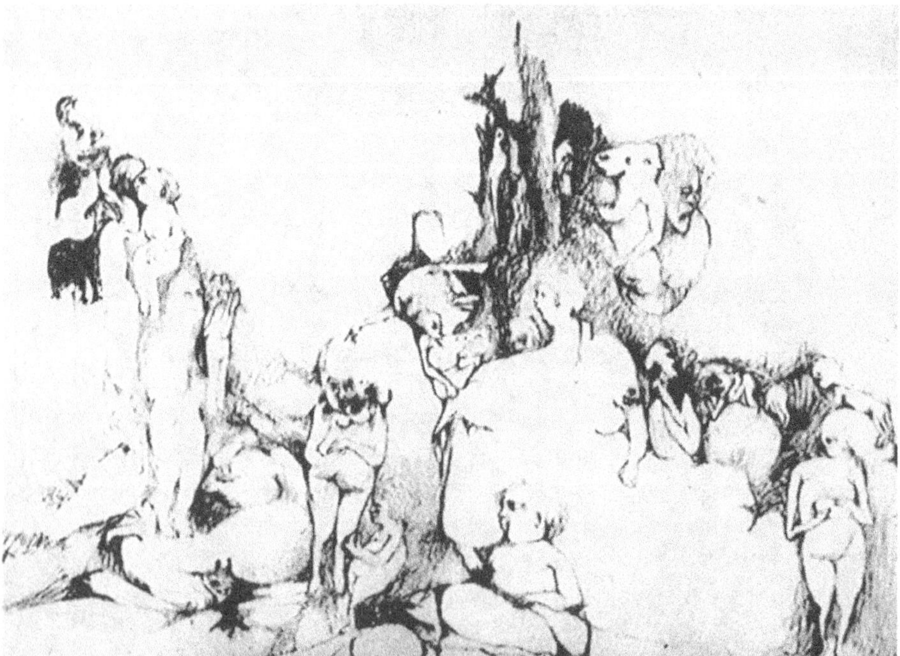

21

For Product Safety Concerns and Information please contact our EU representative GPSR@taylorandfrancis.com
Taylor & Francis Verlag GmbH, Kaufingerstraße 24, 80331 München, Germany

www.ingramcontent.com/pod-product-compliance
Lightning Source LLC
LaVergne TN
LVHW011111300926
849160LV00008B/341
* 9 7 8 1 1 3 8 8 7 1 5 5 7 *